Instructor's Manual and Testbank to Accompany Taylor, Lillis, and LeMone's

Fundamentals of Nursing

THE ART AND SCIENCE OF NURSING CARE

Instructor's Manual and Testbank to Accompany
Taylor, Lillis, and LeMone's

Fundamentals of Nursing

THE ART AND SCIENCE OF NURSING CARE

FOURTH EDITION

INSTRUCTOR'S MANUAL
Marilee LeBon, BA
Journalist
Mountaintop, Pennsylvania

TESTBANK
Karen L. Cobb, RN, EdD
Assistant Professor of Nursing
Instructor, Family Health Nursing
Indiana University School of Nursing
Indianapolis, Indiana

Anita K. Reed, RN, MSN
Instructor of Nursing
St. Elizabeth School of Nursing
Lafayette, Indiana

Geralyn M. Valleroy-Frandsen, RN, MSN
Assistant Professor of Nursing
Maryville University
Saint Louis, Missouri

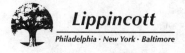
Lippincott
Philadelphia · New York · Baltimore

Ancillary Editor: Doris S. Wray
Printer/Binder: Victor Graphics

4th Edition

ISBN: 0-7817-2821-5

9 8 7 6 5 4 3 2 1

Preface

The instructor's manual portion for the fourth edition of *Fundamentals of Nursing: The Art and Science of Nursing Care* is designed to provide classroom, learning laboratory, and clinical application resources for instructors of Fundamentals of Nursing courses. The manual provides content and teaching/learning activities for each chapter of the book. Objectives and activities are written to encompass the cognitive, psychomotor, and affective domains, based on the belief of the authors that student learning is increased when a variety of learning experiences are used. This variety of teaching resources will also facilitate adaptation to individualized preferences in teaching methods and learning requirements.

The chapters correlate to those in the text and the format below is used, as applicable. To further supplement your teaching package, a printed Testbank allows testing of students. A computerized version also is available in an automatic test-generating program.

CHAPTER OVERVIEW

The chapter overview is a brief description of the key topics covered in the chapter.

KEY TERMS

The key terms, listed at the beginning of each chapter, are defined within the textbook chapter and in the Glossary at the end of the text. The key term is boldfaced in the textbook the first time it is defined.

KEY TOPICS

The key topics provide a brief topical summary of the chapter and provide information about the major concepts and skills covered in the chapter.

TEACHING–LEARNING ACTIVITIES

The teaching-learning activities are divided into three areas:

- **Group Activities:** The activities include exercises, discussion topics, presentations, experiences, learning laboratory practices, and clinical application. They facilitate student learning through application of chapter content in structured or guided observational experiences.
- **Discussion Questions:** The discussion questions provide recall, application, and analysis of chapter content through verbal discussion. Discussion questions also facilitate practice with critical-thinking and problem-solving abilities.
- **Writing Activities:** The writing activities include a variety of activities designed to assist students in integrating chapter content while improving written expression skills. The emphasis on writing abilities in higher education requires that writing activities be an integral component across the curriculum.
- **Guide to Critical Thinking and Developing Blended Skills:** The critical thinking exercises offer an exciting and practical means of challenging the assumptions students bring to nursing and to stretch their application of new theoretical concepts.

TEACHING–LEARNING PLAN

The teaching–learning plan is a table listing learner objectives, content outline, and the resources available in each chapter.

Contents

Foundations of Nursing Practice

Introduction to Nursing

■ Chapter Overview

Chapter 1 explores the historical background of nursing and its status as an emerging profession and discipline. The major aims of nursing—to promote health, to prevent illness, to restore health, and to facilitate coping—are discussed as they interrelate to facilitate maximum function and quality of life for patients. Educational programs, professional nursing organizations, and guidelines for nursing practice are presented along with current nursing trends and issues.

■ Teaching–Learning Activities

GROUP ACTIVITIES

1. Divide the class into four groups. Give each group of students one of the aims of nursing to explore (ie, promoting health, preventing illness, restoring health, and facilitating coping). Have them write down examples of the aim in practice from their own experience with patients. Share each group's results with the class as a whole.

2. Invite members of the community from different professions (such as, teachers, lawyers, doctors, etc) to participate in a panel discussion of the role of nurses in today's society. Explore these ideas and compare them to the students' views of the nursing profession.

3. Divide the class into three groups. Have each group attend a meeting of a local professional nursing organization (eg, ANA, CAN, ICN) and observe the format, function, and content of the meeting and professionalism of the members. Conduct a classroom discussion of the various professional groups available to nurses and their impact on the nursing professional as a whole.

4. Discuss the social policy statement of the American Nurses Association (1980). Choose student groups to represent the "pros" and "cons" for the policy, and conduct a debate.

5. Invite students who are in nursing education programs at a different level than your class to speak to your students. Ask them to discuss their programs and the reasons they chose them. Compare their experiences with those of the class you are teaching.

DISCUSSION QUESTIONS

1. Discuss the following statement: "All nursing actions focus on the person receiving the care and are a blend of the art and science of nursing." What impact will this statement have on the students in terms of their future nursing careers?

2. How has the historical background of nursing influenced the structure, responsibilities, and aims of nursing today?

3. Discuss the critical nursing issues of the new millennium. How does the increasing elderly population affect a person's career as a nurse? What will be the important ethical questions for a nurse practitioner in the current era?

4. Is nursing a discipline or a profession (or both)? Explain your answer.

WRITING ACTIVITIES

1. Ask students to write a paragraph defining nursing from personal perspectives and experiences.

2. Ask students to research an historical figure in nursing, reporting on that person's accomplishments, contributions to the nursing profession, and effect on the role of nurses in today's society.

3. Ask students to write an essay on the role of nursing throughout the years beginning with Florence Nightingale's contributions to the present time.

GUIDE TO CRITICAL THINKING AND DEVELOPING BLENDED SKILLS

1. Instruct the students to identify a nurse in the media, (television, movies, magazines), and write a

brief essay identifying the roles and functions commonly portrayed by the character. Have the students identify the blended skills (cognitive, technical, interpersonal, and ethical/legal) used by the nurse. Explain why this is or is not a positive portrayal of nursing and in what ways, if any, they would modify the nurse's roles. Use these essays as the springboard for a discussion of how media influence the public's perception of nurses as well as nurses' own self-image. You might want to explore the differences between the portrayal of nurses on made-for-TV dramas or daily soap operas. Did the students see themselves in the nurse they identified? Were the nurse's actions consistent with the broad aims of nursing identified in this chapter?

2. Have students write down the first five words that come to mind when they hear the words "nurse" and "doctor." Write these words on the blackboard and enter the student's responses to them under each heading. Explore the words different students use to describe each profession and how they are similar or different based on their own experiences. Compare descriptors used for nurse and doctor and attempt to explain the differences. Guide students in a discussion of the many variables influencing their choice of descriptors (eg, personal life experience, societal values, media).

TEACHING–LEARNING PLAN: Introduction to Nursing

Learning Objectives	Content Outline	Resources
Define key terms used in the chapter.		Table 1-1: People Important to the Development of Nursing
Describe the historical background, the definitions of nursing, and the status of nursing as a profession and as a discipline.	A. Nursing: An emerging profession and discipline: historical background, nursing in North America, definitions of nursing—a profession or a discipline.	Table 1-2: Nursing Roles in All Settings Table 1-3: Expanded Educational and Career Roles of Nurses
Identify the aims of nursing as they interrelate to facilitate maximum function and quality of life for patients.	B. Aims of nursing: promoting wellness, preventing illness, restoring health, facilitating coping.	Table 1-4: Summary of Types of Educational Program for RNs
Describe the various levels of educational preparation in nursing.	C. Educational preparations for nursing practice: levels of education, practical and vocational nursing education, registered nursing education, diploma, associate degree, baccalaureate, graduate education, continuing education, in-service education.	Examples of Settings for Nursing Care Examples of National Health Promotion and Disease Prevention Objectives
	D. Professional nursing organizations: national nursing organizations, international nursing organization, specialty nursing organizations.	American Nurses Association: Standards of Clinical Nursing Practice
Discuss the effect of nursing organizations, standards of nursing practice, nurse practice acts, and the nursing process on the practice of nursing.	E. Guidelines for nursing practice: standards of nursing practice, nurse practice acts and licensure, nursing process.	Canadian Nurses Association Standards for Nursing Practice Computer Applications in Nursing
Identify current trends in nursing.	F. Nursing in transition: new directions in nursing, changes in patient needs, expanded technology, increasing autonomy.	

Health of the Individual, Family, and Community

■ Chapter Overview

Chapter 2 discusses each level of Maslow's hierarchy of basic human needs and nursing actions necessary to meet these needs. Family concepts, including family roles, structures, functions, developmental stages, tasks, and health risk factors, are addressed as well as aspects of the community that affect individual and family health. Nursing interventions are defined that promote and maintain wellness in the individual as a member of a family and as a member of the community.

■ Teaching–Learning Activities

GROUP ACTIVITIES

1. Divide the class into six groups. Assign a specific disease to each group (such as AIDS, diabetes, heart disease, tuberculosis), and have them individually research the disease using the Internet. After completing their assignment, have the students meet with their groups and discuss what information was available to the public, whether the information was accurate or not, and whether the information addressed the needs of the patient and referred the patient to appropriate medical assistance. Report the findings of each group to the entire class.

2. Divide the class into five groups. Assign one of the following family developmental levels to each group: (a) couple and childbearing family, (b) family with school-aged children, (c) family with adolescents, (d) family with middle-aged adults, and (e) family with older adults. Have each group determine the nursing interventions that promote health and wellness for each family. Compare the health needs of each group, noting similarities and differences.

3. Divide the class into small groups to discuss basic human needs as they apply to each person in the group under different conditions (eg, when studying, ill, or under stress). Identify situations in which higher-order needs took precedence.

4. Ask a social worker or community health nurse to present community influences that are major risk factors for the health of individuals and families.

DISCUSSION QUESTIONS

1. How do roles and structures within today's families differ from those of parents or grandparents? (Explore the roles of family members in single-parent families, blended families, extended families versus traditional families.)

2. What problems do single-parent families face that are different from those faced by the traditional family? (Explore support systems, roles of family members, financial and emotional needs of members.)

3. Are the tasks for family survival and continuity as defined by Duvall appropriate in today's society? What should be added or deleted?

4. How are families portrayed in the media (television, movies, magazines, newspapers)? Are these portrayals realistic and representative of the diversity in family structure found in today's society?

WRITING ACTIVITIES

1. Ask students to develop a list of their basic human needs and prioritize them according to Maslow's hierarchy. Identify any resources available (personal, family, community) to help them meet these needs.

2. Ask students to list five rules learned in their family that promoted good health (eg, "Wash your hands before you eat.").

3. Have students make a list of examples of family functions in the following areas: (a) physical, (b) economic, (c) reproductive, (d) affective and coping, and (e) socialization. Have them describe how their family functions successfully or unsuccessfully in these areas and how this affects society as a whole.

4. Ask individual students to describe their feelings and responses when they experienced the following situations: (a) loss of self-esteem, (b) loss of love or belonging, and (c) loss of self-actualization.

GUIDE TO CRITICAL THINKING AND DEVELOPING BLENDED SKILLS

1. Divide the class into groups and have each group explore the availability of community resources to meet the needs of the following patients:

   • A patient with two new above-the-knee amputations is returning home to his wife and 4-year-old son after an extended stay in a rehabilitation facility. (Discuss home healthcare, occupational therapy, services to modify home setting to accommodate a wheelchair.)

   • A single elderly female patient who has outlived friends and family and who lives in her own home needs radiation therapy three times weekly. (Discuss home healthcare, transportation to therapy sessions, meals-on-wheels, public assistance.)

   • A 15-year-old high school student who is referred for drug and alcohol counseling by his teacher. (Discuss family services, private counseling services, drug testing, counseling for family members.)

   • Parents of a recently discharged premature and developmentally delayed infant. (Discuss home healthcare, respite care, counseling services.)

2. Instruct students to diagram the types of family relationships featured in popular television sitcoms. Describe how the nursing needs of each may differ. Brainstorm with the class!

TEACHING–LEARNING PLAN: Health of the Individual, Family, and Community

Learning Objectives	Content Outline	Resources
Define key terms used in the chapter.		Table 2-1: Family Stages, Tasks, Health Risk Factors, and Nursing Interventions to Promote Health
Describe each level of Maslow's hierarchy of basic human needs.	A. The individual: levels of needs, the individual in health and illness, applying Maslow's theory.	
Discuss nursing actions necessary to meet needs for each level of Maslow's hierarchy.		Research: Research in Nursing: Making a Difference: Promoting Healthy Parenting in Single-Parent Families Headed by Women
Discuss family concepts, including family roles, structures, functions, developmental stages, tasks, and health risk factors.	B. The family: what is a family, family structures, family functions, developmental tasks, the family in health and illness, risk factors, nursing interventions to promote wellness.	Examples of NANDA Nursing Diagnoses: The Family
Identify aspects of the community that affect individual and family health.	C. The community: The community in health and illness, risk factors, nursing in the community	
Describe nursing interventions to promote and maintain wellness in the individual as a member of a family and as a member of the community.		

Culture and Ethnicity

■ Chapter Overview

Chapter 3 presents the concepts of culture and ethnicity and explores the effect of gender roles, language, nutrition, socioeconomic factors, physical and mental characteristics, spiritual characteristics, and family values on healthcare. The chapter includes a discussion of alternative healing methods and guidelines that are useful in practicing transcultural nursing care.

■ Teaching–Learning Activities

GROUP ACTIVITIES

1. Divide the class into pairs and have them assess each other's race, gender, culture, ethnicity, family traditions, socioeconomic factors, and so forth. Discuss similarities and differences between individual pairs and have them share their findings with the class.

2. Invite several recently hospitalized minority group members to talk to the class about their hospital experience. Have them describe the care they received, how they were treated by the healthcare staff, their own reaction to the experience, and if and how they would change the experience to make it more positive.

3. Ask a faculty member or a student of a cultural or racial minority to speak about both positive and negative aspects of life as a member of a minority group.

4. Invite a nurse who speaks a second language to perform a nursing history on a student in that language. Explore the reaction of the student to being addressed in another language and the frustration of the student's inability to respond to the questions. Relate this experience to that of non–English-speaking patients in a hospital setting.

DISCUSSION QUESTIONS

1. What are some examples of stereotyping that are commonly used? How are nurses stereotyped? How can this practice affect healthcare?

2. Discuss the statement: "The healthcare system is a culture." Do you agree or disagree, and why?

3. "Poverty is an increasingly devastating epidemic— one that has evolved into a culture of its own." Discuss the characteristics of poverty cultures, the effect of poverty on healthcare, and how it is passed from generation to generation. What, if anything, can be done to break the cycle of poverty?

4. Discuss the effect of culture shock on individuals. Can feelings on entering nursing school be compared to culture shock? How does "burnout" in practicing nurses compare to culture shock?

5. What blended skills does a nurse need to possess to adequately meet the needs of patients from different cultures and ethnic groups?

WRITING ACTIVITIES

1. Have each student interview and prepare a report on a person of a different minority/cultural group to determine the person's family role, use of folk and/or traditional healthcare, values and beliefs, and any common health problems related to the specific culture. Have students share their reports with their classmates.

2. Ask students to summarize a recent nursing journal article that describes an area of transcultural nursing.

3. Ask students to list the various holidays they celebrate and indicate why these holidays are important to them. Have them describe how the occasions are celebrated and any rituals or customs that are associated with them. Which of these holidays have ethnic origins? Share each student's report with the class.

4. Have students research and write a report on the eating habits of a cultural group focusing on (a) which foods are considered edible and which are not, (b) what times and types of food are considered meals, and (c) with whom the food is eaten. Have them share their results with their classmates and initiate a class discussion about the way nurses can assess and accommodate patients' dietary needs.

GUIDE TO CRITICAL THINKING AND DEVELOPING BLENDING SKILLS

1. Identify cultures that are common within the local community. Divide the class into groups and assign a culture to each one. Have each group report on the beliefs, practices, habits, likes, dislikes, customs, and rituals of the culture that pertain to healthcare. Guide the class in a discussion of related nursing implications.

    You might want to explore the following cultural differences:

    • Race
    • Eating habits
    • Hygiene habits
    • Religious beliefs
    • Hereditary factors

    Related nursing implications could include:

    • Teaching the importance of diet and exercise to health
    • Teaching safety in the home
    • Routine screening of the public for blood pressure
    • Inoculations and routine checkups for children

2. Have students identify ways they have been harmed by cultural, racial, or ethnic stereotyping. Draw on these experiences to explore potential harms that nurses can cause patients and families. Role-play a situation in which one nurse observes another acting in a discriminatory manner and invite students to determine the best manner to respond.

    Examples of ways nurses can harm patients may include:

    • Treating each patient the same regardless of ethnic differences
    • Failure to understand health needs of patients from different cultures
    • Expecting patients to share nurse's values and beliefs

TEACHING–LEARNING PLAN: Culture and Ethnicity

Learning Objectives	Content Outline	Resources
Define key terms used in the chapter.		Table 3-1: Cultural Variations in Health Concept and Promotion
Discuss the concepts of culture and ethnicity.	A. Concepts of culture and ethnicity: culture, ethnicity, race, cultural assimilation.	Table 3-2: Cultural Factors that Affect Nursing Care
Describe cultural and ethnic characteristics that influence healthcare, including gender roles, language and communication, orientation to space and time, food and nutrition, socioeconomic factors, important of family, physical and mental characteristics, spiritual characteristics, and perceptions of illness and health.	B. Factors affecting cultural sensitivity. C. Cultural and ethnic influences on healthcare: gender roles, language and communication, orientation to space and time, food and nutrition, socioeconomic factors, family support, physical and mental health, alternative healing systems.	Through the Eyes of a Student Examples of NANDA Nursing Diagnoses Cultural Norms of the Healthcare System Focused Assessment Guide: Transcultural Assessment: Health-Related Beliefs and Practices
Compare and contrast the culture of the healthcare system with the broad concept of culture.		Research: Research in Nursing: Making a Difference: The Meaning of Staying Healthy in Immigrant Pakistani Families
Identify the factors that affect the interaction of the nurse and the patient in terms of culturally different healthcare values.		
Discuss the guidelines that are useful in practicing transcultural nursing care.	D. Transcultural nursing: the culture of healthcare, cultural imposition and ethnocentrism, providing transcultural care.	
Use knowledge of specific cultural and ethnic factors in providing holistic, individualized, culture-sensitive nursing care to patients.		

CHAPTER 4

Health and Illness

■ Chapter Overview

Chapter 4 discusses the various ways in which the patient receiving care influences the practice of nursing. Factors affecting health and illness are identified, including the human dimensions, basic human needs, and self-concept. Models of health and illness and definitions of health are presented. Health promotion and illness prevention are described, incorporating risk factors, acute and chronic illness, and the effects of illness on the family. Levels of preventive care and the role of the nurse in promoting health are discussed.

■ Teaching–Learning Activities

GROUP ACTIVITIES

1. Set up a health-awareness fair at your school or medical facility. Divide the class into groups and assign one area of health and fitness to each group (eg, nutrition, exercise programs, blood pressure screening, information on specific common diseases, immunization schedules, etc). If possible, invite the public and have the students interact with them and describe their area of expertise.

2. Divide the class into four groups. Ask each group to use one of the health models to illustrate applications for different age groups and illnesses. Provide students with examples, such as a 15-year-old with a fractured arm, a 55-year-old with an ulcer, and a 75-year-old with heart problems. Have each group share results with the class.

3. Divide the class into pairs and have them perform a health appraisal on each other. Be sure to assess for risk factors (age, genetic, physiologic, health habits, lifestyle, environment), and devise a nursing care plan to promote health and prevent illness in these areas. Have students role-play their interviews and the implementation of their care plans.

4. Have students meet in small groups to discuss how experiences as members of a family affected the students' own health status, beliefs, and practices.

DISCUSSION QUESTIONS

1. What are the implications of "holistic" healthcare for nursing in today's society?

2. Discuss the three levels of disease prevention and how nurses can incorporate them into their practice. Make a class list of examples of primary, secondary, and tertiary preventive care.

3. How can the nurse serve as a role model for health? Ask students to identify their own behaviors (eg, diet, exercise, rest and sleep, stress, chemical dependency) that will help patients develop or maintain healthy behaviors.

4. What blended skills do nurses need to promote and restore health and to prevent disease and illness?

WRITING ACTIVITIES

1. Ask students to write a paragraph that describes their personal definition of health. Have them list their behaviors and practices that help them maintain health and prevent illness.

2. As a follow-up to activity 1, have students write down their basic human needs and describe how they are or are not presently being met. If they are not being met, have students develop a plan to help them meet these needs in the future. Have students review each other's plans and help to implement them by acting as fitness trainers for each other.

3. Ask students to make a list of preventive care activities available in the community that are advertised in the telephone book, local newspaper, radio, and television.

4. Have students compare and contrast the following terms: health, wellness, illness, and disease.

GUIDE TO CRITICAL THINKING AND DEVELOPING BLENDED SKILLS

1. Divide the class into six groups and assign one of the human dimensions to each group: physical, emotional, environmental, intellectual, spiritual, and sociocultural. Have each group identify potential patient strengths and weaknesses and related nursing interventions within their assigned dimension. For example, a child with asthma may have loving parents with adequate financial resources who smoke in the home. An environmental weakness is second-hand smoke. A strength is the parents' being committed and financially able to modify the home to meet the child's needs. The related nursing intervention is teaching.

   You may use the following example: a patient with end-stage cancer is seeking hospice care.

   Physical: need for pain relief, IV drugs

   Emotional: needs help accepting loss, family members need counseling

   Environmental: needs safe environment with daily care—hospice care, home healthcare

   Intellectual: needs to understand the situation and modification of health state: teaching, counseling

   Spiritual: needs strength from religious sources—pray with patient, provide spiritual counseling

   Sociocultural: needs strong family ties; encourage family members to visit

2. Have students identify two high-level health goals and invite a fellow student to determine the best means of achieving these goals. Use a log to report on progress toward goal achievement for a 1-month period. Identify variables that facilitate or impede goal achievement.

   High-level health goals may include:

   - Lose weight
   - Quit smoking
   - Eat a healthy diet

TEACHING–LEARNING PLAN: Health and Illness

Learning Objectives	Content Outline	Resources
Define key terms used in the chapter.		Table 4-1: Major Areas of Risk Factors
Describe health and illness.	A. Defining health and illness. Models of health and illness: the health–illness continuum, high-level wellness model, agent–host–environment model, health belief model.	Causes of Diseases Health Style: A Self-Test
Identify the factors influencing health and illness, including the human dimensions, basic human needs, and self-concept.	B. Factors affecting health and illness: factors influencing health–illness status, beliefs, and practices; basic human needs; self-concept.	
Compare and contrast acute illness and chronic illness.	C. Promoting health and preventing illness: risk factors, acute and chronic illness, effects of illness on the family.	
Summarize the role of the nurse in promoting health based on knowledge of risk factors for illness, illness behaviors, and the effects of illness on the family.		
Describe the levels of preventive care.	D. Nursing care as preventive care: levels of preventive care, nurse as role model.	

Theoretical Base for Nursing Practice

■ Chapter Overview

Chapter 5 provides an introduction to the theoretical base for nursing practice. The underlying processes and characteristics of nursing theory as well as the historical background, cultural influences, and value of nursing theory are discussed. Selected models and theories of nursing are described and applied to the care of one patient to illustrate application in clinical practice.

■ Teaching–Learning Activities

GROUP ACTIVITIES

1. The philosophy of each nurse and the philosophies of schools of nursing and healthcare institutions form the basis of giving nursing care. Invite a nurse working in a clinical setting, a nurse manager, and a nursing instructor to share their philosophies of nursing with the students. Conduct a discussion to see how their philosophies compare with those of the students.

2. Divide the class into small groups and assign each group one or two nursing theorists. Ask each group to compose one paragraph describing the beliefs of the nursing theorist(s) assigned. Try to include some theorists who have not been covered in the chapter.

3. As a follow-up to activity 2, have the students identify a theorist whose beliefs most closely represent their own and explain why they have chosen this theorist.

DISCUSSION QUESTIONS

1. Discuss the impact of Florence Nightingale's beliefs and philosophies on the establishment of modern-day nursing theory.

2. Defend the following statement: "Nursing theory improves and facilitates communication in nursing."

3. Explain the following terms: theory, process, concept, and philosophy. Give an example of how each term may relate to the nursing practice.

4. Discuss the following statement: "Every nurse's philosophy, developed through education and practice, forms the basis for giving nursing care." How does your personal philosophy of nursing affect the type of care you provide for your patients?

WRITING ACTIVITIES

1. Ask students to write their own definitions of the four concepts common to nursing theory: person, environment, health, and nursing.

2. Ask students to research a general nursing theory present in nursing journals and related literature. Have them report how the theory they have chosen explains, describes, predicts, and controls desired outcomes of nursing care practice.

3. Ask students to choose one nursing theorist and describe how that person's theory or concepts can be applied to themselves when they are well and when they are ill.

4. Have students describe the relationship between a "philosophy of care" and a "nursing theory."

GUIDE TO CRITICAL THINKING AND DEVELOPING BLENDED SKILLS

1. Divide the class into groups and assign a nursing theorist to each group. Present the class with a case and have each group discuss how their theory/framework would influence the related nursing care. Conclude with a discussion of the advantages and disadvantages of using nursing theory in general and individual theoretical models.

   Example: Use the nursing theory chart in the textbook to discuss the nursing care plan for the following patient:

A 55-year-old woman is recently diagnosed with pancreatic cancer. She has been told she will only have a few months to live. She is scheduled to undergo radiation therapy on an outpatient basis. She is in constant pain and emotionally unprepared for handling her diagnosis. She has a husband who travels frequently for work and a married daughter living close by.

2. Have students write a definition of nursing before reading the chapter and compare their definitions

with current and historical attempts to describe nursing. Guide them in a discussion of the factors that account for the difference.

Explore the possible factors accounting for differences in past and present nursing definitions:

• Insurance issues
• Trend toward ambulatory care and home healthcare
• Teaching wellness promotion

TEACHING–LEARNING PLAN: Theoretical Base for Nursing Practice

Learning Objectives	Content Outline	Resources
Define key terms used in the chapter.		Table 5-1: Key Points of Selected Nursing Theories
Describe the underlying processes and characteristics of nursing theory.	A. Introduction to theory: basic processes in the development of nursing theories, basic characteristics of nursing theory, common components in nursing theories.	
Define the four common components of nursing theory.		
Summarize the historical background, cultural influences, and value of nursing theory.	B. Nursing theory and nursing practice: historical perspectives and influences, evolution of nursing theory, value of nursing theory.	
Discuss selected nursing theories, including definitions, assumptions, beliefs, and applications to nursing practice.	C. Conceptual and theoretical frameworks for nursing: Dorothy E. Johnson: behavioral systems model; Imogene M. King: open systems framework; Madeline Leininger: transcultural care diversity and universality; Myra E. Levine: theory of nursing; Betty Neuman: healthcare systems model; Dorothea E. Orem: self-care model; Martha E. Rogers: nursing—a science of unitary man; Sister Calista Roy: Roy's adaptation model; Jean Watson: nursing—human science and human care. Application of conceptual and theoretical frameworks.	

CHAPTER 6

Values and Ethics in Nursing

■ Chapter Overview

Chapter 6 explores the influence of values on human behavior and the ethical dimensions of nursing practice. Codes of professional ethical conduct for nursing are explored and a process of ethical decision making is highlighted. Principle- and care-based approaches to practicing bioethics are compared and contrasted, and common ethical problems encountered by practicing nurses are presented.

■ Teaching–Learning Activities

GROUP ACTIVITIES

1. Have the students role-play the following situations and then discuss their actions and how they handled the ethical issues involved. Invite comments from the audience about how they might have handled the same situation differently.

   • A young woman scheduled for a mastectomy decides not to have the operation after her husband visits her. She tells you that she is afraid he will not love her anymore after her surgery.

   • A mother refuses to allow an emergency room physician to start a transfusion on her child who was involved in a traffic accident. She states that if her child is going to live it will be because of the will of her God and not because of modern medicine.

   • A student nurse surreptitiously catches her charge nurse taking controlled drugs out of the medication cabinet and putting them in her purse.

   • A physician makes inappropriate sexual comments to a student nurse.

2. Ask students to write down an adage they learned growing up (eg, "an apple a day keeps the doctor away"). Collect the adages and read a portion of each one in class and see if the rest of the class can finish it. Discuss where the sayings came from and the diversity or sameness of the adages collected.

3. Ask students to individually write down the five most important parts of their lives and share them in small groups. Encourage exploration of priorities and choices.

DISCUSSION QUESTIONS

1. How would you use the six-step, ethical problem-solving process to evaluate your actions when an assigned patient says: "I'm afraid I have a venereal disease, but please don't tell anyone."

2. How would your own values influence your nursing care for patients who (a) are injured while under the influence of drugs or alcohol, (b) have AIDS, (c) are addicted to drugs, and (d) are having an abortion.

3. How have family and cultural influences influenced your personal values? Would you be a different person if you had grown up in a different family environment?

4. Should a nurse support the Patient's Bill of Rights, even if he feels his patient has put his or her health in jeopardy by refusing treatment? Defend your answer.

5. Should a recovering alcoholic be allowed to be on the waiting list for a liver transplant? Support your answer with statistics.

WRITING ACTIVITIES

1. Have the students select the three values that are most important to them and the three values that are least important from the list below and write a paragraph explaining their choices.

respect	responsibility	education
glamour	authority	work
drama	creativity	traditions
autonomy	marriage	health
independence	financial status	security

2. Ask students to write down the conversation they would have, based on values clarification and

ethical decision making, if their best friend and fellow student nurse confided: "I can only handle patient care if I smoke pot."

3. Have students pick one essential value (aesthetics, altruism, equality, freedom, human dignity, justice, truth) they feel is a strength for them, and describe how their attitudes and actions exemplify this value when they are working with patients.

4. Have the students write a paragraph about nursing using these words: value, value system, attitude, and belief.

5. Have the students compose a letter to the editor of a newspaper or medical journal concerning a nursing issue about which they feel strongly (eg, organ donation, abortion, the right to die, etc). Allow the students to read their letters to the class and invite comments.

GUIDE TO CRITICAL THINKING AND DEVELOPING BLENDED SKILLS

1. Instruct students to use the seven steps in the valuing process to modify the behavior of a student who is over- or undercommitted to achieving scholastically.

   You might want to lead the students through the following steps in the valuing process:

- Choosing freely: The underachieving student must be able and willing to choose to study.

- Choosing from alternatives: There are two alternatives—study and complete courses or flunk out of school.

- After consideration of alternatives: Teach the student the consequences of each alternative.

- Prizing with pride and happiness: Have the student define what staying in school means to her.

- Prizing with public affirmation: Have the student admit to teachers that she will try harder to improve her grades.

- Acting with incorporation of choice into one's behavior: The student should study and pass her courses.

- Acting with consistency and regularity on the value: The student stays in school and completes her course of study.

2. Have students jointly develop a list of ethical rules and apply these to practical situations. For example, if "never lie to a patient" is on their list of rules, present them with a situation in which some nurses would think lying is justified; for example, when a critically injured and unstable man who drove the car in which his wife was killed asks about his wife as he is being wheeled into the emergency room. Brainstorm with the group!

TEACHING–LEARNING PLAN: Values and Ethics in Nursing

Learning Objectives	Content Outline	Resources
Define key terms used in the chapter.		Table 6-1: Principles of Bioethics
List five common modes of value transmission.	A. Values: development of values, values essential to the professional nurse, value neutrality, values clarification.	Professional Values
Describe seven steps in the valuing process.		Steps in the Valuing Process
		Ethical Agency
Use values clarification strategies in clinical practice		A Patient's Bill of Rights
		Three Codes of Ethics for Nurses
Compare and contrast the principle- and care-based approaches to bioethics. Describe three typical concerns of the nurse advocate.	B. Ethics: professional ethical conduct, examples of ethical problems, nurses and ethics committees.	Reasoning About Ethical Decisions
Describe nursing practice that is consistent with the code of ethics for nursing.		Patient Care Study Using a Five-Step Process for Resolving the Ethical Problem
Recognize ethical issues as they arise in nursing practice.		Ethics Resources
Use an ethical framework and decision-making process to resolve ethical problems.		
Identify four functions of institutional ethics committees.		

Legal Implications of Nursing

■ Chapter Overview

Chapter 7 introduces the learner to basic legal concepts and describes the professional and legal regulation of nursing practice. Crimes and torts related to nursing practice are explained and the purpose of credentialing, suspending, or revoking a license or registration is identified. Legal safeguards for the nurse and nursing roles in malpractice litigation are highlighted. The roles of the nurse as defendant, fact witness, and expert witness are also presented.

■ Teaching–Learning Activities

GROUP ACTIVITIES

1. Have students research newspaper or magazine articles for a medical malpractice suit and summarize the following details: (a) who was involved in the case, (b) the issues surrounding the case, (c) when the case occurred, (d) why the case occurred and why it was covered by the media, and (e) how the case was handled or resolved? Divide the students into small groups and have them share the results of their research with each other. See if the class agrees with the resolution of the suit.

2. Arrange the students into groups of four. Give each member of the group one of the following forms to study: (a) an incident report, (b) an informed consent form, (c) a form for leaving the hospital against medical advice, and (d) a will. Have them review the forms and discuss situations in which they might be used.

3. Ask a representative of your local nursing association to speak to the class about carrying their own liability insurance.

4. Have students role-play obtaining informed consent for HIV testing from a patient. Invite the class to critique the performance of the students.

DISCUSSION QUESTIONS

1. When should a nurse question a physician's order? What is the correct procedure for doing this?

2. After surveying nurses in various clinical settings, discuss the legal issues pertinent to each practice and what nurses can do to limit legal liabilities.

3. What is the difference between an intentional tort and an unintentional tort? Give examples of each type. Should nurses be held equally accountable for both types of torts?

4. What is the legal responsibility of nurses in relation to documenting nursing actions? Do you feel it is important?

WRITING ACTIVITIES

1. Have students review the contract your educational facility has with your clinical agency and list the areas of liability for students, instructors, and nursing staff.

2. Have students describe the role of the nurse when litigation has been initiated.

3. Ask students to describe the four aspects of informed consent (disclosure, comprehension, competence, and voluntarism) and apply them to an assigned case.

4. Ask students to compare and contrast licensure and certification.

5. Have students complete incident reports for the following patients: (a) a witnessed fall, (b) a patient found on the floor.

GUIDE TO CRITICAL THINKING AND DEVELOPING BLENDED SKILLS

1. Present the class with the following situations illustrating areas of potential liability and have them describe appropriate safeguards.

   • A woman insists on keeping money and seemingly expensive jewelry at her bedside, even after she is warned that this is unsafe.

   • A patient's husband threatens to sue you if you don't find a private room for his wife. The only two private rooms are in use by patients with greater needs.

   • You have reason to suspect that a patient who is receiving strong medication for pain is using illegal drugs brought in by a friend.

2. Invite a risk manager or nurse attorney to speak to the class about common areas of nursing liability. Have the class develop strategies for reducing liability.

   Some strategies may include:

   • Obtaining informed consent
   • Keeping accurate patient data
   • Developing nursing diagnoses
   • Individualizing patient outcomes
   • Documenting teaching
   • Documenting goal achievement

TEACHING–LEARNING PLAN: Legal Implications of Nursing

Learning Objectives	Content Outline	Resources
Define key terms used in the chapter.		Table 7-1: Proof of Malpractice
Define law and describe its four sources.	A. Legal concepts: definition of law, litigation.	Table 7-2: Areas of Potential Liability for Nurses
Describe the professional and legal regulation of nursing practice.	B. Professional and legal regulation of nursing practice: credentialing.	Incident Report Sample
Identify the purpose of credentialing, using as examples accreditation, licensure or registration, and certification.		Who Makes Nursing Practice Rules? Checklist to Ensure Informed Consent Privacy and Confidentiality of Healthcare Records
Identify grounds for suspending or revoking a license or registration.		Nursing Malpractice Prevention
Differentiate intentional torts (assault and battery, defamation, invasion of privacy, false imprisonment, fraud) and unintentional torts (negligence).	C. Crimes and torts: intentional torts, unintentional torts.	
Evaluate personal areas of potential liability in nursing.	D. Legal safeguards for the nurse: contracts; competent practice; patient education; executing physician orders; documentation; adequate staffing; professional liability insurance; risk management programs; incident, variance, or occurrence reports; Good Samaritan laws.	
Describe the legal procedure once a plaintiff files a complaint against a nurse for negligence.		
Describe the roles of the nurse as defendant, fact witness, and expert witness. Use appropriate legal safeguards in nursing practice.	E. Student liability.	
Explain the purpose of incident reports.	F. Laws affecting nursing practice: occupational safety and health, national practitioner data bank, reporting obligations, controlled substances, discrimination and sexual harassment, persons with disabilities, wills.	
Describe laws affecting nursing practice.		
	G. Legal issues related to dying and death.	

UNIT II

Promoting Health Across the Life Span

Developmental Concepts

■ Chapter Overview

Chapter 8 explores the principles of growth and development from a theoretical perspective. An overview of developmental theories—including psychoanalytic, psychosocial, developmental tasks, cognitive development, moral development, and faith development—is presented. The applications of growth and development principles and theories to nursing are discussed, including their influence on growth and development and their implications for nurses.

■ Teaching–Learning Activities

GROUP ACTIVITIES

1. Write down each stage in Freud's, Erikson's, Piaget's, Kohlberg's, and Havighurst's developmental theories on index cards (one stage or level per card). Assign students to represent each of the following age groups: infant, toddler, preschooler, school-aged child, adolescent, and adult. Distribute the index cards to the class and have them match the stage or level with the appropriate age group.

2. As a group, visit a child-care center and an adult-care center. Spend time interacting with individuals, keeping in mind the principles of growth and development. Develop a plan for activities for both groups that reflect these principles.

3. Divide the class into groups and have them develop a teaching plan for a specific family, which includes information about risk factors for each member, knowledge and skills to increase health promotion, risk factors in the environment, and strategies for the prevention of illness and injury.

DISCUSSION QUESTIONS

1. How do family dynamics affect growth and development?

2. Think about your personal concept of the family. What factors influenced your idea of what a family should be? How might this concept affect your treatment of families in your practice? How might you modify your treatment to ensure quality patient care?

3. Discuss what Freud meant by the ego, the superego, and the id.

4. What effect has studying various developmental theories had on your own idea of human development? Which theory best fits your perception of the stages of growth and development?

5. How might nursing implications differ when caring for a 3-year-old child with leukemia as opposed to a 14-year-old with the same illness? How would you modify your plan of care to accommodate these differences?

WRITING ACTIVITIES

1. Have the students choose a child they know personally from friendships or family relationships and describe the stage of development this child is currently experiencing according to the developmental theories of Freud, Piaget, Havighurst, Kohlberg, and Erikson.

2. Ask students to identify and describe examples of ways in which "the rate and pattern of growth and development can be modified."

3. Have students describe the differences and similarities between the theories of moral development developed by Kohlberg and Gilligan. Which theory do they prefer?

4. Instruct the students to think about patients who represent various developmental stages, such as an infant, a toddler, a school-aged child, a teenager, an adult, and an older adult. How would they know whether or not these patients trusted them? Write down the behaviors they should look for in each developmental stage that would indicate a trusting nurse–patient relationship.

■ Guide to Critical Thinking and Developing Blended Skills

1. Divide the class into six groups, and assign each to research a developmental theorist (Freud, Erikson, Havighurst, Piaget, Kohlberg/Gilligan, or Fowler). Convene a panel with a representative from each group, and have them discuss cases from the viewpoint of their respective developmental theorists. Sample cases follow:

   - A mother of a hospitalized 6-year-old boy expresses concern to the nurse that her son is regressing.
   - Parents of a 13-year-old boy express concerns to a school nurse about their once model son's rebellious behavior in school and at home.
   - A successful 33-year-old businessman has a heart attack and expresses anxiety about the meaning of life: "All of a sudden I'm wondering about my priorities...I'm not even married, and until now, all I cared about was making money."
   - An independent and active older adult becomes severely withdrawn and uncommunicative on admission to a nursing home.

   You may want to refer to Table 8-1 in the textbook as a guide to the developmental stages or use the following example for the 6-year-old:

   - Freud: The 6-year-old is between the phallic and latency stages, interested in gender differences and is in conflict with same-sex parent.
   - Erickson: The 6-year-old is achievement oriented; acceptance of peers and parents is important.
   - Havighurst: Developmental tasks include developing physical skills, wholesome attitude about self, peers, sexual roles.
   - Piaget: The 6-year-old is in the preoperational stage; increased language and physical skills.
   - Kohlberg/Gilligan: Moral development is influenced by cultural effects on perceptions of justice in interpersonal relationships. Illness could affect moral development.
   - Fowler: The 6-year-old is in stage 1: intuitive projection; imitates religious gestures without understanding them.

2. Have members of the class visit various healthcare agencies and institutions (eg, day-care center, children's hospital, rehabilitation center, retirement community, nursing home) and analyze whether or not the environments in each are structured so as to support and challenge developmental growth. Have students suggest necessary modifications and describe nursing's role in securing the needed changes.

   They might want to consider whether the environment is:

   - Warm, friendly, homelike
   - Cold, clinical hospital atmosphere

   Modifications could include:

   - Inclusion of plants and pets
   - Initiating cultural events for the patients
   - Arranging social events for the patients
   - Incorporating the patients' belongings into their rooms

TEACHING–LEARNING PLAN: Developmental Concepts

Learning Objectives	Content Outline	Resources
Define key terms used in the chapter.		Table 8-1: Key Points of Developmental Theories
Summarize basic principles of growth and development.	A. The nature of human growth and development: principles of growth and development.	Incorporating Principles and Theories of Growth and Development
Discuss the theories of Freud, Erikson, Havighurst, Piaget, Kohlberg, Gilligan, and Fowler.	B. Overview of developmental theories: psychoanalytic theory—Sigmund Freud; psychosocial theory—Erik Erikson; developmental tasks—Robert J. Havighurst; cognitive development—Jean Piaget; moral development—Lawrence Kohlberg and Carol Gilligan; faith development—James Fowler.	Research Research in Nursing: Making a Difference: Reducing Risk Factors for Altered Growth and Development
Describe the importance of incorporating theories of growth and development in assessing and planning nursing care for individuals and families.		
Describe the role of the family in growth and development.	C. Family influences on growth and development.	
List implications for nursing practice that use a knowledge base of growth and development.	D. Implications for nursing: facilitating effective family functioning, applying growth and development principles.	

CHAPTER 9

Conception Through Young Adult

■ Chapter Overview

Chapter 9 discusses the development of the person from conception through young adulthood, covering the following stages: neonate, infancy, toddlerhood, preschooler, school-age, adolescence, and young adult. Psychological development, cognitive development, psychosocial development, common health problems, and the role of the nurse in healthcare for each stage are presented. Developmental milestones are briefly presented and nursing actions to promote wellness at each developmental level are discussed.

■ Teaching–Learning Activities

GROUP ACTIVITIES

1. Divide the class into six groups and assign an age group to each (neonate, infant, toddler, preschooler, school-aged child, adolescent, young adult). Have them determine the common health problems for each group and develop nursing strategies to promote health and prevent illness in these groups.

2. Ask a panel of nurses representing clinical practice for various age groups to discuss how a knowledge base of normal growth and development is used in safe and holistic patient care.

3. Have the students visit a maternity unit and interview several new mothers about their experiences with their newborns. Observe the mother with the infant and assess for bonding, health problems, and infant reflexes and temperament.

4. Write the following nursing diagnoses on the board. Have the class come up with potential cases that would reflect each diagnosis.
   - Altered Growth and Development related to poor support system
   - Altered Parenting related to unrealistic expectations for child
   - Altered Growth and Development related to perceptual disturbance
   - Altered Growth and Development related to prolonged illness and disability that exhausts coping abilities

DISCUSSION QUESTIONS

1. What problems in growth and development may appear if bonding does not occur or developmental tasks are not met?

2. Describe the environmental and nutritional factors that influence the stages of development from the neonate to young adult.

3. Discuss the following statement and the nurse's role in meeting the challenge to improve the healthcare of the nation's children: "Although the United States is one of the wealthiest nations in the world, each year thousands of children do not receive adequate healthcare."

4. What factors increase the potential for abusive behavior toward children in families?

WRITING ACTIVITIES

1. Ask students to develop a plan for appropriate play activities for infants, toddlers, preschoolers, and school-aged children. Have them describe how the plan would differ for each group in relationship to their development level.

2. Have the students describe the role of the nurse in providing healthcare for the following age groups:

neonate, infant, toddler, preschooler, school-aged child, adolescent, and young adult.

3. Ask students to write a descriptive essay about their childhood and adolescence.

4. Ask students to summarize a nursing or psychology journal article that discusses one of the age groups presented in this chapter.

GUIDE TO CRITICAL THINKING AND DEVELOPING BLENDED SKILLS

1. Have the students interview a new parent, a parent of a toddler, and a parent of a teenager to determine their primary concerns in caring for their child. How do these concerns differ for each age group? Do the parents feel confident in their parenting roles? What behaviors/actions have you observed that could be addressed by nursing's teaching/counseling role?

   You may want to consider the following needs of each age group:
   a. New parent: basic survival concerns
      • Weight
      • Temperament
      • Growth, sleeping through the night
      • Checkups, immunizations
   b. Parent of a toddler
      • Teach childproofing home
      • Need for regular checkups
      • Verbal and physical skills are developing
   c. Parent of a teenager
      • Influence of peer pressure
      • Teach alcohol and drug abuse
      • Teach school safety

• Teach sex education
• Explore teen's mental health: self-esteem, teen suicide

2. Keeping in mind the cognitive development of each age group, how would you explain the need for a surgical procedure to children aged 3, 10, and 15?

   You may want to use the following examples to explain the different factors affecting the patient's understanding of the procedure:
   a. 3-year-old: In Piaget's preoperational stage, preconceptual stage—play activities allow the child to better understand events.
      • Demonstrate the procedure on a doll.
   b. 10-year-old: In Piaget's concrete operational stage—children learn by manipulating concrete or tangible objects; logical thinking is developing.
      • Explain the procedure as simply as possible and demonstrate on child by role-play activities.
   c. 15-year-old: In Piaget's formal operational stage—use of abstract thinking and deductive reasoning.
      • Explain the procedure and the need for it. Demonstrate the procedure on the child.

TEACHING–LEARNING PLAN: Conception Through Young Adult

Learning Objectives	Content Outline	Resources
Define key terms used in the chapter.		Table 9-1: Apgar Scoring Chart
Summarize major physiologic, cognitive, psychosocial, moral, and spiritual developments from conception through young adulthood.	A. Environmental and nutritional influences.	Table 9-2: Promoting Health in Infancy
	B. Conception and prenatal development.	Table 9-3: Recommended Childhood Immunization Schedule United States, January–December 1999
List common health problems of each age period from conception through young adulthood.	C. Neonate (birth to 28 days): physiologic development, common health problems.	Table 9-4: Promoting Health in Toddlerhood
Describe nursing actions to promote wellness at each developmental level.	D. Infant (1 month to 1 year): physiologic development, growth patterns, cognitive development, psychosocial development, common health problems, role of the nurse in healthcare.	Table 9-5: Promoting Health in Preschoolers
		Table 9-6: Promoting Health in School-Aged Children
	E. Toddler (1–3 years): physiologic development, cognitive development, psychosocial development, common health problems, role of the nurse in healthcare.	Table 9-7: Adolescent Sexual Development
		Table 9-8: Promoting Health in Adolescents and Young Adults
	F. Preschooler (3–6 years): physiologic development, cognitive development, psychosocial development, moral and spiritual development, common health problems, role of the nurse in healthcare.	Examples of NANDA Nursing Diagnoses Infancy Through School Age
		Examples of NANDA Nursing Diagnoses Adolescence
	G. School-aged child (6–12 years): physiologic development, cognitive development, psychosocial development, moral and spiritual development, common health problems, role of the nurse in healthcare.	
	H. Adolescent and young adult: physiologic development, cognitive development, psychosocial development, moral and spiritual development, common health problems, role of the nurse in healthcare.	

CHAPTER 10

The Aging Adult

■ Chapter Overview

Chapter 10 focuses on the middle and older adult. Information presented includes adult developmental theories and theories on aging, with a discussion of physiologic and functional status, cognitive development, and developmental tasks specific to adulthood. Meeting the healthcare needs of this age group is discussed, including the awareness of lifestyle risks, chronic illnesses, injuries, and acute care needs. The nurse's role in the healthcare of this age group is outlined.

■ Teaching–Learning Activities

GROUP ACTIVITIES

1. Divide the class into three groups and have each group list the major tasks that must be accomplished during middle adulthood and older adulthood.

2. Ask students to discuss lifestyles, values, and goals with family members and friends who are in their 40s, 50s, 60s, and 70s. Organize a group discussion of the differences and similarities of these age periods.

3. Ask a member of the AARP to discuss services provided for older adults.

4. Divide the class into small groups and have them discuss the health issues related to aging (diabetes, cardiovascular disease, Alzheimer's disease, urinary incontinence, etc) and develop nursing strategies to care for these patients.

DISCUSSION QUESTIONS

1. Is ageism a common problem? If so, what can be done to decrease the prejudice?

2. Discuss the common health problems in middle-aged adults and older adults.

3. Explain why the older adult requires a longer time period to recover from illness or injury.

4. What nursing actions can help maintain orientation and lessen confusion in the hospitalized adult?

5. Discuss what is meant by empty nest syndrome and being caught in a "generation sandwich." If possible, have the students interview adults who are currently experiencing these conditions to discover their feelings and coping mechanisms.

WRITING ACTIVITIES

1. Have students interview an older adult near retirement age to see how he has adjusted to the changes of aging. Have students explore the adult's physical strength and health, retirement plans, health of spouse, social roles, living arrangements, and relationships with peers and record their findings in a report.

2. Ask students to outline modifications that can be made in the homes of older adults to promote comfort and safety.

3. Ask students to write down their feelings about becoming an adult and coping with new responsibilities and tasks. Have them explore how these feelings differ from perceptions they had about adults as children.

4. Have students research aging theories and write a report on any new findings.

GUIDE TO CRITICAL THINKING AND DEVELOPING BLENDED SKILLS

1. Instruct the class to write down the first three words that come to mind when they hear the term "old age." Guide them in a discussion of why their associations are different and what has influenced their perceptions. Explore how these perceptions can influence their professional relationships with older patients. Brainstorm with the class!

2. Poll the class to determine the diversity displayed by their grandparents' life situations. Ask how many have grandparents in each of the following

categories: living independently in their own homes, living with adult children, living actively in a retirement community, living in a nursing home, deceased. Invite the class to explore how their personal experiences with older family members influence their perceptions of old age and inter-actions with older patients. You may want to explore the following:

- The effect of grandparents on the power structure of the family
- The effect of grandparents on the values of the family
- Independent adults versus dependent adults

3. Have each member in the class identify common health problems for which three family members or friends in different stages of adulthood are at risk. Develop a teaching plan to assist each to prevent these problems. You might want to consider the following health problems for adults:

- Middle adulthood: raising children, divorce, work stress
- Older adulthood: end of life issues, retirement issues, living independently versus living in nursing home or with grown children

TEACHING–LEARNING PLAN: The Aging Adult

Learning Objectives	Content Outline	Resources
Define key terms used in the chapter.		Table 10-1: Myths and Realities About Older Adults
Discuss the adult aging theories.	A. Adult aging theories: the genetic theory; the immunity theory, cross-linkage theory, free radical theory	Table 10-2: Promoting Health and Preventing Illness in the Older Adult
Discuss developmental tasks of the older adult as described by Erikson and Havighurst.	B. Middle adulthood (40–50 years): physiologic development; psychosocial development; cognitive, moral, and spiritual development; common health problems; the nurse's role in healthcare.	Physical Changes in the Middle Adult
Summarize major physiologic, cognitive, psychosocial, moral, and spiritual development of middle and older adulthood. Compare physiologic and functional changes that occur with normal aging.		Examples of NANDA Nursing Diagnoses: Middle Adult
		Normal Physiologic Changes of Older Adulthood
Identify socioenvironmental factors in our society that may prevent the older adult from meeting personal needs and realizing potentials.	C. Older adulthood: physiologic development, cognitive changes, developmental theories, Erikson—psychosocial development, Havighurst—developmental tasks.	Using the Nursing Interventions Classification (NIC): Selected Reminiscence Therapy Activities
		Examples of NANDA Nursing Diagnoses: Older Adult
Discuss nursing implications concerning the continued growth and development of the adult.		Research Research in Nursing: Making a Difference
Describe common myths and stereotypes that perpetuate ageism.	D. Paradoxical aging: an adaptive population, ageism, and common stereotypes.	
Describe the healthcare needs of the older adult in terms of chronic illnesses, accidental injuries, and acute care needs.	E. Gerontology and the healthcare system: common health problems of the older adult, the nurse's role in healthcare.	
List family and community resources that can be used to maintain the health and independence of the elderly patient.		

UNIT III

Community-Based Settings for Patient Care

Community-Based Healthcare

■ Chapter Overview

Chapter 11 introduces the reader to the various settings in which healthcare may be provided, including the home, community healthcare settings, ambulatory care settings, long-term care settings, and hospitals. Government healthcare agencies and their services are discussed, and various methods of financing healthcare in the United States and Canada are described. The roles of healthcare members are presented as well as trends and issues affecting the healthcare delivery system such as cost containment, DRGs, managed care, fragmentation of care, and the focus on self-care and wellness.

■ Teaching–Learning Activities

GROUP ACTIVITIES

1. Divide the class into seven groups and assign a specialized care center for each group to research, such as day-care centers, mental health centers, rural health centers, schools, industry, homeless shelters, and rehabilitation centers. Have each group visit the center and report back to the class on (a) the types of services offered, (b) the role of the nurse in each center, (c) the purpose of the center, (d) the type of funding available (private or public) for the center, and (e) the impact of the center on the community.

2. Have the class divide in half and debate the advantages and disadvantages of DRGs.

3. Invite healthcare professionals (physicians, PAs, PTs, RTs, OTs, social workers, etc) to speak to the class about their individual roles and responsibilities in the healthcare system.

4. Divide the class into small groups and have them develop their ideal method for delivering patient care. How does this method differ from the examples in this chapter?

DISCUSSION QUESTIONS

1. Why is home care one of the most rapidly growing areas of the healthcare system?

2. Is healthcare a right or a privilege? Should public funds be provided for the healthcare needs of the homeless population? Do uninsured people deserve the same healthcare treatment as employed, insured people?

3. How do health maintenance organizations promote wellness?

4. What is meant by the phrase "fragmentation of care"? How does this phenomenon affect the patient, especially the patient who is older and chronically ill?

5. What blended skills should you possess to be a nurse in a community-based setting?

WRITING ACTIVITIES

1. Ask the students to list the different types of healthcare settings they have experienced or observed and briefly describe their differences and similarities.

2. Have the students research different methods for financing healthcare (HMOs, PPOs, PPAs, private insurance), noting how each method works and the advantages and disadvantages of each.

3. Have students compare and contrast Medicaid and Medicare, describing who and what each plan covers.

4. Have the students write an essay describing the future practice of nursing.

GUIDE TO CRITICAL THINKING AND DEVELOPING BLENDED SKILLS

1. Assist the class in making a list of the types and varieties of healthcare settings in the local community (eg, hospitals, primary care offices, ambulatory centers, specialized care centers, long-term care centers, and hospice settings). Assign a team of students to visit each type of institution/agency. Have each team report on the nursing needs of patients in each setting and related nursing functions. Poll the class to determine how many would prefer to work in each setting and discuss their reasons.

You might want to include the following nursing roles in your discussion:

- Hospitals: nurses are administrators or managers; assess and monitor patient's health status; provide direct and/or specialized care; plan, implement, and evaluate plans of care; make referrals.
- Primary care offices: nurses make health assessments, perform technical skills, assist physicians, provide health education.
- Ambulatory centers: nurses make assessments of health status; assist primary caregiver; teach patients and families; plan, implement, and evaluate plans of care.
- Specialized care centers: nurses work in day-care centers, mental health centers, rural healthcare centers, schools, industry, homeless shelters, rehabilitation centers.

- Hospices: nurses manage symptoms of patients, give comfort measures, arrange respite care, are liaisons between the patient and healthcare provider.
- Long-term care: nurses work as administrators; coordinate care; give direct care; teach patients and family; plan, implement, and evaluate plans of care and make referrals.

2. Assign groups of students to research current trends and issues in healthcare, noting nursing's role in bringing about needed change. Topics may be broadly presented (Can healthcare costs be contained without sacrificing quality? Is there a healthcare crisis? How do the increasing numbers of frail elderly affect the availability of healthcare for all? Should wealth and fame influence the distribution of scarce organs?). Topics may also be presented as specific challenges (How would you advise a mother who is delaying seeking treatment for a child because she lacks health insurance? How would you respond to a neighbor who tells you that he is unwilling to pay higher taxes to support the uninsured poor? What do you do if your patient is severely depressed and needs a psychiatric consult that is not approved by his third-party insurer?). Brainstorm with the class!

TEACHING–LEARNING PLAN: Community-Based Healthcare

Learning Objectives	Content Outline	Resources
Define key terms used in the chapter.		Competencies for Healthcare Practitioners for 2005
Describe the role of nursing in meeting the challenges of healthcare reform.	A. Healthcare policy and reform: nursing's role in healthcare reform.	Examples of Nursing Activities in Various Healthcare Settings
Compare and contrast the different community-based settings in which healthcare is provided.	B. Types of healthcare settings: the home setting, hospitals, acute care settings, primary care centers, ambulatory care centers and clinics, specialized care centers, long-term care facilities, hospice services, voluntary agencies, religious agencies, government agencies, public health agencies.	
Describe community-based healthcare agencies and services.	C. Agencies providing care: voluntary agencies, religious agencies, government agencies, public health agencies.	
Discuss the elements of managed care, case management, and primary healthcare.	D. Frameworks for care: managed care systems, case management, primary healthcare.	
Describe the roles of members of collaborative healthcare teams.	E. Collaborative care.	
Discuss various methods of financing healthcare in the United States and Canada.	F. Financial aspects of healthcare: federally funded healthcare programs, group plans, health maintenance organizations.	
Discuss trends and issues affecting healthcare delivery.	G. Trends and issues in healthcare delivery: focus on self-care and wellness; consumer movement; cost containment; fragmentation of care; changes in patient care needs; healthcare—a right or a privilege?	

CHAPTER 12

Continuity of Care

■ Chapter Overview

Chapter 12 introduces the learner to the process of maintaining continuity of care between and among patient care settings. The coordination of services provided to patients before they enter a healthcare setting, during the time they are in the setting, and after they leave the setting is discussed. Also, nursing roles and responsibilities in admitting a patient to a healthcare setting, transferring a patient within and between settings, and performing discharge planning for a patient are explored.

■ Teaching–Learning Activities

GROUP ACTIVITIES

1. Divide the class into pairs and have students take turns role-playing each of the following activities: (a) admitting a patient to a hospital unit, (b) admitting a patient to an ambulatory healthcare facility, and (c) discharging a patient from a healthcare agency. Videotape the interactions and critique them together with the class.

2. Have the students take turns preparing a room for an admission. Be sure they include: (a) positioning the bed, (b) opening the bed, (c) assembling necessary equipment and supplies, (d) assembling equipment for vital signs and specimens, and (e) assembling any special equipment and supplies.

3. Divide the class into five groups and have the students discharge a patient with a specific healthcare problem, such as a patient who underwent surgery for a colostomy or a diabetic patient with foot ulcers. Give each group one aspect of the discharge process to handle (medications, procedures and treatments, diet, referrals, health promotion). Have one person in each group record the knowledge and skills necessary to meet this patient's discharge needs and share each group's results with the class.

4. Have students interview the family caregivers of patients recently discharged home after a hospital stay. Have them report on how confident family members feel about providing necessary care and specific ways nursing could be a help.

DISCUSSION QUESTIONS

1. What medical procedures are now being done on an outpatient or same-day basis that traditionally were done on an inpatient basis? What implications does this have for nursing?

2. What can the nurse do to help to alleviate the anxiety a patient and her family may experience when entering and leaving a healthcare setting?

3. Discuss the new roles a patient assumes when entering a healthcare setting.

4. What teaching–learning principles must be used when preparing the patient and family for self-care at home?

5. Discuss what can be done to bridge the gap between hospital care and home healthcare.

WRITING ACTIVITIES

1. Make a list of the nursing diagnoses appropriate for a patient who has had abdominal surgery and who will be dismissed and require pain medications, antibiotics, and dressing changes.

2. List the comfort, safety, and knowledge needs of a patient who is being transferred (a) from an emergency room to a hospital room, (b) from an acute care setting to a long-term care setting, (c) from an acute care setting to a rehabilitation center, and (d) from an ambulatory care setting to an acute care setting.

3. Have the students write a paragraph describing the factors that should be assessed when discharging a patient and how they would approach and question the patient to obtain the following types of information: (a) health data, (b) personal data, (c) caregivers, (d) environment, and (e) financial and support services.

4. Have the students devise a teaching plan for a patient who is being sent home to his family after a myocardial infarction that left him with paralysis of his left side and speech impairment.

GUIDE TO CRITICAL THINKING AND DEVELOPING BLENDED SKILLS

1. Obtain admission and discharge forms from various healthcare institutions and agencies and have the students take turns admitting and discharging one another from these settings using these forms. Discuss the different types of information required in different settings and the helpfulness of the different forms in facilitating both the process and the documentation of admission and discharge.

   You might want to use the following guidelines in your discussion:
   - Hospitals: Staff obtain information on patients in admitting office. Patient records should include name, address, date of birth, physician, gender, marital status, nearest relative, occupation and employer, financial status, religious preferences, date and time of admission, identification number.
   - Ambulatory centers: Nurses should obtain short health history, conduct a physical assessment, and offer patient teaching and referrals.

2. Assign groups of students to explore the availability of needed community resources for the following patients who are ready to be discharged from an acute care setting. Develop strategies to remedy deficiencies in existing resources.

   - Premature infant who was born to, and abandoned by, a cocaine-abusing mother

   - Frail elderly man hospitalized for pneumonia, who is returning to his home where he lives alone and is in need of some assistance with activities of daily living such as food procurement and preparation, bathing, transportation to and from the doctor
   - Teen who unsuccessfully attempted suicide by slashing his wrists who has a history of drug and alcohol abuse and general acting out behaviors and whose parents are utterly frustrated by his behavior and state being "at the end of their ropes"
   - Adult woman who lives alone and is in need of hemodialysis treatments three times weekly and has a long history of being noncompliant with dietary restrictions, medication administration, and other self-care behaviors
   - Older adult who is moving in with daughter and daughter's family following stabilization for a stroke that left her paralyzed on her left side
   - Fifty-four-year-old man with end-stage cancer of the lung who is returning home to his wife expecting to die because his doctors have told him there are no other therapies worth attempting

   You might want to have your students research the following community resources:
   - Home healthcare
   - Child welfare agencies
   - Hospice care
   - Meals-on-Wheels
   - Mental health centers
   - Public transportation
   - Respite care

TEACHING–LEARNING PLAN: Continuity of Care

Learning Objectives	Content Outline	Resources
Define key terms used in the chapter.		Admission Database Sample
Describe the role of the nurse in ensuring continuity of care among patient care settings.	A. The nurse's role in providing continuity of care.	Establishing an Effective Nurse–Patient Relationship
Discuss considerations for establishing an effective nurse–patient relationship when admitting a patient to a healthcare setting.		Focused Assessment Guide: Discharge Planning

Examples of NANDA Nursing Diagnoses: Discharging From a Healthcare Setting |
Compare and contrast patient admission procedures for an ambulatory versus a hospital setting.	B. Admitting a patient to a healthcare setting: admission to an ambulatory healthcare facility; admission to a hospital unit.	
Discuss transfer of patients within and among healthcare settings.	C. Transferring within and between settings.	
Describe the components of discharge planning in providing continuity of care.	D. Discharging from a healthcare setting: leaving the hospital against medical advice; discharge planning.	

Home Healthcare

■ Chapter Overview

Chapter 13 explores the change in the healthcare industry from hospital-based care settings to community-based care, provided by a variety of agencies and healthcare providers. The role managed care has played in the move from the hospital to the home and the types of agencies providing community-based care are discussed. The chapter focuses on the care provided by nurses in the home and the characteristics and roles of the home health nurse. The various phases of the home visit, hospice nursing, and the future of home care are also presented.

■ Teaching–Learning Activities

GROUP ACTIVITIES

1. Divide the class into pairs and have them role-play the entry phase of a home visit with a patient who is on oxygen therapy following treatment for emphysema. Emphasis should be placed on developing a rapport with the patient and family, mutually determining desired outcomes, making assessments, planning and implementing prescribed care, and providing teaching.

2. Have a representative from a local home healthcare agency speak to the class about the nature of the services it offers, primary methods for reimbursement for these services, and the major challenges facing home healthcare nurses.

3. Invite a home healthcare nurse and hospital nurse to share their experiences with the class. Compare and contrast the role of the nurse in both settings.

DISCUSSION QUESTIONS

1. What are the characteristics of a home health nurse? Which of these characteristics do you have and which do you need to improve on?

2. What can nurses do to decrease the legal risk when working with home care patients? What safety issues may arise for a nurse working in a home healthcare setting?

3. How does the role of the family in home care compare to that of the family in hospital-based care? What teaching strategies would you implement to help families care for patients in their homes?

4. What blended skills will you need to possess to meet the healthcare needs of patients and their families in home healthcare settings?

WRITING ACTIVITIES

1. Have each student make a list of all the concerns that would have to be addressed if they were to bring an aging parent with failing health into their present household. Be sure to consider physical resources (availability of an extra bedroom, bathing facilities, environmental safety, cleanliness, meal preparation) and social resources (availability of home care agencies, reactions of family members, people to assist with respite care). Compare the students' lists and discuss differences and similarities.

2. Have students research the history of home healthcare and write a brief report noting the key figures and events leading to the development of home healthcare agencies.

3. Have students list the major components of the preentry and entry phase of the home visit.

4. "The nurse providing care in the home is a patient advocate, coordinator of services, and patient/family educator." Ask the students to write a brief paragraph explaining the roles of the home healthcare nurse listed above.

GUIDE TO CRITICAL THINKING AND DEVELOPING BLENDED SKILLS

1. Have students interview several families taking care of chronically ill family members in their homes. Determine how they are coping with the responsibilities of providing long-term personal care and the increased financial burden. Develop a plan of care for the family that will help to ease the burden of care, facilitate patient and family access to community resources, and assist the family in meeting medical and financial needs. You might want to have the students check if the patient and family qualify for:

   - Home healthcare
   - Respite care
   - Medicare
   - Specialized therapy

2. Describe the role of the hospice nurse when caring for the terminally ill and their families. How does this role differ from other nursing disciplines? What is the focus of the hospice nurse and what skills does this nurse need to be effective? Explore the following roles of hospice nurses:

   - Focus on maintaining quality of life and dignity for the dying person by providing an environment that encourages open communication, symptom management, comfort measures, and support of family during and after the death of the patient.
   - Hospice nurses use cognitive skills, technical skills, interpersonal skills, and legal/ethical skills.
   - Patient advocate

TEACHING–LEARNING PLAN: Home Healthcare

Learning Objectives	Content Outline	Resources
Define home healthcare.	A. Definition of home healthcare.	Table 13-1: Collaborative Roles of Members of the Home Healthcare Team
Outline the history of home healthcare.	B. The history of home care nursing.	
Describe the characteristics and roles of the home health nurse.	C. Nursing and home healthcare: the unique role of the home care nurse, characteristics of the home health nurse, roles of the home health nurse.	Example of a Home Health Plan or Care
		Example of a Home Health Nursing Progress Note
		Through the Eyes of the Family Caregiver
Identify the essential components of the preentry and entry phase of the home visit.	D. The home visit: the preentry phase of the home visit, the entry phase of the home visit.	Examples of NANDA Nursing Diagnoses: Home Healthcare
Compare the role of the family in home care to hospital-based care.	E. The needs of caregivers in the home.	
Describe the purpose of hospice nursing.	F. Hospice nursing in the home.	
	G. The future of home care.	

UNIT IV

The Nursing Process

Blended Skills and Critical Thinking Throughout the Nursing Process

■ Chapter Overview

Chapter 14 defines the four basic skills essential to nursing practice—cognitive skills, technical skills, interpersonal skills, and ethical/legal skills—and presents plans for developing these skills for use in the nursing process. Developing the method of critical thinking by using purpose of thinking, adequacy of knowledge, potential problems, helpful resources, and critique of judgment/decision is also discussed. An assessment tool is included to determine the individual nurse's proficiency in the skills essential to competent use of the nursing process.

■ Teaching–Learning Activities

GROUP ACTIVITIES

1. Divide the class into small groups and have them list the personal qualities and skills a nurse must possess to develop critical thinking skills, keeping the following considerations in mind: (a) purpose of thinking, (b) adequacy of knowledge, (c) potential problems, (d) helpful resources, and (e) critique of judgment/decision. Have them share their results with the class.

2. Invite a panel of nurses from various healthcare settings to discuss critical thinking skills. Explore what critical thinking means to these nurses and how they apply these skills in their practice. Alternatively, invite these nurses to talk about which blended skills are most useful in their practice, and why.

3. Have students role-play treating different types of patients in a manner that respects their human dignity (eg, a mother with a cocaine addiction, an elderly man with Alzheimer's disease, a woman who had an abortion, a homosexual with AIDS, a victim of child abuse, a victim of rape).

4. Divide the class into small groups. Ask the groups to answer the following questions from the text. Have them work together to collectively answer the questions and develop a plan for self-improvement in these areas. Share each group's results with the rest of the class.
   - To what extent does my commitment to securing the human well-being of those in my care dictate my work priorities?
   - How comfortable am I voicing unmet patient needs to other members of the healthcare team?
   - Do other caregivers listen when I present patient concerns because of my successful record of patient advocacy?
   - What system variables (eg nurse–patient ratios, skill mix, availability of resources) need to change for us to meet the human needs of our patients adequately?
   - In what ways must I change for my patients to be able to rely on me to respond to their needs in a responsible manner?

DISCUSSION QUESTIONS

1. What resources are available to student nurses to help remedy deficiencies in their blended skills?

2. How can student nurses help themselves master intricate procedures that involve working with technical equipment?

3. Discuss the following questions about human dignity and respect:
   - What do I see in my patients that obligates me to respect them?
   - Are all patients equally deserving of my respect?
   - What strengths and weaknesses do I possess when it comes to respecting patients?
   - Which patients in my practice are a challenge to my ability to respect their dignity, and how can I overcome this deficiency?

4. What does it mean to "hold oneself accountable for the human well-being of patients entrusted to your care"?

WRITING ACTIVITIES

1. Have the students choose a procedure from their textbook and become familiar with each step. Have them interview five experienced nurses to see how they perform the same procedure and report the following information: (a) What does each nurse do differently/the same? (b) What actions will you incorporate into your method of performing the procedure? (c) Which method was the easiest, most effective, safest, most efficient, or most beneficial to the patient?

2. Have the students research recent nursing journals for articles concerning critical thinking skills and write a brief report/critique. Share each student's report with the class.

3. Have students write a brief paragraph on the four types of skills essential to nursing practice: (a) intellectual, (b) interpersonal, (c) technical, and (d) ethical/legal.

GUIDE TO CRITICAL THINKING AND DEVELOPING BLENDED SKILLS

1. Have the students choose a problem presented to them in their clinical practice and use the considerations outlined in the textbook to attempt to solve the problem using critical thinking competencies.

   You might want to explore the following critical thinking considerations:
   - Purpose of thinking
   - Adequacy of knowledge
   - Potential problems
   - Helpful resources
   - Critique of judgment

2. Explore the type of message you may be sending your patients when you walk into their room. Does your demeanor communicate a caring attitude, a "drop dead" attitude, or an indifferent attitude? What can you do to improve your ability to communicate a caring attitude through looks, speech, and touch? Brainstorm with the class!

TEACHING–LEARNING PLAN: Blended Skills and Critical Thinking Throughout the Nursing Process

Learning Objectives	Content Outline	Resources
Define key terms used in the chapter.		Table 14-1: Overview of the Nursing Process
Describe the four basic skills essential to nursing practice.	A. Defining the four basic skills: cognitive skills, technical skills, interpersonal skills, ethical/legal skills.	Table 14-2: The Four Domains of Critical Thinking
Use a model of critical thinking when making clinical judgments and decisions.	B. Developing critical thinking skills: purpose of thinking, adequacy of knowledge, potential problems, helpful resources, critique of judgment/decision.	Through the Eyes of a Student

Example of the Nursing Process in Action

Checklist for Evaluating Your Use of the Nursing Process |
| Identify four habits that assist in the development of technical skills. | C. Developing technical skills. | Developing Critical Thinking Skills |
| Describe a personal plan to develop the interpersonal skills essential to quality care. | D. Developing interpersonal skills: promoting human dignity and respect, establishing caring relationships, enjoying the rewards of mutual interchange. | Applying Learning to Practice: Human Dignity: How Who I Am as a Caregiver Affects Others

Through the Eyes of a Patient |
| Explain the relationship between a nurse's sense of accountability and patient well-being. | E. Developing ethical/legal skills: holding oneself accountable. | Applying Learning to Practice: Accountability |
| Identify personal strengths and weaknesses in light of nursing's essential knowledge and skills. | F. Reporting incompetent, unethical, or illegal practice: whistle-blowing. | Take the Challenge |

CHAPTER 15

Assessing

■ Chapter Overview

Chapter 15 introduces the unique focus of nursing assessment: the systematic and continuous collection, validation, and communication of patient data. Types of data, characteristics of data, data collection methods, and sources of data are discussed, as well as methods for interviewing the patient to obtain a nursing history and performing a nursing examination to collect data. Techniques for validating, communicating, timing, and documenting data are also presented.

■ Teaching–Learning Activities

GROUP ACTIVITIES

1. Have two students role-play an interview with a patient to obtain a nursing history. Divide the class into two groups and ask one group to write down all the subjective data obtained through the interview and the other group to write down all the objective data. Compare the two lists and conduct a discussion on the importance of each type of data and how they are different.

2. Divide the class into five groups. Give one member of each group a slip of paper with a description of a health problem that she will role-play during the exercise (eg, risk for self-harm, altered comfort, dysfunctional grieving). Have the rest of the group conduct an interview with the patient to determine a patient diagnosis. Note the type of questions that were asked by the group and how the patient's responses helped formulate a diagnosis.

3. Divide the class into small groups. Supply each group with a completed nursing health history form found in a patient's medical record. Have each group analyze the form, identifying the basic components of the nursing history, any data not identified that are pertinent to the case, the data sources that were used in the health history, and the nature of the data supplied (subjective versus objective data). After reviewing the forms, have the students develop their own health history forms that would incorporate the information listed above.

4. Invite an experienced nurse to conduct an interview with a student volunteer about a health problem he has experienced. Videotape the interview and replay it to the class. Conduct a discussion on the technique of the interviewer, the phases of the interview, and the data obtained.

DISCUSSION QUESTIONS

1. Discuss patient variables that may negatively influence a patient interview and suggest nursing responses to these variables.

2. Discuss potential sources of data a nurse may use when preparing a patient assessment (patient, support people, patient record, other healthcare professionals, nursing and other healthcare literature).

3. What are the differences and similarities between a nursing assessment and a medical assessment?

4. Why is the validation of information important? When must data be verified?

5. Discuss the various data collection methods and when they should be used in practice (observation, interview, physical assessment techniques).

WRITING ACTIVITIES

1. Have students write a paragraph on one phase of the interview process (preparatory phase, introduction, working phase, termination) and all the nursing actions and responsibilities that occur in the phase chosen. Choose a student from the class to represent each phase and role-play a patient interview using their paragraphs as guidelines.

2. Ask students to write a paragraph describing the critical elements in each phase of the nurse–patient interview.

3. Have each student write down the components of a nursing history and how each type of information may be obtained.

4. Have students describe how each of the following factors may influence the type and amount of data that should be collected for a patient: (a) the patient's health orientation, (b) the patient's developmental stage, and (c) the patient's need for nursing.

GUIDE TO CRITICAL THINKING AND DEVELOPING BLENDED SKILLS

1. Have two students role-play a nurse interviewing a young woman in high school who has missed three periods and is terrified that she may be pregnant. Instruct the class to individually list the objective and subjective data gathered during the interview. Use an in-class discussion to compare their data lists and explore reasons for the differences. Identify variables that may impair a nurse's ability to gather data that are complete, accurate, factual, and relevant.

   You might want to explore the following patient variables:
   - Patient anxiety
   - Patient's pain
   - Language difficulties
   - Unrealistic expectations of healthcare professionals

2. Divide the class into groups and assign a work setting/specialty to each group (eg, well-child clinic, planned parenthood center, detox unit, nursing home, burn unit, orthopedic unit). Have students identify the type of data that nurses would need to gather for a comprehensive database, then obtain the assessment tools used in their assigned setting. Assess how well they were able to identify critical data and suggest necessary modifications for the prepared assessment tools.

   You might want to discuss the following:
   - Comprehensive versus focused data assessment
   - Assessment priorities
   - Health orientation
   - Developmental stage
   - Need for nursing
   - Practical considerations

TEACHING–LEARNING PLAN: Assessing

Learning Objectives	Content Outline	Resources
Define key terms used in the chapter.		Table 15-1: Comparison of Objective and Subjective Data
Describe the purpose of the initial nursing assessment and of ongoing nursing assessments.	A. Unique focus of nursing assessment.	Table 15-2: Patient Variables That Can Negatively Influence an Interview and Suggested Nursing Responses
Distinguish between a nursing assessment and a medical assessment.		Table 15-3: Common Problems of Data Collection, Possible Causes, and Suggested Remedies
Distinguish between objective and subjective data. Describe the purpose of nursing observation, interview, and physical assessment.	B. Data collection: types of data, characteristics of data, data collection methods, sources of data.	Through the Eyes of a Student
Obtain a nursing history using effective interviewing techniques.	C. Planning data collection: comprehensive versus focused data collection, assessment priorities, structuring the assessment, problems related to data collection.	Medical-Surgical-Critical Care Admission Assessment
Identify five sources of patient data useful to the nurse.		Through the Eyes of a Student
Distinguish between comprehensive admission assessments and focused assessments.		Legal Alert
Plan patient assessments by identifying assessment priorities and structuring the data to be collected systematically.		
Identify common problems encountered in data collection, noting their possible causes.		
Explain when data need to be validated and several ways to accomplish this.	D. Data validation.	
Describe the importance of knowing when to report. Keep significant patient data and proper documentation.	E. Data communication: timing, documentation.	
Obtain complete, accurate, factual, and relevant patient data.		

CHAPTER 16

Diagnosing

■ Chapter Overview

The interpretation and analysis of data gathered from the nursing assessment is the focus of Chapter 16: diagnosing. The identification of actual and potential problems in the way the patient responds to health or illness and the identification of etiologies and patient strengths are discussed. The distinction between nursing diagnosis versus collaborative problems is highlighted, as well as the interpretation and analysis of data. Guidelines for writing, prioritizing, and documenting diagnoses conclude the chapter.

■ Teaching–Learning Activities

GROUP ACTIVITIES

1. Divide the class into small groups. Ask them to use a case study to write several possible nursing diagnoses (using the NANDA list) and collaborative problems. Discuss how these diagnoses differ from medical diagnoses.

2. Ask the students to use the same case study to cluster groups of data that were used to develop the nursing diagnoses. Would they change any previously made diagnoses? If so, explain why.

3. Invite a panel of experienced nurses to visit the class. Place several case studies on the board and have the nurses and students write a diagnosis for each case. Share each nurse's diagnosis with the class and discuss similarities and differences. Invite the students to share their diagnoses and discuss any changes they may decide to incorporate into their diagnoses.

4. Divide the class into three groups. Present the following case study and have each group make a list of one of the following areas: (a) patient strengths, (b) patient problem areas, and (c) potential patient problems. Share the results with the class.

Case Study: A 16-year-old girl delivers her baby at home in her bedroom. Her parents find her and bring the mother and baby to the ER. The baby is premature and in respiratory distress and the mother has uncontrolled bleeding. The mother blames her situation on her daughter's boyfriend, a fellow classmate, who denies any responsibility for the baby.

DISCUSSION QUESTIONS

1. Discuss the cognitive, technical, interpersonal, and ethical/legal skills you will need as a nurse to meet the everyday diagnostic challenges of patients.

2. Explain the statement: "The etiology of the problem directs the nursing interventions."

3. Discuss the difference between nursing diagnoses and collaborative problems.

4. What factors should be considered when prioritizing nursing diagnoses and documentation?

WRITING ACTIVITIES

1. Ask students to describe the difference between an actual health problem and a potential high-risk health problem.

2. Have students summarize a recent nursing journal article that discussed nursing diagnoses.

3. Have students write nursing diagnoses for five patients to whom they have been assigned in their clinical practice.

4. Ask students to describe how nursing diagnosis is related to assessing.

GUIDE TO CRITICAL THINKING AND DEVELOPING BLENDED SKILLS

1. Present the class with a brief assessment of a patient and instruct students to individually construct a three-part nursing diagnosis. Once students have completed their diagnostic statements, compare their responses and determine which statement best identifies the patient's problem, etiologic factors, and pertinent signs and symptoms.

   - Describe the health state or health problem of a patient as clearly and concisely as possible.

   - Discuss the meaning of the words: altered, impaired, depleted, deficient, excessive, dysfunction, disturbed, ineffective, decreased, increased, acute, chronic, intermittent.

   - Discuss the following etiologic factors: physiologic, psychological, sociologic, spiritual, and environmental.

2. The process of diagnosing is not unique to nursing. Instruct students to review a patient medical record to find examples of medical diagnoses and diagnostic statements recorded by other health professionals. Use their findings to initiate a discussion of the purposes of different types of diagnoses, highlighting nursing's unique focus. Explore the differences between:

   - Actual problems
   - Potential problems
   - Possible problems

TEACHING–LEARNING PLAN: Diagnosing

Learning Objectives	Content Outline	Resources
Define key terms used in the chapter.		Table 16-1: A Comparison: Nursing Diagnosis, Collaborative Problem, Medical Diagnosis
Describe the term nursing diagnosis, distinguishing it from a collaborative problem and a medical diagnosis.	A. Unique focus of nursing diagnosis: nursing diagnosis versus medical diagnosis, nursing diagnosis versus collaborative problems.	Table 16-2: Diagnosing
Describe the four steps involved in data interpretation and analysis.	B. Data interpretation and analysis: recognizing significant data, recognizing patterns or clusters, identifying strengths and problems, reaching conclusions.	Table 16-3: Formulation of Nursing Diagnosis Statements Table 16-4: Common Errors in Writing Nursing Diagnoses and Recommended Corrections
Use the guidelines for writing nursing diagnoses when developing diagnostic statements. Describe means to validate nursing diagnoses.	C. Formulating and validating nursing diagnoses: writing nursing diagnoses; what is not a nursing diagnosis; actual, potential (high-risk), and possible nursing diagnoses; wellness diagnoses; validating nursing diagnoses.	Table 16-5: What a Nursing Diagnosis Is Not, and Why NANDA-Approved Nursing Diagnoses An Example of NANDA Diagnoses With Definition, Defining Characteristics, and Risk Factors or Related Factors
Develop a prioritized list of nursing diagnoses using identifiable criteria.	D. Prioritizing nursing diagnoses and documentation: Maslow's hierarchy of human needs, patient preference, anticipation of future problems.	
Describe the benefits and limitations of nursing diagnoses.	E. Nursing diagnosis: a critique.	

Planning

■ Chapter Overview

Chapter 17 introduces the learner to the planning stage of the nursing process. During this stage, the nurse works with the patient and family to develop patient goals and identify the nursing interventions most likely to assist the patient in achieving these goals. The various elements of planning are presented, including writing goals, developing evaluative strategies, selecting nursing measures, and writing nursing care plans. Problems related to planning and their possible causes and remedies are also discussed.

■ Teaching–Learning Activities

GROUP ACTIVITIES

1. Allow the students to work in small groups to read the situation below and respond to the three questions that follow:

   Ann Rogers is a 49-year-old housewife seen in the emergency room to rule out fractures. She states that she lost her balance and fell down her cellar stairs. Her husband is constantly at her side and she appears fearful. You recall previous admissions for lacerations, bruises, and a fracture.

   • How would you develop and prioritize the patient's nursing diagnoses?

   • What would be an appropriate long-term goal and a short-term goal for the priority nursing diagnosis?

   • What would be appropriate nursing orders for the priority nursing diagnosis?

2. Divide the class into small groups and have them review a nursing care plan for a selected patient in a healthcare facility. Ask the students to (a) identify the three stages of planning (initial, ongoing, discharge), (b) review the prioritized list of nursing diagnoses to see if they are correctly ranked, (c) determine what goals/outcomes are derived from these diagnoses, (d) note which goals are long-term

and short-term, and (e) list the nursing interventions derived from the nursing diagnoses.

3. Have students compare nursing care plans from different healthcare settings (eg, hospitals, clinics, home healthcare, day care) and note how they are similar and different for each setting. How may the plans have been modified to meet the individual needs of patients in various healthcare settings?

4. Have students imagine that a friend or relative has been hospitalized for an operable brain tumor. Ask them to develop a nursing care plan for this person, taking into consideration their friend's or relative's individual needs and potential nursing problems.

DISCUSSION QUESTIONS

1. What are the critical elements of an accurately written patient goal? What are some of the pitfalls to avoid when writing patient goals?

2. Why is it important to establish priorities of patient problems before planning patient care?

3. What is the unique focus of nursing planning? How is the plan of care supportive of nursing's broad aims—to promote health, prevent disease and illness, promote recovery, and facilitate coping with altered functioning?

4. What essential knowledge and skills must nurses possess to design a plan of care that results in the prevention, reduction, or resolution of patient health problems?

WRITING ACTIVITIES

1. Have students write long- and short-term goals for a patient who is recovering from a stroke with paralysis on the left side and who will be discharged to her daughter's home.

2. Have students use the terms "initial," "ongoing," and "discharge planning" to write a paragraph describing the planning step of the nursing process.

3. Have the student use the words listed below to write goals/outcomes for patients in their clinical practice:

define	identify	list
describe	explain	apply
use	demonstrate	prepare
verbalize	perform	choose

4. How would you include the family when planning care for a 14-year-old boy with AIDS acquired from blood transfusions who presented in the emergency room with pneumonia? Devise several goals for this patient and his family.

GUIDE TO CRITICAL THINKING AND DEVELOPING BLENDED SKILLS

1. Provide students with a sample standardized plan of care and four case scenarios of patients for whom the plan would be appropriate but most successful if modified to meet the patient's unique needs. Lead the class in a discussion of the importance of individualizing plans of care so that they respond to the unique needs of individual patients. Have the students consider the following competencies when individualizing care plans:

- Cognitive: know information, know pertinent standards of care, think critically about individual patient needs.

- Technical: research literature, document and communicate the plan.

- Interpersonal: establish trusting nurse–patient relationship, show empathy, work collaboratively with healthcare team, communicate respect and worth to patient.

- Ethical/legal: show personal commitment to the patient, be a patient advocate, use legal safeguards.

2. Pair students and have them role-play a nurse and patient working together to develop a plan of care to childproof a home for an active toddler. The objective is to maximize the parent's involvement in identifying valued goals and the interventions most likely to secure these goals. Videotape the role-play sessions and have the students critique each others' performances, identifying the students who were most successful in securing the parent's involvement, and why they were successful. Brainstorm with the class!

TEACHING–LEARNING PLAN: Planning

Learning Objectives	Content Outline	Resources
Define key terms used in the chapter.		Table 17-1: Examples of Goals to Relieve Problems
Describe the purposes and benefits of planning.	A. Unique focus of nursing planning.	Examples of Long- and Short-Term Goals
Identify three elements of comprehensive planning.	B. Comprehensive planning.	Evaluative Statement
Prioritize patient health problems and nursing responses.	C. Establishing priorities.	Structured Care Methodology and Characteristics
Describe how patient goals/expected outcomes and nursing orders are derived from nursing diagnoses.	D. Writing goals/outcomes and developing evaluative strategies: deriving goals/outcomes from nursing diagnoses; long-term versus short-term goals/outcomes; cognitive, psychomotor, and affective goals; guidelines for goal/outcome writing; common errors.	Standardized Plan of Care
Develop a plan of nursing care with properly constructed goals/outcomes and related nursing orders.		Student Care Plan
Use criteria to evaluate planning skills.	E. Developing evaluative strategy.	
	F. Selecting nursing interventions: deriving nursing interventions from nursing diagnoses, identifying and selecting options, consulting, nursing orders.	
	G. Writing the plan of nursing care: institutional/agency plans of care, student plans of care.	
Describe five common problems related to planning, their possible causes, and remedies.	H. Problems related to planning.	

CHAPTER 18

Implementing

■ Chapter Overview

The focus of Chapter 18 is the implementing step of the nursing process, in which all the nursing actions developed during the planning step are carried out. Assisting the patient to achieve desired health goals, promoting health, preventing disease/illness, restoring health, and facilitating coping with altered functioning are discussed. Nursing skills necessary for carrying out the plan of care and variables that influence goal achievement are also presented. The chapter concludes with a guide for student nurses organizing their nursing care for a clinical day and an introspective look at the art of "nursing oneself."

■ Teaching–Learning Activities

GROUP ACTIVITIES

1. Provide students with a case study that includes independent, interdependent, and dependent nursing interventions. Divide students into small groups to discuss the rationale of, expected effect of, possible side effects of, and possible adverse reactions to the interventions.

2. Divide students into small groups and have them visit different healthcare settings to determine how the nursing staff divides nursing care time. Discuss how much time is spent on independent, dependent, and collaborative nursing and what nursing care tasks are delegated to assistants.

3. Invite a nurse from a critical care unit and one from a long-term facility to visit the class to discuss (a) the amount of time spent with each patient, (b) the type of skills needed to care for their patients, (c) the type of interventions performed on their patients, and (d) expected goals/outcomes for their patients. Conduct a discussion of similarities and differences in each setting and patient variables that affect nursing care.

4. Divide the class into small groups and have them make a list of what factors need to be considered before delegating nursing care for the following patients:
   - Burn patient who needs bandages changed
   - Comatose patient who needs a sponge bath
   - Patient with a feeding tube who needs medication administered
   - New mother who is having difficulty breastfeeding her infant

DISCUSSION QUESTIONS

1. Discuss the advantages of having a standard classification of nursing interventions.

2. Explain how protocols and standing orders may expand the scope of nursing practice. Give examples of each.

3. Describe the role of the nurse as coordinator of healthcare for a patient. How does this role affect the patient and other healthcare professionals?

4. Discuss the role of teaching, counseling, and advocacy in promoting self-care for patients.

5. Discuss the type of variables (patient, nurse, healthcare system) that might adversely affect the implementation process.

WRITING ACTIVITIES

1. Have the students list factors that contribute to patient noncompliance and possible nursing interventions to improve a patient's outlook on illness.

2. Have students research a new nursing strategy that has proven effective and write a paragraph about how they will incorporate this strategy into their own nursing practice.

3. Have students develop a list of guidelines they should follow before implementing a nursing intervention. For example, students should consider the rationale of the action, the expected effect, possible side effects, possible adverse reactions, whether the intervention is still valid, whether the intervention needs to be changed, and so forth.

GUIDE TO CRITICAL THINKING AND DEVELOPING BLENDED SKILLS

1. Invite students to make a list of the personal qualities and skills/abilities that will enable them to work independently, interdependently, and dependently as well as those personal factors that may prove to be problematic in each of the above domains. Instruct the students to use this information to develop a self-improvement plan focused on their development of professional behaviors. For example, a student who is a great team player, but who fears working independently, may plan to assume more responsibility for independently managing select aspects of care.

   You might want to discuss the following competencies necessary for working successfully in the nursing profession:

   • Cognitive competencies: knowledge of what is needed to implement a plan

   • Technical competencies: ability to use equipment and techniques competently

   • Interpersonal competencies: communication skills, trusting nurse–patient relationship

   • Ethical/legal competencies: commitment to do whatever is necessary to implement plan of care; commitment to legal standards and being a patient advocate

2. Ask students to reflect on how their own human needs are being fulfilled and how this affects their ability to focus on their patient's needs. Have them discuss ways to increase self-confidence by developing an awareness of the importance of self-esteem, self-knowledge, satisfying interpersonal relationships, environmental mastery, positive body image, sense of humor, and ability to enjoy life. Brainstorm with the class!

TEACHING–LEARNING PLAN: Implementing

Learning Objectives	Content Outline	Resources
Define key terms used in the chapter.		Table 18–1: Professional Nursing Relationships: Role Responsibilities and Related Competencies
Distinguish independent, interdependent or collaborative, and dependent nursing interventions.	A. Unique focus of nursing implementation: types of nursing implementation, the nursing intervention taxonomy structure, protocols and standing orders, the nurse as coordinator.	Table 18-2 NIC Taxonomy
List the advantages of having a standard classification of nursing interventions.		Using NIC to Implement Care for a Patient/Family Requiring Assistance With Home Maintenance
Use cognitive, interpersonal, technical, and ethical and legal skills to implement a plan of nursing care.	B. Carrying out the plan of care: prerequisite nursing skills; determining the need for assistance; delegating nursing care; promoting self-care—teaching, counseling, advocacy; assisting patients to meet health goals; responding to the noncompliant patient; guide for students.	Through the Eyes of the Family Caregiver
Describe six variables that influence the way a plan of care is implemented.		When Implementing Nursing Care...
		Through the Eyes of a Student
Use seven guidelines for implementation.		Developing Critical Thinking Skills
		Organizing Student Clinical Responsibilities
Use ongoing data collection to direct revision of the plan of care.	C. Continuing data collection.	
	D. Nursing oneself.	

CHAPTER 19

Evaluating

■ Chapter Overview

The evaluating step of the nursing process is the focus of Chapter 19. The reader is introduced to methods of evaluating the patient's achievement of goals/outcomes specified in the plan of care, including collecting evaluative data, documenting evaluation, and determining factors that influence goal achievement. Modification of the plan of care and the use of quality assurance programs and nursing audits are also discussed. The chapter concludes with a student guide to evaluate personal skill in using the nursing process.

■ Teaching–Learning Activities

GROUP ACTIVITIES

1. Invite a nurse who is responsible for quality assurance in a healthcare setting to discuss her role and responsibilities with the class.

2. Divide the class into three groups and have each group work on developing a strategy to measure patient achievement of the following types of goals: (a) cognitive goals, (b) psychomotor goals, and (c) affective goals. Share group results and discuss how the type of patient data collected to support goal achievement evaluation is determined by the nature of the goal.

3. Ask students to examine the plan of care on their unit for evaluative statements. In small groups, have students discuss their findings.

4. Have individuals from other professions or industries speak to the class about the evaluation process they use to measure business results. Compare these techniques with those used by nursing professionals, and discuss the unique focus of the nursing evaluation.

DISCUSSION QUESTIONS

1. What is the difference between criteria and standards? How do they relate to nursing evaluation? How can patient goal/outcome achievement be measured?

2. Discuss the following approaches to quality healthcare—inspection and opportunity—and how they affect the healthcare system.

3. What three options are available to the nurse when using the evaluation process?

4. What is the role of the student nurse in the ANA quality assurance model?

5. Discuss the three options available to the nurse after evaluating a patient's expected outcomes: (a) terminating the plan of care, (b) modifying the plan of care, and (c) continuing the plan of care. How should a nurse decide which option to implement?

WRITING ACTIVITIES

1. Have students list examples of data that would validate the attainment of cognitive, psychomotor, and affective goals.

2. Have students describe how a patient, nurse, or healthcare variable may contribute positively or negatively to patient goal/outcome achievement.

3. Ask students to summarize a recent nursing journal article that discusses quality assurance or nursing audits.

4. Have the students write a brief paragraph describing how a nurse would know when a patient achieved the following goals: (a) cognitive goals, (b) psychomotor goals, and (c) affective goals.

GUIDE TO CRITICAL THINKING AND DEVELOPING BLENDED SKILLS

1. Instruct students to keep a log in which they record how they use their daily clinical experiences to develop self-awareness of their clinical strengths and weaknesses. At the end of a set period of time, have students submit their logs with a plan for self-improvement. Guide the class in a discussion of the value of reflection and self-awareness. Poll the class to determine how many students believe we owe it to our patients to be the best nurses we can be— and the implications of what we believe.

   You might want to discuss the importance of the evaluation of goal achievement in the student's plan for self-improvement and which student goals are involved:

   • Cognitive goals
   • Psychomotor goals
   • Affective goals

   Discuss the importance of a time frame when setting goals.

2. Have the class interview two practicing nurses and two patients to determine what they believe are the components of quality care. Use a class discussion to explore differences in the components of quality care listed by nurses and patients. Explore the role of patient satisfaction in evaluating quality.

   You might want to explore the variables that may distract from quality nursing care, such as:

   • Patient variables: a capable patient giving up self-care and refusing to cooperate with treatment, a patient passively accepting treatment and seldom communicating needs or dissatisfaction
   • Nurse variables: nurse burnout, nurse with overwhelming outside concerns
   • Healthcare system variables: understaffing, insensitivity to nursing demands within the institution

TEACHING–LEARNING PLAN: Evaluating

Learning Objectives	Content Outline	Resources
Define key terms used in the chapter.		Table 19-1: Patient, Nurse, and Healthcare System Variables That May Detract From Quality Nursing Care
Describe evaluation, its purpose, and its relation to other steps in the nursing process.	A. Unique focus of nursing evaluation.	
	B. Evaluation criteria and standards.	Table 19-2: Common Problems Noted During Evaluation of the Nursing Process
Evaluate the patient's achievement of goals/outcomes specified in the plan of care.	C. Measuring patient goal/outcome achievement: collecting evaluative data, documentation evaluation.	Using Four Types of Goals in the Plan of Nursing Care
Manipulate factors that contribute to the patient's success or failure in goal/outcome achievement.	D. Factors that influence goal/outcome achievement.	Steps in Performance Improvement
		National Quality Initiatives
Use the patient's responses to the plan of care to modify the plan as needed.	E. Modifying the plan of care.	Selected Web Resources for Patients and Families
Explain the relation between quality assurance/quality improvement programs and excellence in healthcare.	F. Evaluative programs: quality assurance, from quality assurance to quality improvement, nursing audit.	
Value self-evaluation as a critical element in developing the ability to deliver quality nursing care.	G. Self-evaluation.	

CHAPTER 20

Documenting, Reporting, and Conferring

■ Chapter Overview

Chapter 20 introduces the reader to the guidelines for effective communication of patient care through documentation, reporting, and conferring. The purposes of patient records, methods of documentation, formats for documentation, and potential legal problems in documentation are highlighted in this chapter. Methods of reporting care—including change-of-shift reports, telephone reports and orders, transfer and discharge reports, and reports to family members—are discussed. A section pertaining to the use of consultations and referrals, nursing care conferences, and nursing care rounds concludes the chapter.

■ Teaching–Learning Activities

GROUP ACTIVITIES

1. Have students listen to a change-of-shift report and discuss what they learned, what information was most and least helpful, and what they would have done differently.

2. Divide the class into six groups. Give each group a sample documentation form for recording patient information according to the following formats: (a) source-oriented records, (b) problem-oriented records, (c) PIE charts, (d) focus charting, (e) charting by exception, and (f) case management model. Have the students record a sample patient case according to their method and then switch groups until they have used each method. Conduct a discussion of the various methods of documentation available, the method they found most effective, and why.

3. Have the students role-play reporting care for a sample patient, using the following methods: (a) change-of-shift report, (b) telephone report, (c) transfer and discharge report, and (e) report to family members. Videotape the sessions and have the students critique each others' performances.

4. Divide the class into small groups and give each group a sample format for recording nursing data, such as the initial nursing assessment, Kardex and patient care summary, plan of nursing care, critical/collaborative pathways, progress notes, flow sheets, discharge and transfer summary, and home healthcare and long-term care records. Let each group develop a sample case study and record the information on the appropriate forms.

DISCUSSION QUESTIONS

1. What are the potential legal problems that might accompany the documentation of patient information?

2. Discuss the various methods of communicating among healthcare professionals and their advantages and disadvantages.

3. What are consultations and referrals and when and why should they be used by healthcare professionals?

4. Discuss the information a healthcare team would need to provide quality care for the following patient: A 5-year old child is brought to the ER with a broken arm and multiple contusions. When you examine the child, she tells you she fell down the steps. The mother appears anxious and worried about the child and asks you about women's shelters. After examining the child's record, you realize she has been brought to the ER with lacerations and bruises on two other occasions.

WRITING ACTIVITIES

1. Have the students write a paragraph describing nursing care rounds and nursing care conferences.

2. Ask students to list the critical elements in nursing documentation.

3. Have students describe the purpose of a flow sheet and why it is an important patient record.

4. Have the students write an essay describing the purposes of patient records (communication, care planning, quality review, research, decision analysis, education, legal documentation, reimbursement, historic documentation).

5. Have students summarize an article on documentation from a nursing care journal. How could the findings be used when documenting nursing care?

GUIDE TO CRITICAL THINKING AND DEVELOPING BLENDED SKILLS

1. Prepare three end-of-shift reports on the same patient, which basically provide the same information about the patient's physical condition and needs, but which introduce different subjective estimates of the kind of person the patient is and why the patient is demonstrating certain behaviors. Guide the students in a discussion of how the words used to "report off" on a patient may influence another nurse's opinion of the patient and interactions with that patient.

You might want to discuss the basic information that should be reported in a change-of-shift report:
- Basic identifying information
- Current appraisal of each patient's health status
- Current orders
- Summary of newly admitted patients
- Report of discharged or transferred patients

2. How would you respond to the following situation: A mother-to-be who is visiting a clinic for a checkup confides to you that she has been using cocaine during her pregnancy and is afraid it may affect her baby. She asks you not to tell anyone else because her husband is unaware of her behavior. Does this patient have a right to confidentiality? Should this information be shared with the doctor or her husband (or both)? Should this information be recorded on the patient record? What actions should be taken to protect the baby? Brainstorm with the class!

TEACHING–LEARNING PLAN: Documenting, Reporting, and Conferring

Learning Objectives	Content Outline	Resources
List the guidelines for effective communication.		Table 20-1: Abbreviations and Symbols Commonly Used by Health Practitioners
Identify the abbreviations and symbols commonly used for charting.	A. Documenting care: guidelines for effective documentation, purposes of patient records, methods of documentation, formats for nursing documentation, potential legal problems in documentation.	Table 20-2: Examples of Forms and Information in Source-Oriented Patient Records
Describe the purposes of patient records.		Table 20-3: Organization of the Problem-Oriented Patient Record
Compare and contrast different methods of documentation: source-oriented record, problem-oriented record, PIE charting, intervention, evaluation, focus charting, charting by exception, case management model, and computerized records.	B. Reporting care: change-of-shift reports, telephone orders, transfer and discharge reports, reports to family members and significant others.	Table 20-4: Advantages and Disadvantages of Different Documentation Formats
		Table 20-5: Common Methods of Communication Among Healthcare Professionals
Describe the purpose and correct use of each of the following formats for nursing documentation: nursing assessment, nursing care plan, critical/collaborative pathways, progress notes, flow sheets, discharge summary, and home care documentation.		Sample Activity Flow Sheet With Narrative Patient Care Notes
		Sample of Problem-Oriented Patient Record
		Sample of Focus Patient Care Notes
Document nursing intervention completely, accurately, concisely, and factually—avoiding legal problems.		Sample of PIE Patient Care
		Sample of Charting by Exception
		Sample of Collaborative Pathway Flow Sheets That Accompany the Collaborative Pathway
Describe nursing's role in communicating with other healthcare professionals by reporting and conferring.	C. Conferring about care: consultations and referrals, nursing care conference, nursing care rounds.	Graphic Record That Accompanies the Collaborative Pathway
		Documentation Guidelines
		Safe Computer Charting
		Potential Legal Problems in Documentation

UNIT V

Roles Basic to Nursing Care

CHAPTER 21

Communicator

■ Chapter Overview

Chapter 21 introduces the learner to the communication process, including its forms, influencing factors, and use in the nursing process and helping relationship. The development of therapeutic communication skills is discussed and effective communication techniques, interpersonal skills, and assertive skills are highlighted. Techniques for communicating with patients with special needs and communicating in groups are also presented.

■ Teaching–Learning Activities

GROUP ACTIVITIES

1. Divide the class into pairs and have them role-play communicating the following information to each other: (a) telling a 60-year-old woman she needs bypass surgery, (b) telling a deaf child he must be admitted to the hospital for tests, (c) telling a friend she needs help with an alcohol problem, and (d) letting an unconscious person know you are changing IV lines.

2. Ask students, working in pairs, to interview each other for basic information and videotape the interview. Ask the class as a whole to critique each session to identify effective and ineffective communication techniques. Use the same interview to identify verbal and nonverbal methods of communication. As a follow-up to this activity, invite a local journalist who specializes in feature stories to speak to the class about his or her interviewing techniques.

3. Place students in small groups and devise a list of "blocks to communication." Have the class work together to solve the communication problems listed by each group.

4. Arrange for students to interview a patient and, with the patient's permission, videotape the session. Play back the videotape—the first time with only the sound, a second time with only the video, and a third time with sound and video. Note any differences in the message received when each new component of communication is added.

DISCUSSION QUESTIONS

1. What is the difference between a helping relationship and a social relationship? How can communication be used in the helping relationship?

2. Discuss the following statement: "Active listening is hard work."

3. Discuss your plans for improving your verbal and nonverbal communication techniques.

4. How do gait, posture, and general appearance serve as methods of nonverbal communications?

5. Discuss communication skills necessary in special situations, such as when patients are visually impaired, hearing impaired, or unconscious, or speak a language different from that of the listener.

WRITING ACTIVITIES

1. Have students describe the three phases of the helping relationship.

2. Have students list the clues to a person's identity that can sometimes be determined by learning a person's occupation.

3. Have students describe the role of communication in each step of the nursing process.

4. Ask students to list the roles of group members in each of the following categories: (a) task roles, (b) maintenance roles, and (c) self-serving roles.

5. Have students reflect on the silences that occur during communication. Ask them to describe their feelings and reactions to such silences.

GUIDE TO CRITICAL THINKING AND DEVELOPING BLENDED SKILLS

1. Make up postcards with a patient situation listed on each card (eg, a patient who is depressed, a patient who received good news from test results, a patient who is diagnosed HIV positive, a patient who is entering a hospice with end-stage cancer, an elderly patient in a nursing home who recently lost his spouse, a new mother who is terrified of holding her baby, etc). Ask the students to take turns picking a card and communicating the situation to the class using both verbal and nonverbal communication. Conduct a group discussion on the factors influencing communication and how they will apply this knowledge to their own practice. Explore the blended skills that are needed to communicate effectively with a patient. Brainstorm with the class!

2. Divide the class into groups of 10 students. Invite one student from each group to come forward and give her a message about a hypothetical patient. For example, Mrs. Jones is scheduled for a CT scan in the morning. She appears anxious about her test results and wishes to speak to someone about possible outcomes. Have each student communicate the message to one person in the group, who then communicates the message to the next person and so on. Have the last person to receive the message communicate it to the class. Use this experience to initiate a discussion of the importance of clear communication and skillful listening. Identify variables that may have distorted the original message.

You might want to discuss the variables that may distort a message:
- Developmental considerations
- Gender
- Sociocultural differences
- Roles and responsibilities
- Space and territoriality
- Physical, mental, and emotional states
- Values
- Environment

3. Use an in-class role-play to demonstrate a nursing interview that takes place when a student comes to the student health center because of increasing depression and suicidal ideation. Invite the class to determine how both the nurse and patient used verbal and nonverbal communication techniques. Identify ways in which the nurse's communication was both effective and problematic, and discuss strategies for modifying the problem.

You might want to explore the nonverbal communication portrayed by the student's:
- Body language
- Touch
- Eye contact
- Facial expressions
- Posture
- Gait
- Gestures
- Physical appearance
- Modes of dress and grooming
- Sounds
- Silence

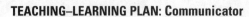

TEACHING–LEARNING PLAN: Communicator

Learning Objectives	Content Outline	Resources
Define key terms used in the chapter.		Table 21-1: Characteristics of Effective and Ineffective Groups
Describe the communication process, identifying factors that influence communication.	A. The communication process: forms of communication, factors influencing communication.	Table 21-2: Summary of Patient Goals for the Three Phases of the Helping Relationship
List at least eight ways in which people communicate nonverbally.		Table 21-3: Examples of Assertive and Nonassertive Speech
Describe the interrelationship between communication and the nursing process.	B. Using communication in the nursing process.	Communication Challenges
Identify patient goals for each phase of the helping relationship.	C. Using communication in the helping relationship: phases of the helping relationship, factors promoting effective communication, blocks to communication.	Using the Nursing Interventions Classification (NIC): Selective Cognitive Stimulation Activities
Use each of the effective communication techniques when interacting with patients from different cultures.		Relating to Patients From Different Cultures
		Through the Eyes of a Patient
Evaluate self in terms of the interpersonal skills needed in nursing.	D. Development of therapeutic communication skills: effective communication techniques, interpersonal skills, assertive skills.	Through the Eyes of a Student
		Focus on the Older Adult
Describe how each of the ineffective communication techniques hinders communication.		Communicating With Patients With Special Needs
Establish therapeutic relationships with patients with impaired verbal communication who are assigned to your care.	E. Impaired verbal communication (NANDA).	Research Research in Nursing: Making a Difference: Family Presence During Invasive Procedures and Resuscitation
Compare and contrast effective and ineffective groups.	F. Communicating in groups: types of groups, purpose of groups, roles of group members.	

CHAPTER 22

Teacher and Counselor

■ Chapter Overview

The professional nursing role of teacher/counselor is explored in Chapter 22. The aims of teaching and counseling—promoting health, preventing illness, restoring health, and facilitating coping—are discussed, and teaching strategies are presented. The learner is also introduced to the three types of counseling needed to assist patients through crises or motivate them to work toward health promotion.

■ Teaching–Learning Activities

GROUP ACTIVITIES

1. Group students in pairs. Have one student assume the role of nurse/teacher/counselor for Mrs. Green (student's partner) in the following situation. Then reverse roles. The situation should take 5 to 10 minutes for each part.

   - Sara Green is an 80-year-old woman who slipped in the bathtub and fractured her hip. She will be discharged from the hospital soon and wants to return to her home. Mrs. Green lives alone and says she will manage. She refuses to talk to her daughter about placement in a nursing home.
   - Jane Radke is Mrs. Green's only daughter. Mrs. Radke works full-time to support her family. Her husband is recovering from a heart attack and her two children will be going to college next year.
   - Mrs. Radke realizes her mother will not be able to take care of herself at home. She wants to abide by her mother's wishes, but she has many family responsibilities.
   - Both Sara Green and her daughter need help identifying their options and selecting the best choice.

2. Have two student volunteers role-play teaching an obese patient about diet and exercise. Divide the class into five groups and have each group identify and discuss the following factors: (a) the patient's readiness and willingness to learn, (b) the patient's learning and counseling needs, (c) the teaching environment, and (d) available resources for education. Have each group share its results with the class as a whole.

3. Ask a nurse who regularly performs patient teaching (eg, with diabetic patients or in a prenatal clinic) to present a topic to the class. Have the class identify the methodology and organization used by the nurse. Conduct a discussion of the importance of formulating learning objectives, outcome criteria, and teaching interventions when educating a patient.

4. Ask students to work in pairs to develop a teaching plan for diabetes counseling for a 65-year-old, a 30-year-old, a 13-year-old, and a 5-year-old. Have them share their projects with the class and discuss the importance of considering age-related variables when planning teaching for a patient.

DISCUSSION QUESTIONS

1. Have the class discuss how the following statement might influence their choice of teaching strategies for future patients: "We reportedly remember 10% of what we read, 20% of what we hear, 30% of what we see, 50% of what we see and hear, and 80% of what we say and do."

2. What are some of the problems that time constraints place on the nurse when planning patient care?

3. What is the difference between formal and informal teaching? Give examples of each type of teaching. Do you feel that one method is more effective than another?

4. Define teaching and learning. Does teaching automatically mean learning has occurred?

5. How does the role of nurse as a teacher compare to the role of nurse as a counselor?

WRITING ACTIVITIES

1. Have students describe how they would evaluate the following types of learning for a patient: (a) cognitive domain learning, (b) affective domain learning, and (c) psychomotor domain learning.

2. Have students formulate a teaching plan for the following patients:

   • A woman recovering from a stroke needs to learn how to take her pulse before being discharged.

   • A diabetic patient needs to know the effects of diet on his condition.

   • A patient needs to be able to self-inject medication.

   • A new mother needs to learn how to bathe her infant before going home from the hospital.

   • A patient needs to learn exercises to strengthen a weak arm.

3. Ask students to recall time spent with a patient during routine care. Have them identify how they could have used this time for patient education.

4. Have students analyze their own learning style and describe teaching/learning methods that are most effective for them.

5. Ask students to write a paper that identifies the counseling needs of patients newly diagnosed as HIV positive and suggests related nursing strategies.

GUIDE TO CRITICAL THINKING AND DEVELOPING BLENDED SKILLS

1. Divide the class into small groups and assign each group one of the nursing situations described below. Instruct the students to identify learning needs and factors that may influence the patient's ability and readiness to learn. Highlight developmental considerations. Determine which teaching strategies are likely to be most effective. Use an in-class discussion for groups to report to the class at large. Be sure to discuss the following factors:

   • The patient's readiness to learn: emotional and experiential

   • The patient's ability to learn: physical condition, cognitive ability, acuity of senses, developmental considerations, level of education, literacy, communication skills, primary language

   • The patient's learning strengths: past success, above average psychomotor skills, high motivation, strong network, adequate financing

   Nursing situations:

   • Women at a shelter for abused women

   • Older adults at a senior center

   • Couples at a natural childbirth class

   • High school students in a class on eating disorders

   • 8- to 12-year-olds in summer camp, learning first aid

2. Instruct the students to write a brief essay describing a time in their lives when they were in need of motivational counseling (eg, underachievement in school, sports; unsatisfactory relationships with friends or family; spiritual or emotional distress). Invite the students to identify a person who was supportive and helpful to them during this time, describing the personal qualities and counseling strategies that were most effective. Use an in-class discussion to develop a list of qualities and counseling strategies that will equip nurses to counsel effectively. Brainstorm with the class!

TEACHING–LEARNING PLAN: Teacher and Counselor

Learning Objectives	Content Outline	Resources
Define key terms used in the chapter.		Table 22-1: An Analysis of Nursing Responses in Common Counseling Situations
Describe the teaching–learning process, including domains, developmental concerns, and specific principles.	A. Aims of teaching and counseling.	Topics for Health Teaching and Counseling
Describe factors that should be assessed for the learning process.	B. The nurse as teacher: teaching–learning process, assessing the patient's learning needs, diagnosing the patient's learning needs, planning, implementing the teaching plan, evaluating teaching–learning, documenting.	Steps in the Teaching–Learning Process
Formulate diagnoses for identified learning needs.		Assessment Parameters: Factors That Affect Learning
Explain how to create and implement a teaching plan for a patient.		Sample Teaching Plan
Name three methods for evaluating learning. Identify the information that should be included in the documentation of the teaching–learning process.		Verbs That Can Be Used When Writing Learner Objectives
		Suggested Teaching Strategies for the Three Learning Domains
Discuss the nurse's role as a counselor.	C. The nurse as counselor: three types of counseling.	Sample Patient Education Materials for Managing Cancer Pain: Pain Control Plan
Summarize the way in which the nursing process is used to assist patients in problem solving.		What to Do if You Have One or More Heart Attack Warning Signs
Describe how to use the counseling role to motivate a patient toward health promotion.		Example of a Contractual Agreement Between a Nurse and Patient
		Research: Research in Nursing: Making a Difference: Promoting Active Roles in Health Education
		Documentation Using a Problem-Oriented Progress Note to Meet a Learning Need
		Promoting Lifestyle Changes
		Short-Term Counseling: An Example of Problem Solving That Follows the Nursing Process

CHAPTER 23

Leader, Researcher, and Advocate

■ Chapter Overview

In Chapter 23 the learner is introduced to the role of the nurse as a leader, researcher, and advocate. As a leader, the nurse directs or motivates others toward the achievement of predetermined goals. The role of researcher entails expanding nursing's body of knowledge to learn improved ways to promote and maintain health. As an advocate, it is the nurse's responsibility to protect and support the patient's rights. Chapter 23 explores how these roles enhance the basic caregiver role of the nurse.

■ Teaching–Learning Activities

GROUP ACTIVITIES

1. Divide the class into four groups and assign a leadership style listed in the textbook to each group. Have the groups work together to determine a method for solving the following problem according to the leadership style they have been assigned. Conduct a discussion on leadership styles and compare and contrast problem-solving methods developed in each group.

   Problem: Head nurse Nancy White is in charge of scheduling for a busy cardiac unit. One of the nurses assigned to her unit is constantly switching shifts with other colleagues, frequently calls in sick, and has been late for work on several occasions. You know that she has a 3-month-old baby and has just recently returned to the work force.

2. Have the class attend a hospital staff meeting and observe the person conducting the meeting. Ask them to rate the leader on (a) communication skills, (b) problem-solving skills, (c) management skills, and (d) self-evaluation skills and explain how they might have handled any situations discussed in the meeting differently.

3. Invite a nurse in a management position (in education or in practice) to discuss styles of leadership and effective leadership skills involving groups.

4. Ask a nurse researcher to present a study, completed or in progress, and discuss its implications. Conduct a discussion on identifying researchable problems, relating research in practice, and protecting the rights of subjects. In conjunction with this activity, have the class attend a research day at your school or community. Explore the presenter's research project, research methods, findings, and the relevancy of the research to clinical practice.

DISCUSSION QUESTIONS

1. Discuss the reasons people resist change and methods for overcoming this resistance.

2. How has consumerism influenced nursing research?

3. What is meant by the term mentor? What type of nurse would you select to be your mentor and why?

4. What is the role of nurse advocate when representing patients, promoting self-determination, and being politically active? What blended skills would a nurse need to be an advocate for patients?

WRITING ACTIVITIES

1. Have the students write a report on how they would go about changing a system of reporting in their clinical practice from one method to another. Have them note how they would present their ideas and how they would handle people who resisted their changes.

2. Have students write their reactions to the following statement: "No one is born a leader; people develop leadership qualities through observations, knowledge, and experience."

3. Ask students to reflect on the portrayal of nurses in the media and describe how they, as nurse practitioners, would institute changes in the public experience of nurses.

4. Have students choose a type of knowledge (traditional, authoritative, scientific) and summarize examples of this knowledge as it appears in nursing journals.

GUIDE TO CRITICAL THINKING AND DEVELOPING BLENDED SKILLS

1. Divide the class into groups of seven or eight and assign each group a task. For example, have students as a group decide whether or not all nurses should be prepared to offer suicide assistance and then develop a strategy to persuade their class to write a resolution to send to the local nursing society. After a set time, invite the students to discuss who assumed leadership in the group, how, and why. Have students identify and critique the roles of different group members. Conclude by inviting students to describe what they have learned about their ability to participate in professional groups and their need to develop leadership and group skills. You might want to discuss the following skills of a leader:

- Communication skills
- Problem-solving skills
- Management skills
- Self-evaluation skills

2. Use a class discussion to identify time-honored rituals in nursing, for example, the procedure for giving a bed bath, mandatory vital signs of certain frequencies, back rubs in the evening, always carrying bandage scissors, or routine nursing procedures. Instruct groups of students to discover whether or not any research supports the effectiveness of these activities. Use their findings to communicate the contribution research makes to practice. Explore the necessity of the staff nurse to contribute to nursing research by:

- Observing nursing care to find areas that need improvement
- Questioning one's own practice to see if the rationale behind caregiving activities is sound
- Participating in patient care research done by colleagues or nurse researchers
- Making suggestions for specific topics to be researched

TEACHING–LEARNING PLAN: Leader, Researcher, and Advocate

Learning Objectives	Content Outline	Resources
Define key terms used in the chapter.		Planned Change: An Eight-Step Process
Identify the qualities, four skills, and three styles of leaders.	A. The nurse as leader: leadership dynamics, leadership and management, models of patient care delivery, effecting change through leadership, the nurse caregiver's leadership skills, areas of leadership, support for leadership training.	Checklist for the Beginning Nurse Who Wishes to Develop Leadership, Research, and Advocacy Skills
List the four managerial functions.		
Summarize the steps in the process of change.		Evolving Models of Nursing Care Delivery . . . Evolving Accountability
Describe areas in which the beginning nurse can develop leadership skills that enhance the caregiver role.		Advantages of Having an Effective Mentor
Compare the strengths and limitations of three sources of nursing knowledge.		Ethical Principles in the Conduct, Dissemination, and Implementation of Nursing Research
Describe three ways the beginning nurse can use research to enhance the caregiver role.	B. The nurse as researcher: professionalism, roots of knowledge, consumerism, the nurse caregiver's research skills.	A Model for Evidence-Based Practice

Internet Links |
| Explain different ways nurse caregivers can be advocates for patients. | C. The nurse as advocate: patient's bill of rights, the nurse caregiver's advocacy skills. | Research
Nursing Research Resources |
| Describe the nurse advocate's role in situations requiring ethical decision making. | | |
| Explain how two types of advance directives promote patient dignity and well-being. | | |

UNIT VI

Actions Basic to Nursing Care

CHAPTER 24

Vital Signs

■ Chapter Overview

Chapter 24 provides a thorough discussion of vital signs: body temperature, pulse, respiration, and blood pressure. Physiologic factors, normal and abnormal findings, assessment methods, and assessment sites are described for each vital sign. The proper uses and care of equipment used for each assessment are also discussed.

■ Teaching–Learning Activities

GROUP ACTIVITIES

1. Assemble different types of thermometers, blood pressure apparatus, and stethoscopes on a table. Have students take turns selecting an instrument and demonstrating its use to the class.

2. Ask each student to work with a partner to assess and record oral body temperature, radial pulse, apical pulse, respirations, and blood pressure.

3. Assign students to take a complete set of vital signs on an assigned patient and record the findings in the patient's medical record. Discuss these findings and compare them with those recorded on the patient's admission to the healthcare setting.

4. Invite a home healthcare nurse to visit the class to discuss vital sign assessments taken in the home setting. Have the class note how the healthcare setting may affect frequency of assessments, equipment used, procedures followed, and so forth.

5. Set up a blood pressure screening session at your school for students to practice taking blood pressure under your guidance. Have them develop a teaching plan for any classmates who have high blood pressure.

DISCUSSION QUESTIONS

1. Discuss how the following factors affect body temperature: circadian rhythms, age, gender, stress, and environmental temperatures.

2. If you take your neighbor's blood pressure three times and each time it is 152/92, what will you do next?

3. How would you explain hypertension and its effect on the body to a patient?

WRITING ACTIVITIES

1. Ask students to describe the vital signs that would be expected in the following situations:
   - A young woman is brought to the emergency room with severe lacerations.
   - An elderly man has just mowed his yard in 95° heat.
   - A teenage girl faints.
   - A baby is sleeping.

2. Have students compare and contrast the causes and effects of hypothermia and hyperthermia.

3. Ask students to research, using nursing journals, the common causes of pyrexia and its resolution. Have them summarize any new information on the treatment of pyrexia and share this information with the class.

4. Have students research the effect of the following medications on vital signs and list the possible complications that can occur when a patient is taking these medications:
   - Warfarin
   - Atenolol
   - Enalapril
   - Glyburide
   - Ritalin

GUIDE TO CRITICAL THINKING AND DEVELOPING BLENDED SKILLS

1. Take students to any practice setting (hospital, clinic, nursing home, mall) and have them take a complete set of vital signs on at least five people. Instruct students to be sensitive to how individual

patient characteristics influence the method they use to take the vital signs (eg, the patient's anxiety may dictate a more supportive nursing presence or the patient's body size may require a smaller or larger blood pressure cuff). Explore patient variables that may affect the readings students take (eg, a physically fit patient who works out daily will usually have a lower pulse rate and blood pressure than a sedentary patient). Be sure to discuss the following factors that affect blood pressure:

- Age
- Time of day
- Gender
- Eating a meal
- Exercise
- Weight
- Emotions
- Position

2. Bring the different types of equipment used to obtain temperature readings to class. Guide the class in a discussion of the advantages and disadvantages of each, citing specific situations when it is appropriate to use each. Next present the class with different scenarios and invite students to describe what method they would use to obtain a temperature reading, noting the site and equipment. Include the following equipment:

- Glass thermometer
- Electronic thermometer
- Tympanic membrane
- Disposable single-use thermometers
- Temperature-sensitive patches
- Automated monitoring device

TEACHING–LEARNING PLAN: Vital Signs

Learning Objectives	Content Outline	Resources
Define key terms used in the chapter.		Table 24-1: Age Related Variations in Normal Vital Signs
	A. Frequency of vital signs.	Table 24-2: Mechanisms of Heat Transfer
Discuss nursing responsibilities in assessing temperature, pulse, respirations, and blood pressure.	B. Body temperature: regulation of temperature, normal and abnormal body temperature, equipment, assessment sites and methods, care of equipment.	Table 24-3: Equivalent Centigrade and Fahrenheit Temperatures
Compare normal and abnormal vital sign assessments, including causes, effects, and implications of abnormal findings.		Table 24-4: Average Normal Temperatures for Healthy Adults at Various Sites
	C. Pulse: regulation of pulse, normal and abnormal pulses.	Table 24-5: Patterns of Respiration
Describe the equipment necessary to assess vital signs.	D. Respiration: regulation of respiration, normal and abnormal respiration, assessment methods.	Table 24-6: Recommended Bladder Sizes for a Blood Pressure Cuff
Identify sites for assessing temperature, pulse, and blood pressure.	E. Blood pressure: regulation of blood pressure, normal and abnormal blood pressure, equipment, assessment sites and methods, care of equipment.	Table 24-7: Normal Pulse Rates per Minute at Various Ages
		Table 24-8: Pulse Rhythms
		Table 24-9: Pulse Amplitude
Provide information to patients about taking temperature, pulse, and blood pressure at home.	F. Teaching about vital signs for home care.	Table 24-10: Blood Pressure Classification
		Table 24-11: Korotkoff Sounds
		Table 24-12: Blood Pressure Assessment Errors and Contribution Causes
		Terms and Definitions for Types of Fevers
		Using the Nursing Interventions Classifications: Fever Treatment
		Guidelines for Nursing Care: Taking an Apical-Radial Pulse
		Guidelines for Nursing Care: Using a Doppler Ultrasound to Assess Pulse and Blood Pressure
		Procedure 24-1: Assessing Body Temperature
		Procedure 24-2: Assessing the Respiratory Rate
		Procedure 24-3: Assessing the Pulse
		Procedure 24-4: Assessing the Blood Pressure

CHAPTER 25

Health Assessment

■ Chapter Overview

Chapter 25 presents the components of the nursing assessment, including the health history, physical assessment, assessment of body systems, and documentation of data. General guidelines provide information on the instruments used for assessments, the proper patient positioning and draping, and the preparation of the environment and patient. The assessment of each body system follows a discussion of the techniques of assessment (inspection, palpation, percussion, and auscultation).

■ Teaching–Learning Activities

GROUP ACTIVITIES

1. Divide the class into five groups. Present the class with the findings of a sample health assessment. Have each group work on one of the following purposes of a health assessment—establish nurse–patient relationship, gather patient data, identify patient strengths, identify actual and potential health problems, and establish a base for the nursing process—to decide whether these goals have been met. If they have not been met, have each group develop a plan for performing a more effective assessment on the patient.

2. Assemble the instruments needed to perform a physical assessment. Have students volunteer to describe the instrument and demonstrate its use. Conduct a discussion on the proper care of the instruments and why they should be readily accessible, clean or sterile, in proper working order, and organized in sequence of use.

3. Demonstrate the four techniques of physical examination (inspection, palpation, percussion, and auscultation) and have each student practice these techniques with a partner.

4. Demonstrate and ask each student to practice selected segments of a physical assessment and record findings. Include a general survey; skin, head, and neck; thorax and lungs; cardiovascular and peripheral vascular; abdomen; and neurologic assessments.

DISCUSSION QUESTIONS

1. How are the findings from nursing assessment used as part of the nursing process?

2. Discuss the variety of positions used during a physical assessment and why it is important to consider the patient's age, physical condition, energy level, and need for privacy when choosing a position.

3. Discuss the type of sounds that may be heard when using percussion to assess the location, shape, size, and density of tissues. Have students practice using this technique with a partner.

4. Discuss the various techniques used to assess a patient's mental status. Have students develop a list of questions that would be appropriate to assess the following conditions: orientation, level of consciousness, memory, abstract reasoning, language.

5. Discuss the effect cultural patterns have on the process of data collection. Give examples of cultural differences represented in your geographic area and how these differences affect the nurse–patient relationship. Brainstorm with the class to develop nursing strategies to deal with these differences.

WRITING ACTIVITIES

1. Have students describe how they would prepare the environment for a physical assessment. What allowances would they make for the following patients: an infant, a confused patient, and a comatose patient.

2. Have students describe how they would assess a patient for edema and dehydration.

3. Ask students to choose one of the cranial nerves and describe assessment techniques.

4. Ask students to complete a written documentation of a health history for a classmate. Then assign to the student a patient in a clinical setting and have her interview the patient, complete a health history, and document the information on the patient's chart.

GUIDE TO CRITICAL THINKING AND DEVELOPING BLENDED SKILLS

1. Instruct the class individually or collectively to describe how nurses should respond in the following situations:

   • A patient who is newly admitted for care refuses to be examined by the nurse.

   • A nurse initiates a physical examination, but discovers in the middle of it that he lacks the technical skill to complete one portion of the examination.

   • The daughter of an alert and competent older adult insists on answering all the nursing history questions directed to the older adult.

   • A child begins crying and pulling away from the nurse during the examination; the child's mother asks if this is necessary and holds the child in a way that is interfering with the examination.

   • An adult patient starts to complain that "This is taking too long, can't you speed it up?"

   Brainstorm with the class!

2. The text directs students to ensure patient privacy and meet patient's physical and psychological needs. Guide the class in a practical discussion of what this means and have them independently list specific suggestions for how this can be accomplished. Place on the board the following three headings: ensure privacy, meet physical needs, and meet psychological needs. Use an in-class discussion to make a master list from the student's individual lists. Be sure to discuss the various positions used during a physical assessment:

   • Sitting
   • Supine
   • Dorsal recumbent
   • Sims
   • Prone
   • Lithotomy
   • Knee–chest
   • Standing

   Discuss the factors that help determine the position used:

   • Age
   • Physical condition
   • Energy level
   • Privacy

TEACHING–LEARNING PLAN: Health Assessment

Learning Objectives	Content Outline	Resources
Define key terms used in the chapter.		Table 25-1: Characteristics of Masses Determined by Palpation
Identify the purposes of the health assessment.	A. Health history.	Table 25-2: Percussion Tones
Describe the techniques used during a health assessment.	B. Physical assessment: general guidelines, preparing the environment, preparing the patient, techniques, general survey.	Table 25-3: Metropolitan Life Insurance Company Height and Weight Table
Discuss methods of patient preparation for a health assessment.		Table 25-4: Skin Color Assessment
	C. Assessment of body systems.	Table 25-5: Basic Types of Skin Lesions
Identify equipment used in performing a health assessment.	D. Integument: skin.	Table 25-6: Common Grading System for Heart Murmurs
Describe positioning used for each body system assessment.	E. Head and neck: skull, face, eyes and ears, nose and sinuses, mouth and pharynx, neck.	Table 25-7: Glasgow Coma Scale
	F. Thorax and lungs.	Table 25-8: Cranial Nerves
Conduct a health assessment in a systematic manner, identifying normal and abnormal findings.	G. Cardiovascular and peripheral vascular system: heart, peripheral vascular system.	Table 25-9: Normal Responses of Commonly Tested Reflexes
Document significant health assessment findings in a concise, descriptive manner.	H. Breasts and axillae.	Table 25-10: Grading of Reflexes on a 0–4+ Scale
	I. Abdomen.	Table 25-11: A Guide to Common Laboratory and Diagnostic Procedures
	J. Male and female genitalia.	
	K. Rectum and anus.	American Cancer Society CAUTION Model
	L. Musculoskeletal system.	
Describe nursing responsibilities before, during, and after diagnostic procedures.	M. Neurologic system: mental status; cranial nerve function; motor, sensory, and reflex function.	Guidelines for Nursing Care: Obtaining Height and Weight With an Upright Balance Scale
	N. Documenting the data.	Focused Assessment Guide: Internal Eye
	O. The nurse's role in diagnostic procedures.	Documentation of a Health Assessment
		Outline of a Head-to-Toe Physical Assessment

CHAPTER 26

Safety

■ Chapter Overview

Chapter 26 focuses on the factors affecting safety and the assessment of the patient and environment for safety. The learner is provided with the problem-solving tools needed to address safety issues—such as falls, fires, and poisoning—which occur in the home, clinical setting, and workplace with alarming regularity. The nursing process is discussed as a facilitator of the nurse's ability to recognize, assess, diagnose, and plan the nursing interventions that will effectively ensure safety for all ages in all environments.

■ Teaching–Learning Activities

GROUP ACTIVITIES

1. Place students in small groups to discuss nursing interventions to ensure the safety of the following patient: Mr. Jackson is a 73-year-old stroke patient, recovering in a home healthcare setting. He has right-side paralysis and has fallen once when trying to go to the bathroom alone. His daughter lives with him, but works during the day.

2. Arrange the class into three groups. Have each group assess sample patients for hazards that could result in suffocation, fire death, and poisoning. Share the groups' results with the class.

3. Have students work in groups to fill out a sample incident report for a postoperative patient who has fallen out of bed trying to open a window in her room.

4. Invite a representative of a poison control center or a fire chief to discuss prevention measures for different age groups.

5. Invite representatives of equipment companies to speak to the class about using their products safely in the hospital environment.

DISCUSSION QUESTIONS

1. How do you feel about using restraints on patients to ensure their safety? What alternative methods could be used instead of restraints? Discuss the guidelines for nursing actions when caring for a patient who is in restraints.

2. Provide students with copies of accident reports that have been filed in the institution in which they will be practicing. Have them go through the reports and determine which accidents were due to negligence and what could have been done to prevent them. Note the nature of the accidents and see if there is a pattern of unsafe practice that could be corrected.

3. Identify high-risk candidates for falls in the healthcare setting and discuss appropriate interventions.

4. Discuss the statement: "Teaching is an important factor in accident prevention and health promotion."

WRITING ACTIVITIES

1. Have students develop nursing care plans that would ensure the safety of the following patients: (a) a patient with mobility limitations, (b) a patient who is unable to communicate, (c) a patient who is confused or disoriented, and (d) a patient with an alteration in sensory perception.

2. Have students summarize a nursing or hospital management journal article that discusses environmental safety.

3. Have students describe the assessment of an assigned patient using either "Home Care Considerations: Preventing Falls," "Checklist: Prevention of Falls in the Healthcare Facility," or "Checklist: Fire Safety in the Home" (provided in textbook).

4. Have students write nursing diagnoses and patient goals related to safety for patients in their clinical practice.

5. Have students interview healthcare providers from various agencies to find out what measures they take to provide a safe environment for their patients. Have them find out if the needs of hospital-based patients differ from those who are in long-term facilities and draw up a plan of safety that they will use when dealing with patients in their own practices.

GUIDE TO CRITICAL THINKING AND DEVELOPING BLENDED SKILLS

1. Have students describe what changes would be needed in their family homes if they were being safety proofed for a toddler, a disabled adult using a wheelchair, or a frail elderly adult. Be sure to discuss:
   - Toddler
       Electrical outlets
       Childproofing cabinets
       Preventing suffocation/drowning
       Fire safety
       Removing chemicals/medications from reach
       Making steps/stairs safe
       Checking child equipment: car seats, infant chairs, cribs, high chairs, and so forth

   - Disabled adult
       Railings
       Toilet seat raised
       Ramps
       Check loose carpets and clutter in hallways
   - Frail elderly
       Remove loose carpets
       Fire safety, fire alarms
       Check lighting in home
       Keep environment free of clutter

2. Bring in several types of restraints and have students apply them to one another. Explore their feelings about being restrained and use this experience to initiate a discussion about the benefits and harms associated with restraints and possible alternatives to the use of restraints. Explore the following:
   - Patient's rights
   - Facility policies
   - Use as a prescription device
   - Patient criteria
   - Sizes
   - Proper use and length of wear
   - Patient monitoring

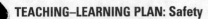

TEACHING–LEARNING PLAN: Safety

Learning Objectives	Content Outline	Resources
Define the terms used in the chapter.		Table 26-1: Deaths and Death Rates Due to Accidents in the United States for 1995
Identify factors that may be safety hazards in the patient's environment.	A. Factors affecting safety.	
		Table 26-2: Common Agents in Childhood Poisoning
Describe ways in which the patient's safety can be promoted in the home and healthcare setting.	B. Assessing safety: the patient, the environment, specific risk factors.	Table 26-3: Developmental Considerations and Safety Topics to be Taught to Parents
Identify patients at risk of falling.	C. Diagnosing.	
Describe preventive strategies to decrease the incidence of falls.	D. Planning: expected outcomes.	Promoting Health: Safety in the Community
Identify alternatives to using restraints.	E. Implementing: teaching to prevent accidents, orienting the person to surroundings, preventing falls, preventing fires and maintaining fire safety, preventing poisoning, preventing suffocation, preventing injury from firearms, preventing equipment-related accidents, preventing procedure-related accidents, filing an incident report.	Physical and Behavioral Manifestations of Child Abuse
Identify nursing diagnoses associated with patients in unsafe situations.		Checklist: Prevention of Falls in the Healthcare Facility
Describe nursing responsibilities for fire safety.		Developing Critical Thinking Skills
		Home Safety Checklist
Identify teaching strategies that should be included in a safety program to prevent poisoning and suffocation.	F. Evaluating.	Decreasing Equipment-Related Accidents
		Focus on the Older Adult
		Research: Research in Nursing: Making a Difference: Using an Educational Seminar to Alter Staff Attitudes Toward the Use of Restraints
		Choosing Alternatives to Restraints
		Procedure 26-1: Applying Restraints

CHAPTER 27

Asepsis

■ Chapter Overview

Chapter 27 introduces the learner to aseptic techniques in infection prevention and control. The involvement of the nurse in identifying, preventing, controlling, and teaching the patient about infection is discussed. The need for consistent application of the nursing process to break the chain of infection is explained, and techniques are offered to achieve this goal. Controlling infectious agents by sterilization and disinfection, surgical asepsis and isolation, and barrier techniques are also presented in this chapter.

■ Teaching–Learning Activities

GROUP ACTIVITIES

1. Demonstrate and have students practice the following procedures: handwashing; putting on sterile gloves; using sterile forceps; opening, maintaining, and adding supplies to a sterile field.

2. Role-play the following situation in which three players will be needed: the patient and his wife and the nurse. Videotape the session and critique the students' performances with the class adding their input and suggestions.

   Example: Mr. Sanchez is a newly admitted patient who has just arrived from Mexico. He has been placed on enteric isolation precautions. His wife and five children are requesting a visit; he needs to go to radiology for a chest x-ray. What will you say to his wife? What precautions do you need to take? How will you transport him to radiology? Conduct a discussion about anticipated concerns Mr. Sanchez may express regarding his isolation precautions and the student's response to being assigned to care for Mr. Sanchez.

3. Invite several patients who have experienced isolation precautions in a hospital setting to describe their experiences to the class. Discuss nursing actions that had a negative or positive effect on the patients.

4. Have students role-play entering and leaving an isolation unit, wearing a cap, mask, gown, and gloves.

5. Invite an infection control nurse to speak to the class about his role, the methods used for controlling infection in his facility, and the use of isolation and universal precautions as safety measures.

DISCUSSION QUESTIONS

1. Discuss the factors that influence an organism's potential to produce disease and factors that affect a patient's susceptibility to infection.

2. Discuss the role of the nurse in controlling or treating infection in each stage of the nursing process.

3. Discuss the factors that should be considered when selecting sterilization and disinfection methods.

4. Compare and contrast medical and surgical asepsis.

5. Discuss the personal protective equipment and supplies necessary to minimize or prevent exposure to infectious material.

WRITING ACTIVITIES

1. Have students research diseases to determine their means of transmission. Include diseases that are transmitted by direct contact, indirect contact, vectors, and the airborne route.

2. Have students describe the four stages of infection: incubation period, prodromal stage, full-stage illness, and convalescent period. Have them interview patients in each stage and record patient data observed in each stage.

3. Have students summarize an article in a nursing journal that pertains to nosocomial infections and their causes, modes of transmission, and methods of prevention.

4. Have students summarize CDC guidelines for category-specific and disease-specific isolation procedures.

GUIDE TO CRITICAL THINKING AND DEVELOPING BLENDED SKILLS

1. After students learn the different types of category-specific isolation systems, present them with diverse patient situations in a simulation lab and have them set up and demonstrate the appropriate isolation precautions for the following situations:

   • Need to suction a patient who has AIDS

   • Need to assist with a bed bath for a patient with active tuberculosis

   • Need to obtain a bed for a child admitted with asthma, when the only bed available is in a double room with a child admitted with severe impetigo

   • Need to obtain a stool specimen from a patient with viral hepatitis

Lead the class in a discussion of:

   • Isolation techniques: category-specific isolation, disease specific isolation, universal precautions, body substance isolation

   • URE guidelines

   • OSHA regulations

2. Have students interview several practicing nurses and ask each to identify the nursing care appropriate for patients on isolation precautions. Use an in-class discussion to determine how many of the interviewed nurses listed meeting a patient's psychosocial needs as a priority and determine if this is consistent with the standards for good practice. Invite the class to determine what these psychosocial needs are and how nurses can best meet them. Guide the class into a discussion concerning:

   • Minimizing psychological trauma of feeling unclean and undesirable

   • Sensory deprivation

   • Loss of self-esteem

   • Loss of visitation

TEACHING–LEARNING PLAN: Asepsis

Learning Objectives	Content Outline	Resources
Define key terms used in the chapter.		Table 27-1: Organisms Capable of Causing Disease
Explain the infection cycle.	A. Infection prevention and control.	Table 27-2: Methods of Sterilization and Disinfection
Describe nursing interventions used to break the chain of infection.	B. Assessing.	Focus on the Older Adult: Predisposition for Infection
List the stages of an infection.	C. Diagnosing.	Laboratory Data Indicating an Infection
Identify patients at risk for developing an infection.	D. Planning: expected outcomes.	
Identify factors that reduce the incidence of nosocomial infection.		Practicing Basic Principles of Medical Asepsis in Patient Care
Identify situations in which handwashing is indicated.		Practicing Basic Principles of Surgical Asepsis
Identify nursing diagnoses associated with a patient who has an infection or is at risk of developing an infection.		Applying Learning to Practice: Promoting Health
Compare CDC guidelines for standard and transmission-based precautions with category-specific, disease-specific, universal, and the body substance isolation systems.	E. Implementing: teaching about infection control, using medical asepsis, controlling infectious agents by sterilization and disinfection, using surgical asepsis, using isolation and barrier techniques for infection prevention and control.	Summary of CDC Recommended Practices for Standard and Transmission-Based Precautions
		Latex Allergy Summary
		Through the Eyes of a Student
Describe the recommended techniques for medical and surgical asepsis.		Procedure 27-1: Handwashing
		Procedure 27-2: Preparing a Sterile Field
		Procedure 27-3: Donning and Removing Sterile Gloves
		Procedure 27-4: Using Personal Protective Equipment

CHAPTER 28

Medications

■ Chapter Overview

Chapter 28 provides the learner with the knowledge base required to accurately prepare and administer medications. Drug names, preparations, classifications, adverse effects, and physiologic factors affecting drug action are discussed in this chapter. Protocols for assessing the medication history, preparing nursing diagnoses, and planning expected patient outcomes are presented, along with guidelines for implementing, documenting, and evaluating medication administration.

■ Teaching–Learning Activities

GROUP ACTIVITIES

1. Demonstrate and have students practice the following procedures:
   - Reading and understanding medication orders, including abbreviations, symbols, and dosage conversions
   - Administering oral medications in both solid and liquid forms
   - Selecting sizes for needles and syringes and assembling equipment using sterile technique
   - Withdrawing solution from an ampule and a vial
   - Preparing and using prefilled cartridges
   - Mixing medications in one syringe
   - Locating correct sites for intradermal, subcutaneous, and intramuscular injections
   - Administering IV medications by piggyback, by bolus, by controlled-volume sets, and by heparin lock
   - Instilling eyedrops, eardrops, and ointments
   - Administering an intradermal, subcutaneous, and intramuscular injection
   - Irrigating the eye and ear
   - Inserting a rectal suppository
   - Documenting medication administration

2. Have students work in groups to complete the following activity on oral and topical medications:
   Example: Mary Scott is a 70-year-old woman admitted to your unit. Her medical diagnoses include congestive heart failure and pneumonia. She is to receive the following medications:

   > Lasix 20 mg p.o. o.d.
   > Lanoxin 0.125 mg p.o. daily
   > Ampicillin 500 mg p.o. q.i.d.
   > Transderm-nitro patch 5 mg daily
   > Milk of Magnesia 30 mg h.s. p.r.n. constipation

   - Discuss the principles followed for the safe preparation of oral and topical medications.
   - Simulate the administration of these medications for Mary Scott.
   - Discuss variables that might influence drug action for Mary Scott.
   - List the subjective and objective data you would use to evaluate Mary Scott's response to the medications she has received.
   - Describe the teaching that should accompany the initial administration of these medications.

3. Have students observe the dispensing of medications by different methods used in the healthcare system (eg, stock supply system, individual supply system, unit dose system). Conduct a discussion on the various types of supply systems and compare their advantages and disadvantages.

4. Have students take turns locating the intramuscular injection sites on a mannequin and describe the appropriate patient position for each site. Describe situations that might make one site more preferable than another.

5. Assemble the equipment necessary for administering IV medications. Have students choose a piece of equipment and explain when it may be indicated for use, demonstrate its use, and describe any precautions that should be observed with its use.

6. Invite a pharmacist to discuss laws and regulations governing the administration of controlled substances.

DISCUSSION QUESTIONS

1. Discuss the ways in which the following factors influence the absorption of a drug: route of administration, drug solubility, pH, local conditions at the site of administration, drug dosage.

2. Discuss the following types of drug orders prescribed by a physician and the types of medications that would fall into each category: (a) standing orders, (b) single order, (c) stat order, and (d) p.r.n. order.

3. Under what situations should a medication order be questioned by a nurse?

4. Discuss the recommended techniques to help reduce discomfort when injecting medications subcutaneously or intramuscularly.

5. Discuss different types of drug side effects. What assessments would indicate their occurrence?

6. Describe methods of calculating drug dosages for adults and for children.

WRITING ACTIVITIES

1. Have students research and summarize their findings on a drug, using at least three sources of information (eg, experienced nurse, the *Physician's Desk Reference*, pharmacist, textbook).

2. Have students consult the *Physician's Desk Reference* to identify three types of parenteral medications and list examples and dosages of each.

3. Have students describe how the following factors would affect the type of equipment a nurse would choose for an injection: (a) route of administration, (b) viscosity of the solution, (c) quantity to be administered, (d) body size, and (e) type of medication.

4. Ask students to list the information that should be recorded when medicine has been administered to a patient.

GUIDE TO CRITICAL THINKING AND DEVELOPING BLENDED SKILLS

1. Have students describe how they would respond in the following situations:
   - A patient with a high blood pressure reading refuses to take the ordered antihypertensive medication because he doesn't like the way the medicine makes him feel.
   - Another student tells you that she inadvertently gave medications to the wrong patient but is afraid to tell your instructor.
   - You just realized that you forgot to bring a patient a medication that she was supposed to get 3 hours ago.
   - You suspect that a patient may be having a negative reaction to an antibiotic you administered.
   - An elderly woman whom you are preparing for discharge tells you that she has no idea how she will ever be able to keep all her pills straight once she gets home.

2. Have someone demonstrate multiple scenarios of administering medications, some of which are performed according to procedure and others of which incorporate errors of various types. Have students independently write down each error they observe and what should have been done differently. Alternately have teams of students see which team can identify and correct the greatest numbers of errors first. Be sure to discuss the factors affecting drug actions:
   - Developmental considerations
   - Weight
   - Gender
   - Genetic and cultural factors
   - Psychological factors
   - Pathology
   - Environment
   - Time of administration

TEACHING–LEARNING PLAN: Medications

Learning Objectives	Content Outline	Resources
Define key terms used in the chapter.		Table 28-1: Common Types of Drug Preparations
Discuss drug legislation in the United States and Canada.	A. Drug legislation.	Table 28-2: Routes for Administering Drugs
		Through the Eyes of a Student
Describe drug names, types of preparations, and types of drug orders.	B. Introduction to pharmacology: drug preparations, classifications, mechanisms of drug action.	Focus on the Older Adult: Altered Drug Response in Older People
Identify drug classifications and actions.	C. Factors affecting drug action.	Research in Nursing: Making a Difference: Medications
		Communicating Effectively About Medications With Culturally Diverse Patients
Discuss adverse effects of drugs, including allergy, tolerance, cumulative effect, idiosyncratic effect, and interactions.	D. Adverse drug effects.	Focused Assessment Guide: Medications
		Applying Learning to Practice: Medications
Obtain patient information necessary to establish a medication history.		Nursing Responsibilities for Administering Drugs
Calculate drug dosages using the various systems of equivalents.	E. Assessing the medication history.	Guidelines for Nursing Care: Instilling Eyedrops
	F. Diagnosing.	Guidelines for Nursing Care: Instilling Ear Drops
Describe principles used to safely prepare and administer medications orally, parenterally, topically, and by inhalation.		Guidelines for Nursing Care: Instilling Nose Drops
	G. Expected outcomes for medication administration: medication orders, medication supply systems, dosage calculations, using safety measures while preparing drugs, administering oral medications, administering parenteral medications, administering topical medications, administering medications by inhalation, documenting medication administration, teaching about medications and abuse.	Guidelines for Nursing Care: Inserting Vaginal Suppository or Cream
Develop teaching plans to meet patient needs specific to medication administration.		Guidelines for Nursing Care: Applying Transdermal Patches
		Developing Critical Thinking Skills
		Procedure 28-1: Administering Oral Medications
		Procedure 28-2: Removing Medication From an Ampule
		Procedure 28-3: Removing Medication From a Vial
		Procedure 28-4: Mixing Insulins in One Syringe
		Procedure 28-5: Administering an Intradermal Injection
		Procedure 28-6: Administering a Subcutaneous Injection
		Procedure 28-7: Administering an Intramuscular Injection
	H. Evaluating the patient's response to medications.	Procedure 28-8: Adding Medications to an IV Solution Container
		Procedure 28-9: Adding a Bolus IV Medication to an Existing IV
		Procedure 28-10: Administering IV Medications by Piggyback, Volume-Control Administration Set, or Mini-infusion Pump
		Procedure 28-11: Introducing Drugs Through a Heparin or Intravenous Lock Using the Saline Flush
		Procedure 28-12: Administering an Eye Irrigation
		Procedure 28-13: Administering an Ear Irrigation

CHAPTER 29

Perioperative Nursing

■ Chapter Overview

Chapter 29 introduces the reader to the surgical experience and describes the phases of the perioperative period and related nursing care provided in the preoperative phase, intraoperative phase, and postoperative phase. The classification of surgical procedures, use of anesthesia, and informed consent are discussed along with the use of the nursing process in all the phases of the perioperative period.

■ Teaching–Learning Activities

GROUP ACTIVITIES

1. Ask a panel of nurses working in the holding area, operating room, and postanesthesia recovery to discuss nursing roles and patient care.

2. Divide the students into small groups and ask them to discuss their experiences with surgery, either for themselves or for family members. Was their experience positive or negative? What actions did the nurses perform to hasten recovery and facilitate coping with the situation? Were family and friends included in the recovery process? Was discharge planning thorough and complete?

3. Divide the students into pairs and have them help each other practice turning, coughing, deep-breathing exercises, and leg exercises.

4. Have students interview several nurses about operative positions, comparing their advantages and disadvantages.

5. Have students observe postoperative patients and record assessments on a postoperative checklist.

DISCUSSION QUESTIONS

1. What is the role of the nurse in meeting the psychological needs of surgical patients?

2. What is the role of the nurse in preventing postoperative complications?

3. What type of blended skills does a nurse need to safely care for patients undergoing surgical experiences?

4. Discuss the role of the nurse in preparing patients for each phase of the surgical experience.

WRITING ACTIVITIES

1. Have students research several surgical procedures and describe the sensations patients will be experiencing during the perioperative period. Have them develop a teaching plan for patients undergoing this type of surgery.

2. Have students research and describe the following alternative methods of pain control: TENS and PCA.

3. Have students develop a nursing care plan for a postsurgical patient that incorporates coughing, incentive spirometry, deep breathing, leg exercises, and turning in bed.

4. Ask students to develop a nursing care plan for a patient with a colostomy that includes interventions to facilitate coping and acceptance by the patient and family of changes in body structure or function.

GUIDE TO CRITICAL THINKING AND DEVELOPING BLENDED SKILLS

1. Have students interview several people who have had surgical procedures performed, asking them what was positive and negative about the care they received. Use the responses students elicit to develop a master list of helpful nursing interventions. These interventions may include:

   • Providing information and emotional support necessary to successful recovery from surgery: address fear of unknown, fear of pain or death, fear of changes in body image or self-concept

   • Identifying support system: spiritual beliefs, family support, other support system

   • Identifying sociocultural needs: health beliefs, economic factors, cultural background

2. Have students interview surgical nurses to determine what lifestyle factors affect postoperative recovery and rehabilitation. Use the negative factors to identify patients who are at risk and design preventive nursing strategies. Lifestyle factors include:

   • Nutrition
   • Use of alcohol or nicotine
   • Activities of daily living
   • Occupation

TEACHING–LEARNING PLAN: Perioperative Nursing

Learning Objectives	Content Outline	Resources
Define the terms used in the chapter.		Table 29-1: Classification of Surgical Procedures
Describe the surgical experience, including perioperative phases, postanesthesia phases, categories of surgery, types of anesthesia, informed consent, and advanced directives.	A. The surgical experience.	Focus on the Older Adult: Physiologic Changes With Aging That Increase Surgical Risk
	B. Preoperative nursing care: nursing history, physical assessment, screening tests.	Preoperative Physical Assessment
Conduct a preoperative nursing history and physical assessment to identify patient strengths as well as factors that increase surgical and postoperative complication risk.	C. Diagnosing. D. Planning: expected outcomes.	Sample Preoperative Teaching: Activities and Events for In-Hospital Surgery
Teach preoperative exercises: deep-breathing, coughing, and leg exercises.		Research Research in Nursing: Making a Difference: Protecting the Skin Integrity of Patients in the OR
Prepare a patient physically and psychologically for surgery.	E. Implementing: preparing the patient psychologically, preparing the patient physically, preparing the patient the day of surgery.	Through the Eyes of a Student Pneumatic Compression Devices
Identify assessments specific to the prevention of complications in the immediate postoperative phase.	F. Evaluating.	Procedure 29-1: Preoperative Patient Care: Hospitalized Patient
Use the nursing process to knowledgeably develop an individualized plan of care for the surgical patient during each phase of the perioperative period.	G. Intraoperative care: assessing, diagnosing, implementing, evaluating.	Procedure 29-2: Postoperative Care When Patient Returns to Room
Provide information to patients and caregivers for self-care at home.	H. Postoperative care: immediate postoperative care, ongoing postoperative care, preventing postoperative complications, promoting a return to health, helping the patient cope, providing ambulatory surgery postoperative care, dressing for a draining wound, changing dressings in special situations, teaching for home care of a wound. I. Evaluating.	

UNIT VII

Promoting Healthy Psychosocial Responses

CHAPTER 30

Self-Concept

■ Chapter Overview

Chapter 30 introduces the learner to self-concept: its dimensions, its formation, and key factors affecting self-concept. Practical interview guides are offered for assessing self-concept, and strategies for enhancing the self-esteem of nurses are explored. Examples of nursing diagnoses and goals are presented, along with specific nursing strategies for helping patients meet self-concept goals.

■ Teaching–Learning Activities

GROUP ACTIVITIES

1. Divide the class into six groups. Assign each group one of the following factors affecting self-concept: (a) developmental considerations, (b) culture, (c) internal and external resources, (d) history of success and failure, (e) stressors, and (f) aging, illness, or trauma. Have the groups discuss the ways each factor affects self-concept and share their ideas with the class.

2. Divide the class into pairs. Have each student discuss with her partner how she would answer the following questions:
   - What are my basic unmet needs and how can I meet them?
   - Do I schedule time each day to meet my needs?
   - Can I describe my physical strengths accurately?
   - Have I developed a realistic plan to achieve goals for personal growth and development?
   - Can I accurately assess feedback from others on self-esteem?

3. Ask students to interview as many parents as they can to learn how they helped to instill self-confidence in their children. Conduct a discussion of their findings and have them reflect on what their own parents did to shape their children's self-confidence.

4. Invite a panel of junior high and high school counselors to discuss adolescent self-concept and the influence of peer pressure.

DISCUSSION QUESTIONS

1. How can nurses develop self-esteem in relation to their professional practice?

2. Discuss how nurses can help patients maintain a sense of self and worth.

3. What are the steps involved in the development of self-confidence?

4. What strategies would you use to teach parents about the psychological conditions that foster healthy development of self in children?

5. Identify specific threats to an older person's self-concept. How can society in general and professional caregivers specifically be more responsive to the self-concept needs of older adults?

WRITING ACTIVITIES

1. Have students describe how they would record a self-concept assessment using their personal lifestyle as an example.

2. Have students make a list of interview questions they would use to assess a patient's self-concept in the following areas: (a) personal identity, (b) patient strengths, (c) body image, (d) self-esteem, (e) role performance, (f) power, (g) competence, and (h) virtue.

3. Have students interview a hospitalized patient to assess self-concept and find out how the experience may have affected the patient's self-image. Have them record and document their findings.

4. Have students describe a childhood or adolescent learning experience that made them feel good about themselves and motivated them to continue to want to learn.

GUIDE TO CRITICAL THINKING AND DEVELOPING BLENDED SKILLS

1. Have students explore their self-concept by writing answers to the following questions:

   - How do I perceive myself? Who am I? What makes me the way I am?

   - How do others see me?

   - Do I respect and like myself as I am?

   - Are there ways I need to change to achieve my desired self-image?

   - What are my goals for self-improvement?

   - What does all this have to do with my professional practice?

   Direct students to share their responses with a close friend, specifically noting differences in the way individuals perceive themselves versus the way friends perceive them. Encourage student self-introspection.

2. Instruct the class to identify ways in which the following factors might influence a patient's self-concept positively and negatively: family, peers, culture, history of success and failure, health/illness state, and stressors. Guide the class in a discussion of ways self-concept may influence a patient's response to illness and injury and have them describe related nursing responses.

   Discuss the following high-risk factors for self-concept disturbances:
   - Personal identity disturbance
   - Body image disturbance
   - Self-esteem disturbance
   - Altered role performance

TEACHING–LEARNING PLAN: Self-Concept

Learning Objectives	Content Outline	Resources
Define key terms used in the chapter.		Table 30-1: Developmental Changes Affecting Self-Concept
Identify three dimensions of self-concept—self-knowledge, self-expectation, self-evaluation (self-esteem).	A. Overview of self-concept: dimensions of self-concept, formation of self-concept, threats to self-concept.	Applying Learning to Practice: The Nurse as a Role Model
Describe major steps in the development of self-concept.		Focused Assessment Guide: Self-Concept
Differentiate positive and negative self-concept and high and low self-esteem.		Applying Learning to Practice: Promoting Health
Identify six variables that influence self-concept.	B. Factors affecting self-concept: developmental considerations, culture, internal and external resources, history of success and failure, stressors, aging, illness or trauma.	Nursing Diagnoses for Common Problems: Disturbances in Self-Concept
Use appropriate interview questions and observations to assess a patient's self-concept.		Using the Nursing Interventions Classification (NIC): Selected Self-Awareness Enhancement Activities
	C. The nurse as role model. Assessing: personal identity, body image, self-esteem, role performance.	Exploring and Developing the Positive Building Self-Esteem in Children
Develop nursing diagnoses to correctly identify disturbances in self-concept (body image, self-esteem, role performance, personal identity).	D. Diagnosing.	Focus on the Older Adult: Nursing Strategies to Promote Self-Esteem in Older Adults
	E. Planning: expected outcomes.	
Describe nursing strategies that are effective in resolving self-concept problems.	F. Implementing: helping patients identify and use personal strengths, helping high-risk patients maintain a sense of self, changing a negative self-concept, developing a positive body image, teaching adults how to develop self-esteem in children and adolescents, developing self-esteem in older adults.	Applying Learning to Practice: Patient Care Study
Plan, implement, and evaluate nursing care related to select nursing diagnoses for disturbances in self-concept.		Research Nursing Research: Making a Difference: Promoting Enhanced Self-Concept Through Social Support
	G. Evaluating.	Nursing Plan of Care
	H. Nursing process in clinical practice: self-concept disturbance, patient care study.	

CHAPTER 31

Stress and Adaptation

■ Chapter Overview

Chapter 31 discusses basic concepts of homeostasis, stress, and adaptation. Physiologic and psychological responses to stress are described, including mind–body interaction, local adaptation syndrome, and coping mechanisms. The effects of stress on the individual and the family are addressed. Nursing actions to promote stress reduction and specific stress management techniques are also presented. The chapter concludes with a discussion of stress management for nurses and a patient care study on stress.

■ Teaching–Learning Activities

GROUP ACTIVITIES

1. Show a videotape of a situation comedy to the class, stopping it whenever a stressful situation for one of the characters occurs. Have the class discuss how they would resolve the situation and then play the tape to see how the character resolved the problem. Be sure to note any examples of adaptation, the use of defense mechanisms, or anxiety displayed by the characters. Discuss whether the character's reaction was healthy or unhealthy, a positive or negative experience, and effective or ineffective.

2. Divide the class into small groups. Present each group with an example of a patient experiencing stress (eg, a woman awaiting a hysterectomy operation). Instruct the class to discuss how the patient would manifest: (a) mild anxiety, (b) moderate anxiety, (c) severe anxiety, or (d) panic.

3. Ask a mental health nurse to lead students in stress reduction activities.

4. Have students visit crisis intervention centers to see how counselors help patients deal with their problems. Conduct a discussion of the techniques used by the counselors.

5. Have students work in groups to explore self-help groups in their community and the effectiveness of their treatments. Share each group's results with the entire class.

DISCUSSION QUESTIONS

1. Discuss why humans must maintain psychological homeostasis to remain healthy.

2. Does stress ever have a positive impact on individuals? Give some examples.

3. Discuss family responses to the stress of illness.

4. Discuss how high levels of stress may precipitate cardiovascular disease, gastrointestinal disorders, and cancer.

5. What is the difference between developmental stress and situational stress?

6. Discuss the following statement: "Not only is stress a part of everyday experience, but a person's responses to stress are also necessary to life."

WRITING ACTIVITIES

1. Have students reflect back to a time in their lives when they resorted to one of the following coping mechanisms to reduce stress: (a) attack behavior, (b) withdrawal behavior, or (c) compromise behavior. Ask them to write down the feelings they experienced at that time and the effectiveness of the coping mechanism they used. Could they have chosen a more effective or healthier method of dealing with the stress they were experiencing?

2. Have students research defense mechanisms and give examples of the following mechanisms from their research or practical experience: (a) compensation, (b) denial, (c) displacement, (d) introjection, (e) projection, (f) rationalization, (g) regression, (h) reaction formation, (i) repression, (j) sublimation, and (k) suppression.

3. Ask students to research and summarize stress reduction methods not listed in the textbook. Share students' reports with the entire class.

4. Provide students with a sample crisis situation and have them write a report on the techniques they would use to help resolve the crisis.

5. Have students research new methods of dealing with stress and anxiety, including both pharmacologic and nonpharmacologic methods. Have them develop a nursing care plan for a patient suffering from panic attacks using this new knowledge.

GUIDE TO CRITICAL THINKING AND DEVELOPING BLENDED SKILLS

1. Have the class identify a common stressor (academic jeopardy, illness, failed relationship, divorce, being prepared for new clinical responsibilities) and contrast their individual responses to the stressor and effective and ineffective coping strategies. Use these descriptions to lead the class in a discussion of how patients respond differently to the stress of illness and the reasons an effective coping strategy for one patient may be ineffective for another. Discuss the implications for nursing care. Be sure to include the following responses to stress in your discussion:

- Physiologic responses to stress
   Local adaptation syndrome: reflex pain response, inflammatory response
   General adaptation syndrome
- Psychological responses to stress
   Anxiety
   Coping mechanisms
   Defense mechanisms

2. Have students interview family members or friends who have recently been hospitalized and ask which nursing interventions were most helpful in reducing stress. Similarly, ask which nursing interventions caused greater stress. Brainstorm with the class!

TEACHING–LEARNING PLAN: Stress and Adaptation

Learning Objectives	Content Outline	Resources
Define key terms used in the chapter.		Table 31-1: Homeostatic Regulators of the Body
Describe the mechanisms involved in maintaining physiologic homeostasis.	A. Physiology of stress and adaptation: homeostasis, adaptive responses to stress, effects of stress.	Examples of Physical Illnesses Associated With Stress
Explain the interdependent nature of stressors, stress, and adaptation.	B. Factors affecting stress and adaptation: sources of stress, types of stressors.	Physiologic Indicators of Stress Effects of Stress on Basic Human Needs
Compare and contrast developmental and situational stress, incorporating the concepts of physiologic and psychosocial stressors.	C. The nurse as role model. D. Assessing stress: nursing history, physical assessment.	Research Research in Nursing: Making a Difference: Stress, Social Support, and Health in Rural Older Adults
Describe the physical and emotional responses to stress, including mind–body interaction, local adaptation syndrome, general adaptation syndrome, and coping and defense mechanisms.	E. Diagnosing. F. Planning: expected outcomes. G. Implementing: teaching healthy activities of daily living, encouraging use of support systems, encouraging use of stress management techniques, providing crisis intervention, addressing stress in nursing profession.	Focused Assessment Guide: Assessing Anxiety Nursing Diagnoses for Common Problems: Stress Guidelines for Nursing Care: Reducing Anxiety in the Patient Entering the Healthcare Setting
Discuss the effects of short- and long-term stress on basic human needs, health and illness, and the family.	H. Evaluating. I. Nursing process in clinical practice: anxiety.	Applying Learning to Practice: The Nurse as Role Model Promoting Health: Stress and Adaptation
Integrate knowledge of healthy lifestyle, support systems, stress management techniques, and crisis intervention into hospital-based and community-based care.	J. Patient care study: assessment findings, essential knowledge and skills, documentation.	Developing Critical Thinking Skills Applying Learning to Practice: Patient Care Study
Recognize and effectively cope with stress unique to the nursing profession.		Nursing Plan of Care

CHAPTER 32

Loss, Grief, and Dying

■ Chapter Overview

Chapter 32 provides the learner with an overview of loss, grief, and death. The responses to death and dying, the impact of terminal illness, signs of impending death, and ethical and legal responsibilities are presented. The factors that affect loss, grief, and dying—including developmental considerations, family, socioeconomic factors, cultural influences, religious influences, and causes of death—are discussed. The chapter concludes with an overview of the nurse's role in developing a trusting nurse–patient relationship and the presentation of a patient care study.

■ Teaching–Learning Activities

GROUP ACTIVITIES

1. Invite the class to work in small groups to discuss the feelings they had when someone close to them died. Did they experience the stages of dying outlined by Kübler-Ross? How were they affected by the death and what coping mechanisms did they use?

2. Conduct a discussion with the class about the role of the nurse in preparing a terminally ill patient for the diagnosis and prognosis. Who is responsible for deciding what and how much the patient should be told? What information should be discussed with the patient? How should the family be involved? What are the roles of other healthcare professionals in these cases? Group students in pairs and have them role-play preparing a patient and the patient's family to respond to the diagnosis of a terminal illness.

3. Invite an experienced nurse to address the class regarding do-not-resuscitate, slow-code, and no-code orders. Discuss the role of the nurse in these situations and any legal implications.

4. Have students interview experienced nurses who have worked with dying patients and ask them the following two questions: (a) "How could you

improve the quality of care for a terminally ill patient for whom you are caring?" and (b) "If you were a member of the patient's family, what would you want the nurse to do for you?"

5. Ask the director of a hospice program to discuss the objectives and services of the program.

DISCUSSION QUESTIONS

1. What does the term "managed death" mean to you?

2. Should assisted suicide and direct voluntary euthanasia be legalized?

3. Discuss how students would react to a patient who said the following to a nurse: "Nurse, please help me die."

4. What is the nurse's role in developing a trusting nurse–patient relationship with a dying patient? What human needs is a nurse entrusted to meet for a dying patient?

5. How can The Dying Person's Bill of Rights be used when caring for the patient who is dying?

WRITING ACTIVITIES

1. Have students describe the clinical signs of impending death and describe how a nurse could use this information to prepare family caregivers of a patient dying at home.

2. Have students research the following types of advance directives and describe how these directives can help to protect a patient's end-of-life treatment preferences and benefit families: (a) living wills, and (b) durable power of attorney.

3. Ask the students to write nursing goals for sample patients who are terminally ill.

4. Have students write a list of nursing responsibilities after a patient dies.

GUIDE TO CRITICAL THINKING AND DEVELOPING BLENDED SKILLS

1. Have each member of the class prepare an advance directive listing their end-of-life treatment preferences, should they become unable to speak for themselves. Explore the different options selected and the reasons for these differences. Use the class experience to initiate a discussion of how nurses can be most helpful to patients preparing advance directives.

    Be sure to discuss:

    • Advance directives: living wills, durable power of attorney for healthcare

    • Patient self-determination act: nurses can be helpful by developing policies that ensure patients are encouraged to talk to family, significant others and healthcare professionals about treatment preferences.

2. Identify major cultures and religions within the local community and divide the class into groups to research how each views death and dying and related traditions and rituals. Invite the groups to report on how nurses can care for the dying and their families in a manner respectful of cultural and religious differences.

    Explore with the class:

    • Judaism: Sabbath

    • Christianity: prayer, faith healing, laying on of hands

    • Islam: women not allowed to make independent decisions

    • Eastern philosophies

    • Native Americans

TEACHING–LEARNING PLAN: Loss, Grief, and Dying

Learning Objectives	Content Outline	Resources
Define key terms used in the chapter.		Grief and Death Reactions
Differentiate the types of loss.	A. Loss and grieving: loss, grieving.	Grieving
Describe the grief process and the stages of grief.	B. Dying and death: responses to death and dying, impact of terminal illness, signs of impending death, definitions of death, ethical and legal responsibilities.	The Dying Person's Bill of Rights
Describe Kübler-Ross' stages of dying.		Research Research in Nursing: Making a Difference: Promoting Quality End-of-Life Care
Compare and contrast three definitions of death.		
Identify ethical and legal issues concerning end-of-life care.		Five Principles of Palliative Care Decisional Conflict
Identify six factors that affect loss, grief, and dying.	C. Factors that affect loss, grief, and dying: developmental considerations, family, socioeconomic factors, cultural influences, religious influences, cause of death.	Internet Resources for End-of-Life Care
Describe physiologic, psychological, and spiritual care of dying patients and their families.		Selected Dying Care Activities Advance Directives
Use the nursing process to plan and implement care for dying patients and their families.	D. The nurse as role model. E. Assessing. F. Diagnosing.	Assisted Suicide and Direct Voluntary Euthanasia: Arguments for and Against
Articulate and defend a personal response to a patient's plea, "Please help me die."	G. Planning: expected outcomes.	Applying Learning to Practice: Promoting Health
List the clinical signs of approaching death.	H. Implementing: developing a trusting nurse–patient relationship, teaching self-care and promoting self-esteem, teaching family members to assist in care, meeting the needs of dying patients, responding to requests for suicide assistance, providing postmortem care.	Competencies Necessary for Nurses to Provide High Quality Transition at the End of Life
Outline nursing responsibilities after death.		Focused Assessment Guide: The Experience of Loss, Grief, Dying and Death
Discuss the role of the nurse in caring for a patient's family.		Nursing Diagnoses for Common Problems
	I. Evaluating.	
	J. Nursing process in clinical practice.	Using the Nursing Intervention Classification (NIC)
	K. Patient care study.	Through the Eyes of a Student
		Applying Learning to Practice: Patient Care Study
		Nursing Plan of Care

CHAPTER 33

Sensory Stimulation

■ Chapter Overview

Chapter 33 introduces the learner to the sensory experience: its components and conditions, arousal mechanisms, and alterations. Examples of nursing diagnoses describing the effects of altered sensory functioning on other areas of human functioning are provided, along with specific patient goals for preventing and managing sensory alterations. Specialized nursing interventions for vision- or hearing-impaired, confused, or unconscious patients and a patient care study conclude the chapter.

■ Teaching–Learning Activities

GROUP ACTIVITIES

1. Have students work in small groups to develop a list of conditions, both physical and psychological, that might place a patient at high risk for sensory deprivation. Have each group develop a nursing care plan to provide sensory stimulation to high-risk patients. Share each group's results with the class.

2. Have students observe patients on their nursing unit for the effects of sensory overload. Conduct a class discussion on the subject and ask students to relate their findings. What measures can nurses take to help eliminate or modify sensory overload?

3. Divide the class into three groups to determine how to provide sensory stimulation for the following age groups: (a) infant, (b) adult, and (c) elderly. Have them share their results with the class as a whole.

4. Have students work in pairs. Have one student feed a bowl of cereal to a blindfolded partner. Ask students to discuss their feelings as both patient and nurse.

5. Invite a speech therapist to class to discuss the hearing-impaired person.

DISCUSSION QUESTIONS

1. What does the term "cultural care deprivation" mean to you? How can nurses be sensitive to a patient's cultural needs for acceptable stimuli?

2. What focused interview questions can be used to assess sensory function?

3. Identify nursing diagnoses appropriate for disturbances in sensory/perceptual function.

4. Discuss nursing interventions and teaching specific to patients who are visually impaired, hearing impaired, confused, or unconscious.

5. Discuss the various factors affecting sensory stimulation including developmental considerations, culture, personality and lifestyle, stress, illness and medication, and develop nursing strategies to promote healthy sensory functioning for patients experiencing these conditions.

WRITING ACTIVITIES

1. Ask the students to describe the following effects of sensory deprivation: (a) perceptual responses, (b) cognitive responses, and (c) emotional responses.

2. Have students describe how they would provide sensory stimulation for an elderly patient receiving home healthcare who lives alone in a small, cramped, and somewhat barren apartment.

3. Have students describe how they would communicate with the following patients: (a) a hearing-impaired patient, (b) a visually impaired patient, (c) a confused patient, and (d) an unconscious patient.

4. Show several videotaped commercials to the class with the audio turned off. Ask the students to describe what the commercials were selling and the nature of the sales pitch. Then show the commercials with the audio turned on and see how accurate their appraisals were. Conduct a discussion of the hearing-impaired patient and necessary modifications in the communication process.

5. Have students close their eyes for 2 minutes and describe the sounds, smells, and sensations they receive during that time.

GUIDE TO CRITICAL THINKING AND DEVELOPING BLENDED SKILLS

1. Present the class with the following patient situations and have them describe or role-play the appropriate nursing response:
   - A visually impaired adult man is being admitted to a same-day surgery unit for a biopsy.
   - A nurse is bathing an unconscious patient in a critical care unit.
   - A nurse is preparing to change the linens on the bed of a patient who has severe burns on both legs.
   - A resident in a nursing home again refuses to eat, complaining "It doesn't taste or smell like anything I once enjoyed eating."

   Brainstorm with the class!

2. Divide the class into small groups and assign a sensory/perceptual alteration to each group. Invite members in the group to attempt to experience the alteration (or to interview persons with these alterations) so that they can report on the feelings and needs of these patients. Instruct the groups to identify as many types of persons at risk for these alterations as they can and related nursing interventions.

   Explore with the students the following sensory/perceptual alterations:
   - Sensory deprivation
   - Sensory overload
   - Sleep deprivation
   - Cultural care deprivation

TEACHING–LEARNING PLAN: Sensory Stimulation

Learning Objectives	Content Outline	Resources
Define key terms used in the chapter.		Table 33-1: Overview of Sensory Deprivation and Sensory Overload
Describe the four conditions that must be met in each sensory experience.	A. The sensory experience: components and conditions, arousal mechanism, sensory alterations.	State of Awareness
Explain the role of the reticular activating system in sensory experience.	B. Factors affecting sensory stimulation: developmental considerations, culture, personality and lifestyle, stress, illness, and medication.	Research Research in Nursing: Making a Difference: Promoting Improved Intensive Care Experiences
Identify etiologies and perceptual, cognitive, and emotional responses to sensory deprivation and sensory overload.		Focus on the Older Adult
	C. The nurse as role model.	Focused Assessment Guide: Sensory Stimulation
Perform a comprehensive assessment of sensory functioning using appropriate interview questions and physical assessment skills.	D. Assessing sensory functioning: assessing the sensory experience, physical assessment.	Focused Assessment Guide: Sensory Perceptual Alteration
	E. Diagnosing.	Nursing Diagnoses for Common Problems: Sensory/Perceptual Alterations
Develop nursing diagnoses that correctly identify sensory/perceptual alterations that may be treated by independent nursing intervention.	F. Planning: expected outcomes. G. Implementing: preventing sensory alteration and stimulating the senses, teaching about sensory experiences, meeting the needs of visually impaired patients, meeting the needs of hearing impaired patients, communicating with a confused patient, communicating with an unconscious patient.	Stimulating the Senses Applying Learning to Practice: Patient Care Study Applying Learning to Practice: Nursing Plan of Care
Describe specific nursing interventions to prevent sensory alterations, to stimulate the senses, and to assist patients with sensory difficulties.		
	H. Evaluating.	
	I. Nursing process in clinical practice: sensory deprivation related to inadequate parenting, chronic sensory deprivation related to effects of aging.	
Develop, implement, and evaluate a plan of nursing care to help patients meet individualized sensory/perceptual outcomes.		
	J. Patient care study.	

CHAPTER 34

Sexuality

■ Chapter Overview

The focus of Chapter 34 is sexuality: the degree to which a person exhibits and experiences maleness or femaleness physically, emotionally, and mentally. Reproductive anatomy and physiology, the sexual response cycles, and factors that affect sexuality are discussed. The learner is introduced to the development of a sexual history as part of a comprehensive patient history and the use of specific interview questions to address a patient with sexual dysfunctions. Specific methods of contraception, teaching self-examination, and correcting sexual myths are also presented. The chapter concludes with a patient care study.

■ Teaching–Learning Activities

GROUP ACTIVITIES

1. Arrange students into groups of three to participate in the following simulation. Students should role-play the characters: a husband and his wife and a nurse.

   Example: Mr. Ruddy is a 55-year-old married African American man who has been hospitalized for a myocardial infarction. Mr. Ruddy is scheduled for discharge tomorrow. You are with Mr. and Mrs. Ruddy at the present time. What are your responses to their questions?

   • "When will we be able to resume sexual activity?"

   • "Can I hurt my husband during sexual intercourse?"

   • "We used to have one cocktail before dinner. Can we still do this?"

   • "I used to take a pill for my blood pressure, and I had difficulty achieving an erection. Will this still happen?"

2. Have students conduct a poll of their colleagues to see if they feel premenstrual syndrome should be allowed as a legal defense for violent behavior in women. Share the results of the polls with the class

and conduct an in-class discussion of the nurse's role in researching premenstrual syndrome and ensuring that women and the public correctly understand its effects.

3. Have students work in small groups to develop a teaching plan for a sexually active teenager who is unaware of contraceptive methods and sexually transmitted diseases (STDs).

4. Ask a nurse who works in a family planning or women's health clinic to discuss teaching to meet sexual and contraceptive needs.

5. Demonstrate and have students practice the following procedures on models:

   • Breast self-examination

   • Testicular self-examination

   • Assisting with a pelvic examination

DISCUSSION QUESTIONS

1. How would you respond to the following patients?

   • You accidentally walk in on a male patient who is masturbating.

   • A female patient with a roommate asks you to provide her with privacy for a sexual liaison with her husband.

   • A patient admits to you that he is a transvestite.

   • A woman confesses that she is having sexual dreams about her physician.

   • A young woman tells you she intends to remain celibate because she is terrified of contracting AIDS.

2. Discuss how the following diseases/altered states may influence a patient's sexuality: (a) diabetes, (b) spinal cord injuries, (c) mental illness, (d) STDs, and (e) cardiovascular disease.

3. What is the role of the nurse in promoting sexual health in patients?

4. When should a sexual history be obtained by a nurse?

5. Discuss sexual orientation. How may the nurse's values and beliefs affect the care of a patient whose sexual orientation is different from the nurse's?

6. How can sexual needs of the hospitalized patient be met?

7. What blended skills does a nurse need to possess to promote sexual health in patients?

WRITING ACTIVITIES

1. Have students conduct research on alternate forms of sexual expression and religious and society norms that affect their practice.

2. Have students research and report on a sexual dysfunction common to men or women or both.

3. Have students develop and write nursing outcomes and related interventions to enhance interactions with patients and promote individual sexual health.

4. Have students describe the age and method in which they learned about male and female sexuality. Did their sex education (formal or informal) help or hinder acceptance of their own sexuality?

5. Have students research factors that affect sexuality and new treatments to alleviate sexual problems. They might want to explore developmental considerations, culture, religion, ethics, lifestyle, and health state.

GUIDE TO CRITICAL THINKING AND DEVELOPING BLENDED SKILLS

1. Invite students to role-play and process the following situations:
   - A female physician routinely makes lewd comments to a male nurse.
   - A nurse frequently touches coworkers in sexually inappropriate ways.
   - A patient reports to you that the night nurse asked her to have sex and that she was terrified when he repeatedly came to her room after she refused.
   - The nurse coordinator suggests that you could have a dream schedule if you'd go out with her.
   - A surgeon routinely makes lewd and inappropriate comments about body parts while patients are under anesthesia.

   Be sure to discuss the following measures to stop sexual harassment:
   - Confrontation
   - Documentation
   - Written complaint
   - Government complaint

2. Assign students to identify the holistic needs of patients with problems related to sexuality. Invite in-class reports of how nurses can effectively meet these needs. Use this discussion to help students explore their own beliefs about sexuality and related potential to discriminate and act unprofessionally with patients and coworkers. Illustrate the harmful effects of discrimination on human well-being.

   Have the students explore the effects of:
   - Sexual dysfunction
   - Altered sexuality patterns
   - Alteration in comfort–pain

TEACHING–LEARNING PLAN: Sexuality

Learning Objectives	Content Outline	Resources
Define key terms used in the chapter.		Table 34-1: Developmental Aspects of Sexuality Through the Life Span
Describe male and female reproductive anatomy and physiology.	A. Physiology: female, male.	Table 34-2: Sexually Transmitted Diseases
Describe the sexual response cycle differentiating male and female responses.	B. Sexual response cycle: excitement, plateau, orgasm, resolution.	Table 34-3: Medications and Their Effects on Sexual Functioning
Identify factors that affect an individual's sexuality.	C. Sexual orientation.	Table 34-4: Sexual Dysfunction and Nursing Assessment
Perform a sexual assessment using suggested interview questions and appropriate physical assessment skills.	D. Sexual expression: masturbation, sexual intercourse, oral-genital stimulation, celibacy, alternative forms of sexual expression.	Table 34-5: Sexual Myths and Facts to Refute Them

Developing Critical Thinking Skills |
| Describe types of sexual dysfunction and assessment priorities for each one. | E. Factors affecting sexuality: developmental considerations, culture, religion, ethics, lifestyle, health state, medications. | Applying Learning to Practice: Promoting Health

Focused Assessment Guide: Sexuality |
| Develop nursing diagnoses identifying a problem with sexuality that may be remedied by independent nursing actions. | F. The nurse as role model: sexual harassment. | Focus on the Older Adult: Talking With Elderly People About Sexuality |
| Describe five areas in which the nurse can provide the patient with education to promote knowledge of sexuality. | G. Assessing: sexual history, sexual dysfunction, physical assessment.

H. Diagnosing.

I. Planning: expected outcomes. | Nursing Diagnoses for Common Problems: Sexuality

Through the Eyes of a Student

Research
Nursing Research: Making a Difference: Promoting Breast Health Education and Screening |
| Plan, implement, and evaluate nursing care related to select nursing diagnoses involving problems of sexuality. | J. Implementing: establishing a trusting nurse–patient relationship, teaching about sexuality and wellness.

K. Evaluating.

L. Nursing process in clinical practice: sexual dysfunction, inhibited sexual desire, altered sexuality patterns, change in sexual expression, knowledge deficit, contraception methods, body image disturbance related to breast removal.

M. Patient care study. | Knowledge Deficit: Contraceptive Methods

Using the Nursing Interventions Classification (NIC): Selected Teaching: Safe Sex Activities

Advocating Patient's Sexual Needs

Model for Counseling Patients With Sexual Problems (PLISSIT)

Applying Learning to Practice: Patient Care Study

Applying Learning to Practice: Nursing Plan of Care |

CHAPTER 35

Spirituality

■ Chapter Overview

Chapter 35 provides the learner with a knowledge base of spirituality. Practical suggestions for performing a spiritual assessment and specific interview questions are presented. Major religions—including Judaism, Christianity, Islam, American Muslim Mission, and Native American religions—are discussed along with various factors affecting spirituality. Sample nursing diagnoses are provided for common problems of spiritual distress, and evaluation guides are offered for patients experiencing spiritual distress related to challenged beliefs and value systems. The chapter concludes with a patient care study.

■ Teaching–Learning Activities

GROUP ACTIVITIES

1. Have students divide into small groups and discuss the following situations:
   - A woman who is terminally ill asks, "How could God let this happen to me?"
   - A patient of a very different faith asks you to pray with him.
   - A patient who is a Jehovah's Witness refuses a needed blood transfusion.

2. Ask a panel of religious leaders to present different religious practices, rituals, and beliefs.

3. Have students interview children to determine their perception of God and preferred forms of prayer or spiritual exercises. Have them discuss their findings in small groups and determine how the age, sex, religion, and personality of the child may have affected the responses.

4. Divide students into small groups to develop interview questions to assess patients for the following types of spiritual distress: (a) spiritual pain, (b) spiritual alienation, (c) spiritual anxiety, (d) spiritual guilt, (e) spiritual anger, (f) spiritual loss, and (g) spiritual despair.

5. Divide the class into pairs and have them perform a spiritual assessment on each other. Instruct them to focus on the student's guide to daily living habits, sources of support, sources of strength and healing, and sources of conflict and what factors affect their spirituality.

DISCUSSION QUESTIONS

1. What are some of the ways that nurses can assist patients to meet their spiritual needs?

2. What is the difference between an atheist and an agnostic? What are their philosophies of living?

3. Discuss how religion's life-affirming influences and life-denying influences may affect an individual's health and well-being.

4. What basic tenets do the religions discussed in this chapter have in common?

5. What role does spirituality play in the practice of holistic nursing care?

6. What blended skills would a nurse need to possess to promote spiritual health in a patient who is agnostic and is dying of cancer.

7. How do you feel about praying with a patient? What type of prayers do you feel comfortable sharing with patients?

WRITING ACTIVITIES

1. Have students research a religion different from their own and report how certain practices generally associated with healthcare may have religious significance for a patient (eg, dietary requirements and restrictions, prayer positions, physical contact).

2. Have students reflect on their own religious faith (or lack of religious faith) to determine if it is a source of support, strength, and healing or a source of conflict. Have them write a report on what their religion means to them and how or if it meets their spiritual needs.

3. Have students research and write a report on a famous religious leader and this person's contributions to society.

4. Have students describe how therapeutic communication skills are used to meet spirituality needs.

GUIDE TO CRITICAL THINKING AND DEVELOPING BLENDED SKILLS

1. Have students interview four or five hospitalized patients or patients in a residential healthcare setting to determine their spiritual needs. What is nursing's responsibility to meet these needs and how can this be best accomplished? Use an in-class discussion to explore how many students feel comfortable addressing spiritual needs and how they can best prepare themselves to do this.

   Use as an example: factors to assess:
   - Spiritual beliefs
   - Spiritual practices
   - Relation between spiritual belief and everyday living
   - Spiritual deficit or distress
   - Spiritual needs
   - Significant behavioral observations

2. Divide the class into small groups and assign each group a religion that is popular in the community. Have students research that religion's beliefs and practices that pertain to healthcare. Distinguish practices and beliefs that are life affirming from those that are life denying. Develop nursing considerations for each religion, describing the specific nursing measures you would use if caring for a patient of this religion.

   Consider the healthcare practices of the following religions:
   - Adventists
   - Christian Scientists
   - Church of Jesus Christ Latter Day Saints
   - Jehovah's Witnesses
   - Unification Church
   - Unitarian Universal Association of Churches and Fellowships
   - Christianity
   - American Muslim Mission
   - Native American religions
   - Religions with Eastern philosophies

TEACHING–LEARNING PLAN: Spirituality

Learning Objectives	Content Outline	Resources
Define key terms used in the chapter.		Table 35-1: Beliefs and Healthcare Practices of Major Religious Traditions in the United States
Identify three spiritual needs believed to be common to all people.		
Describe the influences of spirituality on everyday living, health, and illness.	A. Spirituality and faith: spirituality and everyday living, spirituality, health, and illness.	Six Basic Spiritual Needs of Americans The Center Point That Grounds Us ...
Differentiate life-affirming influences of religious beliefs from life-denying influences.	B. Major religions: religions with a Western philosophy, religions with an Eastern philosophy, Native American religions.	Cultural Care Applying Learning to Practice: The Nurse as Role Model
Distinguish the spiritual beliefs and practices of the major religions practiced in the United States and Canada.	C. Religions and law, ethics, and medicine.	Focused Assessment Guide: Spirituality
Identify five factors that influence spirituality.	D. Factors affecting spirituality: developmental considerations, family, ethnic background, formal religion, life events.	Nursing Diagnoses for Common Problems: Spiritual Distress Using the Nursing Interventions Classification (NIC): Selected Spiritual Support Activities
Perform a nursing assessment of spiritual health, using appropriate interview questions and observation skills.	E. The nurse as role model. F. Assessing spirituality: nursing history, nursing observation.	Using the Nursing Interventions Classification (NIC): Ways to Develop a Relationship With One's Inner World
Develop nursing diagnoses that correctly identify spiritual problems.	G. Diagnosing. H. Planning: expected outcomes.	Nurturing Spirituality Applying Learning to Practice: Patient Care Study
Describe nursing strategies to promote spiritual health and state their rationale.	I. Implementing: offering supportive presence, facilitating the patient's practice of religion, nurturing spirituality, praying with a patient, counseling the patient spirituality, contacting a spiritual counselor, resolving conflicts between treatment and spiritual beliefs.	Nursing Plan of Care Research Research in Nursing: Making a Difference: Promoting Spiritual Health
Plan, implement, and evaluate nursing care related to select nursing diagnoses involving spiritual problems.	J. Evaluating. K. Nursing process in clinical practice: spiritual distress. L. Patient care study.	

UNIT VIII

Promoting Healthy Physiologic Responses

CHAPTER 36

Hygiene

■ Chapter Overview

Chapter 36 introduces the reader to personal hygiene, including the measures for personal cleanliness and grooming that promote physical and psychological well-being. The multiple factors that affect personal hygiene and a practical guide for assessing the adequacy of a patient's hygiene are discussed and samples of nursing diagnoses, collaborative problems, and goals are provided. Descriptions of specific nursing strategies used when performing care of the skin, mouth, eyes, ears, nose, feet, and perineal and vaginal areas are also presented. A patient care study concludes the chapter.

■ Teaching–Learning Activities

GROUP ACTIVITIES

1. Demonstrate and have students practice the following procedures:
   - Making an occupied bed
   - Giving a massage
   - Providing oral care
   - Giving a patient a bed bath

2. Divide the class into four groups. Give each group one of the following situations and have them discuss the nursing care they would be expected to provide for the patient. Share each group's key points with the rest of the class.
   - A comatose patient
   - An elderly female patient with dentures and glasses
   - A 35-year-old male patient who is in a body cast
   - A postoperative female patient who has diabetic foot ulcers

3. Divide the students into two groups. Have one group review nursing documentation for the personal hygiene activities that are most routinely performed and one group review nursing documentation for the personal hygiene activities

that are least routinely performed. Have each group share their results.

4. Have students role-play taking care of the following appliances for a patient: (a) corrective lenses, (b) glass eye, (c) dentures, (d) hearing aid, and (e) contact lenses.

5. Ask for a volunteer to have her hair washed by another student while lying on a hospital bed. Explore how each student felt about the procedure. Conduct a discussion on hair care and have students give suggestions for caring for the following conditions/hair types: (a) dandruff, (b) pediculosis, (c) ticks, (d) kinky hair, and (e) beards/mustaches.

DISCUSSION QUESTIONS

1. Discuss the six major functions of the skin.

2. Have students discuss the following situations:
   - Agency protocol requires a daily bath, but your assigned patient refuses to have one.
   - Mrs. Jane is a 79-year-old diabetic. During morning care she asks you to soak and trim her toenails.
   - Mr. Sal has an artificial eye, but he is unable to provide self-care.
   - Miss Mack was in a motorcycle accident a week ago. Her hair is matted together with old blood.
   - Mr. Toss has an area the size of a quarter on his coccyx that is red and blistered.

3. What is the rationale for the use of antiembolic stockings? Identify clinical situations in which they might be used.

4. What cognitive, technical, interpersonal, and ethical/legal skills would a nurse need to respond to a homeless patient with diabetic foot ulcers who refuses to take off her shoes because she fears that they will be stolen?

5. Have students discuss their daily personal hygiene habits and how they would change if they were suddenly hospitalized and unable to provide self-care.

6. Explore the students' feelings about giving complete physical care to a member of the opposite sex. If they have negative feelings, how can they avoid embarrassing the patient and themselves?

WRITING ACTIVITIES

1. Have students describe how they would clean the following areas for a patient: (a) the ear, (b) the nose, and (c) the eyes.

2. Have students examine each other's skin and write an assessment of their findings.

3. Have students describe how the following factors may influence personal hygiene behaviors: (a) culture, (b) socioeconomic class, (c) religion, and (d) health status.

4. Assemble the equipment necessary for proper nail and foot care. Have students describe the proper use of each article. Perform the same exercise with a pair of dentures and the equipment necessary to care for them.

5. Have students observe the proper technique for bathing an infant and write a teaching plan to teach a new mother how to bathe her infant. Be sure they include special skin care needs that must be addressed when providing infant care.

GUIDE TO CRITICAL THINKING AND DEVELOPING BLENDED SKILLS

1. Present the class with different patient descriptions. Have students identify which patients are at greatest risk for skin alterations by recognizing the factors that place them at increased risk. Alternately, have students review the records of a number of patients in your clinical setting and identify those at greatest risk for skin alterations. Have students describe the nursing measures that are most likely to prevent skin alterations in these patients by anticipating possible complications.

   Be sure to discuss the factors that affect skin alterations:

   • Skin condition: developmental considerations, health state

   • Personal hygiene: culture, socioeconomic class, spiritual practices, developmental level and knowledge level, health state, personal preferences

2. Have all members of the class interview their parents or grandparents about the hygiene practices that are most important to them. Use an in-class discussion to sensitize students to racial, ethnic, and cultural differences. Explore the degree to which nurses are obliged to respect and meet these differences. Brainstorm with the group!

.

.

/

/

/

/

/

/

/

/

/

/

/

/

/

/

/

/

/

/

/

/

/

/

/

/

/

/

/

/

/

/

/

/

/

/

/

/

/

/

/

/

/

TEACHING–LEARNING PLAN: Hygiene

Learning Objectives	Content Outline	Resources
Define key terms used in the chapter.		Table 36-1: Functions of the Skin
List five functions of the skin, three factors influencing the skin's condition, and four basic principles that guide practices of skin care.	A. Physiology of the skin and its appendages: functions of skin and mucous membranes, principles of skin care.	Table 36-2: Factors Placing an Individual at Risk for Skin Alterations
		Table 36-3: Skin Care Problems
Identify factors affecting skin condition and personal hygiene.	B. Factors affecting skin condition and personal hygiene: skin condition, personal hygiene.	Focus on the Older Adult
		Applying Learning to Practice: The Nurse as Role Model: Personal Hygiene
Assess the integumentary system and the adequacy of hygiene self-care behaviors using appropriate interview and physical assessment skills.	C. The nurse as role model.	
	D. Basic skin care and personal hygiene.	Focused Assessment Guide: Hygiene Practices
Develop nursing diagnoses related to deficient hygiene measures.	E. Assessing: nursing history, physical assessment.	Through the Eyes of a Student
Describe the priorities of scheduled hygienic care, early morning care, morning care, afternoon care, and evening care.	F. Diagnosing.	Guidelines for Nursing Care: Flossing
	G. Planning: expected outcomes.	Through the Eyes of a Student
		Using the Nursing Interventions Classification: Ear Care
Identify at least four reasons for including the back massage in daily nursing care.	H. Implementing: cleaning the eyes, caring for the unconscious patient's eyes, providing care of eyeglasses, providing care of contact lenses, providing care of an artificial eye, providing ear care, providing nose care.	Guidelines for Nursing Care: Shaving
Demonstrate techniques used when assisting patients with hygiene measures, including those used when administering various types of baths and those used in cleaning each part of the body.		Guidelines for Nursing Care: Foot Care
		Guidelines for Nursing Care: Hygiene Needs: Adaptations for the Home Environment
	I. Evaluating.	
	J. Oral care.	Applying Learning to Practice: Promoting Health: Feminine Hygiene
Describe agents commonly used on the skin and scalp and precautions to observe in their use.	K. Assessing: nursing history, physical assessment.	Applying Learning to Practice: Patient Care Study
Plan, implement, and evaluate nursing care for common problems of the skin and mucous membranes.	L. Diagnosing.	Nursing Plan of Care
	M. Planning: expected outcomes	Research
	N. Implementing: administering oral hygiene, teaching oral hygiene.	Research In Nursing: Making a Difference: Using Massage to Reduce Agitation
	O. Evaluating: Care of the eyes, ears, and nose.	Procedure 36-1: Giving a Bed Bath
	P. Assessing: nursing history, physical assessment.	Procedure 36-2: Applying Antiembolism Stockings
	Q. Diagnosing. Planning: expected outcomes.	Procedure 36-3: Making an Unoccupied Bed
	R. Evaluating.	Procedure 36-4: Making an Occupied Bed

(continues)

TEACHING–LEARNING PLAN: Hygiene *(Continued)*

Learning Objectives	Content Outline	Resources
	S. Hair care.	Procedure 36-5: Assisting the Patient With Oral Care
	T. Assessing: nursing history, physical assessment.	Procedure 36-6: Providing Oral Care for the Dependent Patient
	U. Diagnosing.	
	V. Planning: expected outcomes.	
	W. Implementing: grooming the hair, shampooing the hair, caring for beards and mustaches, shaving.	
	X. Evaluating.	
	Y. Nail and foot care.	
	Z. Assessing: nursing history, physical assessment.	
	AA. Diagnosing.	
	BB. Planning: expected outcomes.	
	CC. Implementing: providing care of fingernails, providing foot care, providing foot care for the diabetic patient.	
	DD. Evaluating.	
	EE. Perineal and vaginal care.	
	FF. Assessing: nursing history, physical assessment.	
	GG. Diagnosing.	
	HH. Planning: expected outcomes.	
	II. Implementing: providing perineal care, providing vaginal care.	
	JJ. Evaluating.	
	KK. Nursing process in clinical practice: bathing/hygiene self-care deficit, altered oral mucous membranes.	
	LL. Patient care study: essential knowledge and skills.	

CHAPTER 37

Skin Integrity and Wound Care

■ Chapter Overview

Wound care and the treatment of pressure ulcers is the focus of Chapter 37. The development of pressure ulcers, the factors affecting skin integrity, and the prevention of pressure ulcers are discussed. The treatment of pressure ulcers—including cleaning and dressing the ulcer, controlling infection, and providing care in other treatment options—is also presented. The chapter concludes with a patient care study.

■ Teaching–Learning Activities

GROUP ACTIVITIES

1. Have students work in pairs to identify the pressure points on the body most susceptible to the development of a pressure ulcer. Have the students devise positions to alleviate specific pressure ulcers and eliminate the effect of friction and shearing forces.

2. Invite an experienced nurse who works in a critical care unit to speak to the class about assessing skin integrity, preventing pressure ulcers, and treating pressure ulcers.

3. Have students work in small groups to devise a preventive strategy to keep a bedridden elderly patient in a home healthcare setting free of pressure ulcers.

4. Collect a variety of bandages and binders and have the students take turns demonstrating their use by applying them to each other.

5. Have the students visit a postoperative patient in a healthcare setting to assess, diagnose, plan care, and evaluate the patient's surgical wound.

DISCUSSION QUESTIONS

1. What type of information should be collected in a nursing history designed to assess for skin integrity?

2. Discuss the following sentence: "Education is a vital component in the treatment of pressure ulcers." What is the nurse's role in educating the patient and family regarding management and treatment strategies?

3. What are the assessment priorities that should be considered when a pressure ulcer is noted? What are the expected outcomes for a patient with a pressure ulcer?

4. What are the psychological effects of wounds? Be sure to discuss patient pain, anxiety and fear, and alterations in body image.

WRITING ACTIVITIES

1. Have students research nursing articles for new methods of treating pressure ulcers and report any new findings.

2. Have students describe the effect the following factors have on the development of pressure ulcers in patients: (a) mobility and immobility, (b) nutrition and hydration, (c) moisture on the skin, (d) mental status, and (e) age.

3. Have students list the complications that can accompany pressure ulcers and the proper procedure for cleaning and dressing them.

4. Instruct the students to make a list of the type of blended skills they will need to diagnose and treat patients with alterations in skin integrity.

GUIDE TO CRITICAL THINKING AND DEVELOPING BLENDED SKILLS

1. Have students interview experienced nurses in various healthcare settings about their experience with pressure ulcers. Have them answer the following related questions:

   - What types of patients may be predisposed to the condition?
   - What factors contribute to the development of pressure ulcers?
   - What treatment do you find most effective?
   - How do you attempt to prevent pressure ulcers in your patients?
   - Have you incorporated any new methods for treating pressure ulcers in your care plan?
   - What is the psychological effect of pressure ulcers on the patient?

   Have students share their findings in a class discussion.

Be sure to explore the types of patients who are predisposed to pressure ulcers:

- Immobile patients
- Malnourished patients
- Incontinent patients
- Apathetic or confused patients

2. Instruct students to interview someone with a skin alteration about the psychological effects he is experiencing. After preparing a list of possible effects, identify nursing interventions to minimize these complications.

   You might want to discuss the following interventions:

- Assessing the stage of the pressure ulcer
- Eliminating pressure on the area of skin breakdown
- Cleansing the wound with each dressing change
- Applying a moisture-retentive dressing to wound
- Monitoring for possible infection

TEACHING–LEARNING PLAN: Skin Integrity and Wound Care

Learning Objectives	Content Outline	Resources
Define key terms used in the chapter.		Table 37-1: Common Types of Drains
Discuss the processes involved in wound healing.	A. Wound classification: phases of wound healing, wound healing, processes, factors affecting wound healing.	Table 37-2: Types of Tape
Describe factors that affect wound healing.		Table 37-3: Comparison of Stages of Pressure Ulcers
Accurately assess and document the condition of wounds.	B. Wound complications: infection, hemorrhage, dehiscence and evisceration.	Focus on the Older Adult: Factors that Affect Wound Healing in Older Adults
Implement dressing changes for different kinds of wounds.	C. Psychological effects of wounds	Guidelines for Nursing Care: Removing Staples and Sutures
Apply heat and cold effectively and safely.	D. Assessing the wound.	Using the Nursing Interventions Classification (NIC): Incision Site Care
Provide information to patients and caregivers for self-care of wounds at home.	E. Diagnosing in wound care.	Focused Assessment Guide: Skin Integrity
	F. Planning: expected outcomes for wound care.	Measurement of a Pressure Ulcer
	G. Implementing wound care.	Examples of Pressure Ulcer Risk Assessment Tools
	H. Teaching for home care of a wound.	Guidelines for Nursing Care: Preventing Pressure Ulcers
	I. Evaluating wound care.	Effective Irrigation Pressure
Identify patients at risk of developing a pressure ulcer.	J. Pressure ulcers: pathology of ulcer development, factors affecting pressure ulcer developing, pressure ulcer staging.	Developing Critical Thinking Skills
Describe the four stages of pressure ulcers.		Applying Learning to Practice: Patient Care Study
Provide nursing interventions to prevent or minimize pressure ulcers in adults.	K. Assessing the risk for or actual pressure ulcers.	Nursing Plan of Care
Follow guidelines for cleaning and dressing a pressure ulcer.	L. Diagnosing pressure ulcers.	Procedure 37-1: Cleaning a Wound and Applying a Sterile Dressing
Discuss the guidelines for cleaning and dressing a pressure ulcer.	M. Planning: expected outcomes for pressure ulcers.	Procedure 37-2: Collecting a Wound Culture
	N. Implementing interventions to prevent and care for pressure ulcers.	Procedure 37-3: Irrigating a Sterile Wound
	O. Evaluating pressure ulcer care.	Procedure 37-4: Applying an External Heating Device
	P. Applying learning to practice	Procedure 37-5: Applying Warm, Sterile Compresses to an Open Wound

CHAPTER 38

Activity

■ Chapter Overview

Chapter 38 provides the learner with knowledge of the physiology of movement, the principles of body mechanics, and factors affecting body alignment and mobility. Types of exercise, the role of exercise in disease prevention and health promotion, risks related to exercise, and individualized exercise programs are presented. The effect of immobility on body systems is explored, and a practical guide to assessing body alignment and mobility states is offered. The chapter concludes with a patient care study.

■ Teaching–Learning Activities

GROUP ACTIVITIES

1. Divide the class into seven groups and instruct each group to research the effects of mobility and immobility on the following body systems: cardiovascular, respiratory, musculoskeletal, metabolic, gastrointestinal, urinary, and skin. Have them discuss their research in small groups and then report their findings to the class as a whole.

2. Write the different types of movement of the neck, shoulder, elbow, wrist, fingers, hip, knee, ankle, and toes on index cards (eg, hip—hyperextension; toes—adduction; knee—extension). Have students take turns picking a card and demonstrating the movement for the class.

3. Have students role-play moving a patient from (a) one side of the bed to another, (b) a bed to a chair, and (c) a chair to a bed. Demonstrate the correct procedures and discuss safety factors involved in the movements.

4. Have students take turns demonstrating the different types of bed positions, noting the complications to be avoided.

5. Invite a physical therapist to discuss muscle-strengthening exercises and demonstrate crutch walking.

6. Arrange for the students to visit a healthcare facility where many of the patients are immobile. Have them work together in pairs to assist the healthcare professionals with patient exercises and mobility. Discuss in class how the students will use this knowledge in their own practices.

DISCUSSION QUESTIONS

1. What are the health benefits of the following types of exercise: aerobic exercise, stretching exercises, strength and endurance exercises, and movement and activities of daily living? How would you incorporate these types of exercises into a nursing care plan?

2. Why is knowledge of the musculoskeletal system and body mechanics important in nursing?

3. Describe proper body mechanics to prevent possible injury to nurses while caring for patients.

4. Discuss the positive effects of exercise and the negative effects of immobility on physical and psychosocial needs.

5. What blended skills will you need to assist patients with fitness goals and problems related to positioning, activity, or mobility?

6. Discuss the following statement: "The ability to move is closely related to the fulfillment of other basic human needs."

WRITING ACTIVITIES

1. Have students describe the following types of exercises and develop a nursing care plan that incorporates each type into an exercise program for a patient recovering from a transient ischemic attack: (a) isotonic exercise, (b) isometric exercise, and (c) isokinetic exercise.

2. Have students ambulate through a mall with (a) a walker, (b) crutches, and (c) a wheelchair. Ask them to describe how it felt to have their movement restricted and the reaction of other people to their decreased mobility.

3. Have students explain the rationale for the use of a trapeze, trochanter rolls, a footboard, and side rails for an assigned patient.

4. Ask students to write nursing diagnoses appropriate to problems with activity.

5. Have students research medical journals to find new treatments for immobile patients. Then, have them develop a plan of care for a hypothetical patient using this new knowledge.

GUIDE TO CRITICAL THINKING AND DEVELOPING BLENDED SKILLS

1. Invite students to demonstrate routine nursing actions such as positioning, turning, and lifting patients and heavy equipment. Have the class critique the body mechanics of the nurse demonstrating the procedure and offer suggestions. Similarly, have students place other students in different protective positions and invite the class to critique these positions.

Be sure to discuss the following positions and complications to be prevented:

- Fowler's position
- Protective supine position
- Protective side-lying or lateral position
- Protective Sims' position
- Protective prone position

2. Ask students to determine their exercise needs and whether or not they are meeting them. Students should develop a varied exercise program and keep a log that documents their success in meeting exercise goals and the reasons for any noncompliance. The log could also note activities of daily living that contribute to their fitness, such as walking to school instead of riding, using stairs instead of elevators, or dancing at a party instead of hanging out by the bar or refreshment table. Students should conclude the log with a list of reasons they fail to exercise and strategies to overcome these reasons.

TEACHING–LEARNING PLAN: Activity

Learning Objectives	Content Outline	Resources
Define key terms used in the chapter.		Table 38-1: Terms Commonly Used to Describe Body Positions and Movements
Describe the role of the skeletal, muscular, and nervous systems in the physiology of movement.	A. Physiology of movement: skeletal system, muscular system, nervous system, body mechanics.	Table 38-2: Activity Variations Based on Developmental Level
Identify seven variables that influence body alignment and mobility.	B. Factors affecting body alignment and mobility: developmental considerations, physical health, mental health, lifestyle variables, attitude and values, fatigue and stress, external factors.	Table 38-3: Comparison of Effects of Exercise and Immobility on Body Systems
		Table 38-4: Overview of the Physical Assessment of Mobility Status
		Table 38-5: Selected Nursing Diagnoses, Assessment Priorities, Expected Outcomes, and Nursing Interventions
Differentiate isotonic, isometric, and isokinetic exercise.	C. Exercise: types of exercise, effects of exercise and immobility on major body systems, role of exercise in preventing illness and promoting wellness, risks related to exercise.	Table 38-6: Common Bed Positions and Protective Nursing Actions
Describe the effects of exercise and immobility on major body systems.		Applying Learning to Practice: The Nurse as Role Model: Activity
Assess body alignment, mobility, and activity tolerance, using appropriate interview questions and physical assessment skills.	D. The nurse as role model.

E. Assessing: nursing history, physical assessment. | Applying Learning to Practice: Promoting Health

Research: Research in Nursing: Making a Difference: Supporting Positive Self-Care Practices in Older Adults |
| Develop nursing diagnoses that correctly identify mobility problems amenable to nursing therapy. | F. Diagnosing.

G. Planning: expected outcomes. | Focus on the Older Adult: Exercise and Activity

Focused Assessment Guide: Mobility and Exercise |
| Use proper body mechanics when positioning, moving, lifting, and ambulating patients. | H. Implementing: positioning patients, assisting with range-of-motion exercises, moving and lifting the patient, logrolling a patient, using a hydraulic lift, helping patients ambulate, designing exercise programs, teaching exercise benefits to populations at risk. | Nursing Diagnoses for Common Problems

Adaptive Equipment to Assist With Activities of Daily Living

Characteristics of a Successful Exercise Program |
| Design exercise programs. Plan, implement, and evaluate nursing care related to select nursing diagnoses involving mobility problems. | | Using the Nursing Interventions Classification (NIC): Exercise Therapy: Balance |
| | I. Evaluating. | Applying Learning to Practice: Patient Care Study |
| | J. Nursing process in clinical practice: activity intolerance, impaired physical mobility, risk for injury, complications of immobility, altered health maintenance: lack of exercise program. | Applying Learning to Practice: Nursing Plan of Care

Procedure 38-1: Turning a Patient in Bed

Procedure 38-2: Assisting With Passive Range-of-Motion (ROM) Exercises |
| | K. Patient care study: essential knowledge and skills. | Procedure 38-3: Assisting a Patient Up in Bed (Two Nurses)

Procedure 38-4: Transferring a Patient From Bed to Stretcher

Procedure 38-5: Assisting a Patient to Transfer From Bed to Chair

Procedure 38-6: Transferring a Dependent Patient From Bed to Chair (Two Nurses) |

Rest and Sleep

■ Chapter Overview

Chapter 39 provides the learner with knowledge of the functions and physiology of sleep, dreams and dream theories, and factors affecting sleep. Practical suggestions for performing a comprehensive sleep assessment and sample interview questions for a general and focused sleep history are presented. Patient goals and specific nursing strategies for promoting rest and sleep are described, and information on sleep diaries and pertinent physical assessment data are discussed. A patient care study concludes this chapter.

■ Teaching–Learning Activities

GROUP ACTIVITIES

1. Have students interview patients in various healthcare settings regarding their sleep patterns. Ask them to confirm that the patient is getting sufficient rest to provide energy for the day's activities or validate the existence of a sleep disturbance. If there is a sleep disturbance, have students develop a nursing care plan to alleviate the problem.

2. Divide students into small groups to discuss their coping mechanisms when they are unable to fall asleep.

3. Invite experienced nurses to discuss sleep problems they have experienced related to work demands and how they have learned to cope.

4. Divide students into small groups to develop a teaching tool that could be used to teach parents about their children's sleep requirements throughout development. Have them identify factors that may interrupt sleep patterns and measures to provide a restful environment for their children.

DISCUSSION QUESTIONS

1. How would you provide a restful sleep environment for an older patient living at home, in a nursing home, or in the hospital?

2. Discuss interventions appropriate for insomnia.

3. What are the effects of napping on normal sleep patterns?

4. Compare and contrast REM and NREM sleep.

5. Discuss how a nurse could provide a restful environment for a patient with sleep pattern disturbance in a healthcare facility. (eg, preparing a restful environment, promoting bedtime rituals, offering appropriate snacks, promoting relaxation and comfort, scheduling nursing actions, and using medications to promote sleep)

WRITING ACTIVITIES

1. Have students research sleep disorders in nursing journals and report any new findings.

2. Ask students to list the factors a nurse should discover in a sleep history when a sleep disturbance is noted.

3. Have students keep a personal sleep diary for a 2-week period, noting any sleep disturbances that may occur and their potential causes.

4. Ask students to choose five factors that affect sleep (eg, developmental considerations, physical activity, psychological stress, motivation, cultural implications, etc) and write a brief paragraph describing the effect of each factor on sleep and appropriate interventions to promote normal sleep patterns.

GUIDE TO CRITICAL THINKING AND DEVELOPING BLENDED SKILLS

1. Instruct the class to interview three older adults about their sleep/rest patterns, using the focused assessment guide in the text. Use a class discussion to explore the special problems experienced by the elderly, the efficacy of self-help measures they are using to cope, and helpful nursing interventions.

   Be sure to discuss the following factors affecting sleep:

   - Developmental considerations
   - Physical activity
   - Psychological stress
   - Motivation
   - Cultural implications
   - Diet
   - Alcohol and caffeine intake
   - Smoking
   - Environmental factors
   - Lifestyle
   - Illness
   - Medications

2. Instruct the class to interview three practicing nurses who are recent graduates, using the focused assessment guide for rest and sleep found in the text. Ask the interviewed nurses if they believe they are getting adequate rest, what factors are compromising their rest (eg, working double or rotating shifts), how this is affecting their practice, and what self-help measures are indicated. Discuss in class the number of practicing nurses with sleep alterations, the factors that place nurses at risk for sleep alterations, and what the students can learn to lower their risk.

   Examples of interventions may include:

   - Listing a specific number of hours of sleep to obtain each night
   - Getting regular exercise
   - Relaxing 1 hour before bedtime
   - Evaluating the use of stimulants
   - Limiting the number of back-to-back shifts

TEACHING–LEARNING PLAN: Rest and Sleep

Learning Objectives	Content Outline	Resources
Define key terms used in the chapter.		Table 39-1: Characteristics of NREM and REM Sleep
Describe the functions and physiology of sleep	A. Physiology of sleep: circadian rhythms, stages of sleep, sleep cycle, sleep requirements and patterns.	Table 39-2: Developmental Patterns of Sleep
Identify 12 variables that influence rest and sleep.	B. Factors affecting sleep: developmental considerations, physical activity, psychological stress, motivation, cultural implications, diet, alcohol intake, common sleep disorders.	Applying Learning to Practice: The Nurse as Role Model: Rest and Sleep
Describe nursing implications for age-related differences in the sleep–wake cycle.		Research Research in Nursing: Making a Difference: Using Protocols That Enhance Sleep in Hospitalized Elderly Patients.
	C. The nurse as role model	
Perform a comprehensive sleep assessment using appropriate interview questions, a sleep diary when indicated, and physical assessment skills.	D. Assessing rest and sleep: sleep history, sleep diary, physical assessment.	Focused Assessment Guide: Rest and Sleep
		Applying Learning to Practice: Promoting Health
Describe common sleep disorders, noting key assessment criteria.		Nursing Diagnosis for Common Problems: Sleep
Develop nursing diagnoses that correctly identify sleep problems that may be treated through independent nursing intervention.	E. Diagnosing. F. Planning: expected outcomes.	Using the Nursing Interventions Classification (NIC): Sleep Enhancement
Describe nine nursing strategies to promote rest and sleep, and identify their rationale.	G. Implementing: preparing a restful environment, promoting bedtime rituals, offering appropriate bedtime snacks and beverages, promoting relaxation, promoting comfort, respecting normal sleep–wake patterns, scheduling nursing care to avoid unnecessary disturbances, using medications to produce sleep, teaching about rest and sleep.	Focus on the Older Adult: Promoting Sleep
		Developing Critical Thinking Skills
Plan, implement, and evaluate nursing care related to select nursing diagnoses involving sleep problems.		Applying Learning to Practice: Patient Care Study
		Nursing Plan of Care
	H. Evaluating.	
	I. Nursing process in clinical practice: sleep pattern disturbance: insomnia, sleep deprivation.	
	J. Patient care study.	

CHAPTER 40

Comfort

■ Chapter Overview

Chapter 40 provides the learner with knowledge of the pain experience and the factors that influence it, including culture, religion, environment, support people, anxiety, and past pain experience. A detailed guide to assessing alterations in comfort is presented, including specific questions and approaches to use when assessing various pain factors. Specific nursing strategies for promoting comfort and assisting patients to achieve pain management are detailed. The chapter concludes with a discussion of the pain experience, its treatment modalities, patient and family responses to pain, and a patient care study.

■ Teaching–Learning Activities

GROUP ACTIVITIES

1. Instruct students to interview a patient who is experiencing chronic pain and one who is experiencing acute pain. Have them note the intensity and nature of the pain and pain relief measures that have been initiated. Ask them to assess if the method of pain control is effective, and if not, what they would do differently to control the patient's pain. Invite the students to share their experiences with the rest of the class in an in-class discussion.

2. Place students in small groups to discuss patient misconceptions about pain (eg, "The nurse will know when I am in pain and do something about it.") and how they might affect their ability to communicate their pain.

3. Have the students work with a partner to practice the following nonpharmacologic relief measures: (a) distraction, (b) imagery, (c) relaxation techniques, and (d) cutaneous stimulation.

4. Ask nurses from a coronary care unit, an oncology unit, and an acute surgical unit to discuss invasive and noninvasive comfort measures.

5. Ask students in small groups to discuss the use of analgesic agents for the following situations:
   - A newborn infant being circumcised
   - A known drug addict with a fractured femur
   - A young adult with terminal cancer
   - An elderly man with severe rheumatoid arthritis

DISCUSSION QUESTIONS

1. What is the gate control theory of pain? Why is it the basis for selected nursing interventions to promote comfort?

2. What are the characteristics of pain that should be included in a focused assessment?

3. Should placebos be used to satisfy a patient's demand for a drug?

4. Discuss physical, environmental, and psychosocial factors that affect the pain experience.

5. Discuss the possible rationale for research findings that pain of hospitalized patients is undertreated.

6. What blended skills should a nurse possess to meet the comfort needs of a patient with end-stage AIDS who asks for a lethal dose of morphine to end his suffering?

WRITING ACTIVITIES

1. Have students describe the following types of pain, its origins, and comfort measures: (a) chronic pain, (b) acute pain, and (c) intractable pain.

2. Have students list the advantages of patient-controlled analgesia.

3. Have students list the information about pain management that should be shared with the patient.

4. Ask students to briefly describe personal experiences with pain, including physical and emotional responses.

5. Have students summarize a nursing journal article that discusses nursing interventions to meet comfort needs.

GUIDE TO CRITICAL THINKING AND DEVELOPING BLENDED SKILLS

1. Have the class make a list of all the nonpharmacologic pain relief measures they can discover and then assign groups of students to research the origin, rationale, and efficacy of these measures. Where possible, have students talk with people who routinely use these measures and practice using them to gain first-hand experience. Conclude this exercise with an in-class discussion of the advantages and disadvantages of pharmacologic and nonpharmacologic measures and the related nursing care.

   Be sure to discuss the following nonpharmacologic relief measures:

   • Distraction
   • Imagery
   • Relaxation
   • Cutaneous stimulation
   • Transcutaneous electrical nerve stimulation
   • Acupuncture
   • Hypnosis
   • Biofeedback
   • Therapeutic touch

2. One of the reasons people often list for wanting to legalize assisted suicide is a fear of dying in horrible, unrelieved pain. Invite the class to determine whether or not this is a realistic fear, and if it is, what nursing needs to do to change this reality. Brainstorm with the class!

TEACHING–LEARNING PLAN: Comfort

Learning Objectives	Content Outline	Resources
Define key terms used in the chapter.		Table 40-1: Common Pain Syndromes
Describe specific elements in the pain experience.	A. The pain experience: definition; origins of pain; transmission of pain stimuli; perception of pain; modulation of pain; duration, severity, and periodicity of pain; responses to pain; acute versus chronic pain.	Table 40-2: Additional Terms Used by Patients to Describe Pain
Compare and contrast acute and chronic pain.		Table 40-3: Pain Expressions in Selected Ethnocultural Groups
		Table 40-4: Barriers to the Assessment and Treatment of Pain
Identify factors that may affect an individual's pain experience.	B. Factors affecting the pain experience: culture, religious beliefs, environmental and support people, anxiety and other stressors, past pain experience.	Applying Learning to Practice: The Nurse as Role Model: Comfort
		Common Responses to Pain
	C. The nurse as role model.	Applying Learning to Practice: Promoting Health
Obtain a complete pain assessment using appropriate interviewing and physical assessment skills.	D. Assessing the pain experience: misconceptions, components of pain assessment.	Focused Assessment Guide: The Pain Experience
Develop nursing diagnoses that correctly identify pain problems and demonstrate the relation between pain and other areas of human functioning.	E. Diagnosing. F. Planning: expected outcomes: chronic pain.	Research Research in Nursing: Making a Difference: Managing Pain in Children
	G. Implementing: establishing a trusting nurse–patient relationship, manipulating factors affecting the pain experience, initiating nonpharmacologic relief measures, managing pharmacologic relief measures, reviewing additional pain control measures, considering the ethical/legal responsibility to relieve pain, teaching the patient about pain.	Nursing Diagnoses for Common Problems: Pain
Demonstrate the correct use of nonpharmacologic pain relief measures.		Through the Eyes of a Patient
		Using Humor to Help Patients Cope With Pain
Administer analgesic agents safely to produce the desired level of analgesia without causing undesirable side effects.		Addiction, Physical Dependence, and Tolerance
Collaborate with the members of other health disciplines using different treatment modalities to promote pain relief.	H. Evaluating: the pain experience, treatment modalities, patient and family response.	Focus on the Older Adult: Nursing Strategies for Pain Affecting Older Adults
Use the Nursing Interventions Classification.	I. Nursing process in clinical practice: pain: acute postoperative, chronic pain: malignant.	Using the Nursing Interventions Classification (NIC): Patient-Controlled Analgesia (PCA) Assistance
Use teaching and counseling skills to empower patients to direct their own pain management programs.	J. Patient care study.	Guidelines for Nursing Care: Caring for Patients Receiving Epidural Opioids
		The Rights of Patients With Pain
		Applying Learning to Practice: Patient Care Study
		Nursing Plan of Care
		Procedure 40-1: Giving a Back Massage

CHAPTER 41

Nutrition

■ Chapter Overview

Chapter 41 provides the opportunity for the learner to gain a knowledge base regarding basic nutrition theory. The six classes of nutrients, energy balance, choice of an adequate diet, food patterns and habits, and factors affecting nutrition are discussed. Components of simple screening and in-depth nutritional assessments are outlined. Sample nursing diagnoses are presented and patient goals for healthy nutrition are explored. The chapter concludes with a patient care study.

■ Teaching–Learning Activities

GROUP ACTIVITIES

1. Instruct students to work in small groups to develop teaching strategies a nurse may use to achieve compliance with diet instructions. Share the results of each group's discussion with the class.

2. Have students investigate the variety of community services and programs available to provide nutritional support to patients at home.

3. Have students bring to class several boxes, cans, and bottles of various types of food, such as snacks, fruits, vegetables, convenience foods, cereals, and breads. Instruct the students to read the labels and decide which foods are (a) highest in carbohydrates, (b) highest in fat, (c) highest in vitamins, (d) highest in calories, and (e) highest in fiber.

4. Have students work in small groups to devise a diet plan for (a) an overweight teenage girl and (b) an economically disadvantaged family consisting of a single working mother with a 9-month-old infant.

5. Collect various types of feeding tubes. Have students take turns picking a tube, explaining its use, and demonstrating the procedure for insertion.

6. Invite a dietitian from a healthcare agency to discuss special diets and tube feeding formulas.

DISCUSSION QUESTIONS

1. Discuss why water is more vital to life than food.

2. Discuss the effects of anorexia nervosa and bulimia on the patient and family.

3. Discuss contributing factors to the development of obesity.

4. Make a list of low-fat, nutritional substitutes for the following foods: (a) extra-cheese, pepperoni pizza; (b) fast-food cheeseburger, French fries, and milk shake; (c) strawberry cheesecake ice cream; (d) potato chips; (e) bacon and eggs; and (f) steak and baked potato with butter and sour cream.

5. What assessments would be made to monitor for possible complications for the patient who is NPO?

6. What is the health effect of losing and gaining weight in response to fad diets?

WRITING ACTIVITIES

1. Have students describe the difference between a fatty acid and saturated fatty acid, and give examples of each.

2. Ask students to research and summarize dietary recommendations designed to protect the general population from chronic disease.

3. Have students describe how the following behavior modification techniques can help a patient lose weight: (a) planning strategies, (b) changing eating habits, (c) modifying shopping habits, and (d) incorporating lifestyle changes.

4. Using the Food Guide Pyramid, have students prepare a 1-week diet plan for a healthy, 40-year-old male sales executive who has a fairly sedentary lifestyle. Be sure they include the recommended number of daily servings from each food group when planning the menu.

5. Have students write a brief summary of a fad diet they have tried. Why did they stop using that diet?

6. Have students research new dietary guides that are designed to promote healthy weight control and report their findings to the class.

GUIDE TO CRITICAL THINKING AND DEVELOPING BLENDED SKILLS

1. Instruct students to interview the person responsible for food purchasing and preparation in a local economically disadvantaged family. Identify the adequacy of the family's diet, noting risk factors for nutritional deficiencies. What modifications are necessary to reduce their nutritional risks and which of these are feasible? How can nursing help this family?

   Consider the following factors that influence dietary requirements:

   - Developmental considerations
   - Gender
   - State of health
   - Alcohol abuse
   - Medications
   - Megadoses of nutrient supplements

2. Instruct the students to do a 24-hour food recall and analyze their dietary habits. Using the Food Guide Pyramid, determine if they met the daily requirements for each food group. Identify problems with frequency, amount, and types of foods and beverages, the fat content of frequently consumed foods, and their average daily consumption of empty calories. Identify the nutritional deficiencies for which they are at risk and develop preventive strategies. Brainstorm with the class!

TEACHING–LEARNING PLAN: Nutrition

Learning Objectives	Content Outline	Resources
Define key terms used in the chapter.		Table 41-1: Sources, Functions, and Significance of Carbohydrates, Protein, and Fat
List the six classes of nutrients and explain the significance of each.	A. Principles of nutrition: energy balance, energy nutrients, regulatory nutrients.	Table 41-2: Summary of Vitamins
Evaluate a diet using the Food Guide Pyramid.	B. How to choose an adequate diet: Food Guide Pyramid, recommended dietary allowance and recommended nutrient intakes, dietary recommendations, food labeling.	Table 41-3: Summary of Macrominerals and Microminerals Table 41-4: Cultural Variations on Nutrition
Identify risk factors for poor nutritional status.	C. Factors affecting nutrition: physiologic factors that influence nutrient requirements, sociocultural and psychological factors, decreased food intake.	Table 41-5: Clinical Observations for Nutritional Assessment
Describe nutritional implications of growth and development throughout the life cycle.		Methods of Calculating Caloric Requirements
	D. The nurse as role model.	Food Guide Pyramid: Typical Serving Size
Discuss the components of nutritional assessment.	E. Assessing nutritional status: dietary data, medical and socioeconomic data, anthropometric data, clinical data, biochemical data.	Dietary Guidelines for Americans Nutritional Assessment Considerations for Older Adults

(continues)

TEACHING–LEARNING PLAN: Nutrition *(Continued)*

Learning Objectives	Content Outline	Resources
Develop nursing diagnoses that correctly identify nutritional problems that may be treated by independent nursing intervention. Describe nursing interventions to help patients achieve their nutritional goals. Plan, implement, and evaluate nursing care related to selected nursing diagnoses that involve nutritional problems. Distinguish between enteral and parenteral nutrition.	F. Diagnosing. G. Planning: expected outcomes. H. Implementing: teaching nutritional information, monitoring nutritional status, stimulating appetite, assisting with eating, providing nutrition in special situations, providing enteral nutrition, providing parenteral nutrition. I. Evaluating: altered nutrition: more than body requirements obesity, altered nutrition: less than body requirements—iron deficiency anemia, knowledge deficit, new therapeutic diet. J. Patient care study: assessment findings, core competencies.	Applying Learning to Practice: The Nurse as Role Model: Nutrition Applying Learning to Practice: Promoting Health Focused Assessment Guide: Nutrition Biochemical Data with Nutritional Implications Nursing Diagnoses for Common Problems: Nutrition Using the Nursing Interventions Classification (NIC): Nutritional Counseling Focus on the Older Adult: Nursing Strategies for Nutritional Problems Affecting Older Adults Research Research in Nursing: Making a Difference: Using pH and Bilirubin Concentration to Predict Feeding Tube Placement Guidelines for Nursing Care: Measuring pH of Gastric Fluids Through the Eyes of a Student Guidelines for Nursing Care: Preventing Complications in Enteral Feeding Guidelines for Nursing Care: Monitoring Administration of Parenteral Nutrition Applying Learning to Practice: Patient Care Study Nursing Plan of Care Procedure 41-1: Inserting a Nasogastric Tube Procedure 41-2: Administering a Tube Feeding Procedure 41-3: Removing a Nasogastric Tube Procedure 41-4: Irrigating a Nasogastric Tube Connected to Suction Procedure 41-5: Monitoring the Blood Glucose Level

CHAPTER 42

Urinary Elimination

■ Chapter Overview

Chapter 42 provides the learner with knowledge of the physiology of the urinary system and the multiple factors affecting urination. A practical guide to assessing urinary elimination is presented, as well as examples of nursing diagnoses. The learner is also introduced to focused assessment, diagnosis, planning, implementation, and evaluation guides for selecting nursing diagnoses of common urinary problems. These guides illustrate how the nurse's knowledge of the urinary system and urinary pathology is combined with specific nursing interventions to resolve urinary problems successfully. The chapter concludes with a patient care study.

■ Teaching–Learning Activities

GROUP ACTIVITIES

1. Have students interview parents of young children about toilet training. What factors occurred that indicated the child was ready for toilet training? What teaching strategies would you use to prepare parents for training their children? Compare the students' findings in an in-class discussion.

2. Gather as many containers and devices for collecting urine as possible and place them on a table in the classroom. Have the students take turns selecting a device and describing or demonstrating its intended use.

3. Have students work in small groups to develop a list of nursing strategies designed to restore urinary continence and postpone a caregiver's decision to place a family member in a costly healthcare facility.

4. Invite a laboratory technician to discuss and demonstrate diagnostic examinations of urine.

5. Have students interview and develop an appropriate nursing care plan for an assigned patient who has an actual or potential problem with urinary elimination. Share results with the class.

6. Have students work in small groups to develop a teaching plan for a patient being released from the hospital with an indwelling catheter. Be sure they identify support groups and community resources that could be helpful to the patient.

DISCUSSION QUESTIONS

1. What is the role of the nurse in helping patients develop healthy urinary elimination patterns?

2. Discuss how the following factors may influence normal voiding patterns for patients: (a) schedule, (b) privacy, (c) position, (d) hygiene, and (e) fluid intake.

3. What should be taught to patients who have indwelling catheters?

4. Identify the anatomy and physiology of the urinary system.

5. Discuss the psychological variables that influence a person's normal voiding habits.

WRITING ACTIVITIES

1. Have the students describe any special considerations that should be included when performing a nursing history to assess urinary functioning for the following patients: (a) infants and young children, (b) older adults, and (c) people with limited or no bladder control.

2. Ask the students to list nursing interventions that promote normal voiding in a patient.

3. Have students use each of the following words in a sentence: diuretic, hematuria, incontinence, cystoscopy.

4. Have students outline a teaching plan for teaching self-catheterization.

5. Ask students to describe nursing interventions to prevent nosocomial infections in patients who have indwelling catheters.

6. Instruct students to keep a record of their own fluid intake and output for 24 hours. Have them state how their intake affected their output and identify factors in their life that could promote or hinder urinary elimination.

GUIDE TO CRITICAL THINKING AND DEVELOPING BLENDED SKILLS

1. Divide the class into groups and assign to each an area of physical assessment for urinary functioning: kidneys, bladder, urethral meatus, skin, and urine. Instruct each group to report on the method used to examine this component, related diagnostic tests, and abnormal findings. Identify the appropriate nursing response for each abnormal finding.

   Be sure to include the following assessments in your discussion:

- Kidneys
  Palpation
  Contour and size
  Tenderness or lumps
  Costovertebral tenderness
- Bladder
  Palpation when full
  Percussion
- Urethral orifice
  Inspection
  Inflammation
  Discharge
- Skin integrity
  Assessment for color, texture, turgor, excretion of wastes
- Urine
  Assessment for color, odor, clarity, presence of sediment

2. Investigate resources in the community that would be helpful for a patient who had an ileostomy. List the services that these resources can provide. Identify any lifestyle changes this patient may face and how to facilitate coping with altered functioning. Brainstorm with the class!

TEACHING–LEARNING PLAN: Urinary Elimination

Learning Objectives	Content Outline	Resources
Define key terms used in the chapter.		Table 42-1: Characteristics of Urine
Describe the physiology of the urinary system.	A. Physiology: kidneys and ureters, bladder, urethra, act of micturition.	Table 42-2: Common Diagnostic Procedures Used to Study the Urinary Tract
Identify seven variables that influence urination.	B. Factors affecting micturition: developmental considerations, food and fluid, lifestyle, psychological variables, activity and muscle tone, pathologic conditions, medications.	Applying Learning to Practice: The Nurse as Role Model: Urinary Elimination
Assess urinary elimination, using appropriate interview questions and physical assessment skills.		Applying Learning to Practice: Promoting Health
	C. The nurse as role model.	
Execute the following assessment measures: measure urine output, collect urine specimens, determine the presence of select abnormal urine constituents, determine urine specific gravity, and assist with diagnostic tests and procedures.	D. Assessing: nursing history, physical assessment, assessment measures.	Focused Assessment Guide: Urinary Elimination
	E. Diagnosing.	Terms Used to Describe Additional Urinary Problems
	F. Planning: expected outcomes.	

(continues)

TEACHING–LEARNING PLAN: Urinary Elimination *(Continued)*

Learning Objectives	Content Outline	Resources
Develop nursing diagnoses that correctly identify urinary problems amenable to nursing therapy.		Guidelines for Nursing Care: Collecting a Clean-Catch or Midstream Urine Specimen
Demonstrate how to promote normal urination; facilitate use of the toilet, bedpan, urinal, and commode; perform catheterizations; and assist with urinary diversions.	G. Implementing: promoting normal urination, caring for an incontinent patient, catheterizing the patient's bladder, assisting with urinary diversions.	Nursing Diagnosis for Common Problems: Urinary Elimination
		Focus on the Older Adult: Nursing Strategies for Urinary Elimination Problems Affecting Older Adults
	H. Evaluating.	
		Using the Nursing Interventions Classification (NIC): Urinary Retention Care
Describe the nursing interventions that can be used to manage urinary incontinence effectively. Plan, implement, and evaluate nursing care related to select nursing diagnoses associated with urinary problems.	I. Nursing process in clinical practice: altered urinary elimination related to dysuria, altered urinary elimination related to maturational enuresis, urinary retention related to varying etiologies, risk for infection related to indwelling catheter. Patient care study.	Treatment Options for Urinary Incontinence
		Applying Learning to Practice: Developing Critical Thinking Skills
		Research Research in Nursing: Assisting Older Adults to Manage Urinary Incontinence
		Through the Eyes of a Student
		Procedure 42-1: Offering and Removing a Bedpan or Urinal
		Procedure 42-2: Catheterizing the Female Urinary Bladder (Straight and Indwelling)
		Procedure 42-3: Catheterizing the Male Urinary Bladder (Straight and Indwelling)
		Procedure 42-4: Irrigating the Catheter Using the Closed System
		Procedure 42-5: Giving a Continuous Bladder Irrigation
		Procedure 42-6: Applying a Condom Catheter
		Procedure 42-7: Changing a Stoma Appliance on an Ileal Conduit
		Applying Learning to Practice: Patient Care Study
		Nursing Plan of Care

Bowel Elimination

■ Chapter Overview

Chapter 43 provides the learner with knowledge of the physiology of bowel elimination and the multiple factors that influence this process. A practical guide to assess bowel elimination is presented, which includes a description of nursing responsibilities related to diagnostic studies of the gastrointestinal tract. The effects of nutrition, exercise, and medication on bowel elimination are also discussed, and interventions to prevent constipation, diarrhea, and flatulence are presented. Numerous examples of nursing diagnoses and expected patient outcomes are offered. The chapter concludes with a patient care study.

■ Teaching–Learning Activities

GROUP ACTIVITIES

1. Place the students in small groups and have them discuss the techniques for assessing the following body sites for bowel elimination: (a) abdomen, (b) anus, and (c) rectum. Demonstrate the assessments on a mannequin in front of the class and invite questions from students.

2. Have students work in groups of five to outline the responsibilities of the nurse in one of the following diagnostic studies: (a) stool collection, (b) timed specimens, (c) pinworms, (d) direct visualization studies, and (e) indirect visualization studies. Have one member of each group take notes and present a summary of the group's findings for the class.

3. Have students work in small groups to develop nursing guidelines that help promote physical and psychological comfort for the ostomy patient. Share the results of each group with the class.

4. Invite a nurse who is an enterostomal therapist to discuss ostomy care and teaching.

5. Ask a radiologist to discuss barium studies of the lower and upper gastrointestinal tracts.

6. Have students interview a patient who has an actual or potential problem with bowel elimination. Have them each identify an appropriate nursing diagnosis using the PES format, develop a nursing care plan for this patient based on the nursing diagnosis they identified, and implement their nursing plan. Compare the results with the class.

DISCUSSION QUESTIONS

1. What effect does surgery have on peristalsis?

2. What is the role of the nurse in helping patients maintain healthy bowel elimination patterns?

3. What is a bowel training program, and how can it help patients with a history of chronic constipation and impaction and those who are incontinent of stool?

4. Discuss the anatomy and physiology of the large and small intestine, rectum, and anus.

5. Identify developmental, physical, psychological, and illness-related factors that affect bowel elimination.

6. Discuss the effect the following factors have on promoting regular bowel habits: (a) timing, (b) positioning, (c) privacy, (d) nutrition, and (e) exercise.

WRITING ACTIVITIES

1. Have students list nursing interventions designed to promote regular bowel habits.

2. Ask students to describe the nursing interventions they would recommend for a patient with the following gastrointestinal problems: (a) constipation, (b) diarrhea, and (c) flatulence.

3. Have the students list ways in which they can promote the physical and emotional comfort of a patient when meeting bowel elimination needs.

4. Instruct students to research and summarize a new surgical procedure to correct impaired bowel functioning.

5. Have students research the types and uses of enemas.

GUIDE TO CRITICAL THINKING AND DEVELOPING BLENDED SKILLS

1. Present the class with diverse situations in which patients require gastrointestinal studies. Invite individual students to describe the appropriate nursing care before, during, and after the study. Instruct students to address all aspects of required nursing competencies: intellectual, technical, interpersonal, and ethical/legal.

   Explore the following tests and purposes:
   - Esophagogastroduodenoscopy
   - Colonoscopy
   - Sigmoidoscopy
   - Upper gastrointestinal and small-bowel series
   - Barium enemas

2. Invite someone with a bowel diversion to speak to the class about his related experiences. Ask him to specifically address how the diversion influenced self-image, how he learned to cope, what self-care measures he practices, and what type of assistance from healthcare professionals has been most helpful. Enlist his help in preparing a teaching plan for patients with new bowel diversions, which addresses practical concerns, such as where and how to purchase supplies, travel considerations, hygiene concerns, and modifications demanded by recreational activities. Brainstorm with the class!

TEACHING–LEARNING PLAN: Bowel Elimination

Learning Objectives	Content Outline	Resources
Define key terms used in the chapter.		Table 43-1: The Stool: Normal Characteristics and Special Considerations for Observation
Describe the physiology of bowel elimination.	A. Physiology: large intestine, anal canal and anus, act of defecation, normal defecation.	Table 43-2: Common Diagnostic Procedures Used to Study the Gastrointestinal Tract
Identify 10 variables that influence bowel elimination.	B. Factors affecting bowel elimination: developmental considerations, daily patterns, food and fluid, activity and muscle tone, lifestyle, psychological variables, pathologic conditions, medications, diagnostic tests, surgery and anesthesia.	Table 43-3: Classification of Laxatives
Assess bowel elimination using appropriate interview questions and physical assessment skills.		Table 43-4: Commonly Used Enema Solutions
Assist with the following diagnostic measures: stool collection for laboratory analysis and direct and indirect visualization studies of the gastrointestinal tract.		Table 43-5: Nutritional Impact on Ostomies
	C. The nurse as role model.	Warning Signs of Colon Cancer
	D. Assessing: nursing history, physical assessment, assisting with diagnostic studies.	Focus on the Older Adult
Develop nursing diagnoses that correctly identify bowel elimination problems amenable to nursing therapy.	E. Diagnosing.	Applying Learning to Practice: The Nurse as Role Model: Bowel Elimination
	F. Planning: expected outcomes.	Applying Learning to Practice: Promoting Healthy Bowel Elimination
Demonstrate how to (1) promote regular bowel habits (timing, positioning, privacy, nutrition, exercise); (2) provide instruction in the use of cathartics, laxatives, and antidiarrheals; (3) empty the colon of feces (enemas, rectal suppositories, rectal catheters, digital removal of stool); (4) design and implement bowel training programs; and (5) use comfort measures to ease defecation.	G. Implementing: promoting regular bowel habits, teaching about cathartics, laxatives and antidiarrheals, decreasing flatulence, emptying the colon of feces, managing fecal incontinence, designing and implementing bowel training programs, meeting needs of patient with bowel diversions, providing comfort measures.	Focused Assessment Guide: Bowel Elimination
		Guidelines for Nursing Care: Testing for Fecal Occult Blood
		Nursing Diagnoses for Common Problems
		Research
		Research in Nursing: Making a Difference: Managing Chronic Constipation in Long-Term Care Residents
Describe nursing care for a patient with an ostomy.	H. Evaluating.	Guidelines for Nursing: Inserting a Rectal Suppository
Plan, implement, and evaluate nursing care related to selected nursing diagnoses that involve bowel problems.	I. Nursing process in clinical practice: constipation, bowel incontinence, diarrhea.	Using the Nursing Interventions Classification (NIC): Bowel Training
	J. Patient care study.	Applying Learning to Practice: Patient Care Study
		Nursing Plan of Care
		Procedure 43-1: Administering a Cleansing Enema
		Procedure 43-2: Changing or Emptying an Ostomy Appliance

CHAPTER 44

Oxygenation

■ Chapter Overview

The focus of Chapter 44 is the physiology, general purpose, and general factors affecting respiratory functioning. Practical suggestions for performing a comprehensive respiratory assessment are given, and expected outcomes and specific nursing strategies for implementation are described. Sample interview questions for both a general and focused respiratory history are presented, along with information on collecting data from the nursing examination. The chapter concludes with a patient care study.

■ Teaching–Learning Activities

GROUP ACTIVITIES

1. Have students perform a nursing history on a patient with altered respiratory function. Instruct the students to use interview questions to identify (a) current or potential health deviations, (b) patient actions for meeting this need and their effects, (c) contributing factors, (d) use of aids to improve intake of air, and (e) effect on current lifestyle and relationships with others. Have students share the results of their interviews with the class.

2. Have students role-play performing a physical assessment of the lungs and respiratory status on a partner. Guide the students through each sequence of inspection, palpation, percussion, and auscultation by discussing normal and abnormal findings during each phase of the assessment.

3. Invite a respiratory therapist to demonstrate and discuss techniques, supplies, and procedures to improve oxygenation.

4. Demonstrate and have students practice the following procedures:

   • Use of the incentive spirometer
   • Pursed-lip breathing
   • Postural drainage
   • Suctioning

DISCUSSION QUESTIONS

1. What is the role of the nurse when working with patients to initiate changes in health habits that affect respiration?

2. How can nurses teach patients to assess their environment and make adjustments, where necessary, to factors that impair respiratory functioning?

3. Identify normal anatomy and physiology of the respiratory system.

4. Discuss the effects (both active and passive) of cigarette smoking. What environmental controls are being legislated? What are the rights of smokers and nonsmokers?

5. What needs to be taught to promote safety when oxygen is in use?

6. Discuss how the following factors affect respiratory functioning: levels of health, development, opioids, lifestyle, environment, and psychological health.

WRITING ACTIVITIES

1. Have students describe the variations in the respiration process that occur in (a) infants, (b) preschool and school-aged children, and (c) the elderly.

2. Have students develop interview questions to assess a teenager with asthma for respiratory functioning.

3. Instruct students to evaluate their own environments (at home, work, school, or during social activities) for air pollution and describe their findings.

4. Ask students to write nursing diagnoses appropriate for problems with oxygenation.

5. Instruct students to write a paragraph describing how they would perform a physical assessment of respiratory functioning using inspection, palpation, percussion, and auscultation.

6. Have students research diagnostic procedures used to assess respiratory functioning and share their results with the class.

GUIDE TO CRITICAL THINKING AND DEVELOPING BLENDED SKILLS

1. Assemble oxygen administration equipment (nasal cannula, nasal catheter, transtracheal catheter, oxygen masks, and tent) as well as artificial airway equipment (oropharyngeal airway, endotracheal tube, tracheostomy tube, and cuffed endotracheal tube) and invite individual students to select a device and describe the conditions under which it is indicated, the related procedure for insertion, and priorities for nursing care. Invite the class to identify potential problems with the use of each and to strategize about nursing solutions.

Use Table 44-4 in the text to explore the use of the following oxygen administration equipment:

- Nasal cannula
- Nasal catheter
- Transtracheal catheter
- Oxygen masks
- Tent

You might want to explore the use of the following artificial airway equipment:

- Oropharyngeal airway
- Endotracheal tube
- Tracheostomy tube
- Cuffed endotracheal tube

2. Invite the class to identify variables in the local environment (at home, at work, and in general) that predispose to respiratory problems. What can nurses individually and collectively do to promote pollution-free environments? Brainstorm with the class!

TEACHING–LEARNING PLAN: Oxygenation

Learning Objectives	Content Outline	Resources
Define key terms used in the chapter.		Table 44-1: Respiratory Variations in the Life Cycle
Describe the principles of respiratory physiology.	A. Physiology of respiration: the respiratory system, pulmonary ventilation, alveolar gas exchange, transport of respiratory gases, control of respiration, developmental variations.	Table 44-2: Common Diagnostic Procedures Used to Assess Respiratory Functioning
Decsribe age-related differences that influence care of the patient with respiratory problems. Identify six factors that influence respiratory function.		Table 44-3: Medications Used to Improve Respiratory Functioning
	B. Factors affecting respiratory functioning: levels of health, development, opioids (narcotic analgesics), lifestyle, environment, psychological health.	Table 44-4: Oxygen Delivery Systems
		Applying Learning to Practice: The Nurse as Role Model: Oxygenation
	C. The nurse as role model.	Applying Learning to Practice: Promoting Health
Perform a comprehensive respiratory assessment using appropriate interview questions and physical assessment skills.	D. Assessing respiratory functioning: nursing history, physical assessment, common methods of assessing respiratory functioning.	Focused Assessment Guide: Respiration
	E. Diagnosing.	

(continues)

TEACHING–LEARNING PLAN: Oxygenation *(Continued)*

Learning Objectives	Content Outline	Resources
Develop nursing diagnoses that correctly identify problems that may be treated by independent nursing interventions. Describe 11 nursing strategies to promote adequate respiratory functioning, identifying their rationale. Plan, implement, and evaluate nursing care related to select nursing diagnoses involving respiratory problems.	F. Planning: expected outcomes. G. Implementing: establishing a trusting nurse–patient relationship, promoting proper breathing, promoting and controlling coughing, promoting comfort, using nebulizers, providing supplemental oxygen, using artificial airways, assisting ventilation, clearing an obstructed airway, administering cardiopulmonary resuscitation, hyperbaric oxygen therapy. H. Evaluating. I. Nursing process in clinical practice: impaired gas exchange, ineffective breathing pattern, ineffective airway clearance. J. Patient care study.	Nursing Diagnoses for Common Problems: Respiration Focus on the Older Adult: Physiologic Changes and Nursing Strategies for Oxygen Problems Affecting Older Adults Using the Nursing Interventions Classification (NIC): Ventilation Assistance Guidelines for Nursing Care: Using an Incentive Spirometer Guidelines for Nursing Care: Monitoring a Patient With a Chest Tube Guidelines for Nursing Care: Using a Nebulizer Device Guidelines for Nursing Care: Transporting a Patient With a Portable Oxygen Cylinder Guidelines for Nursing Care: Inserting an Oropharyngeal Airway Research Research in Nursing: Making a Difference: Family Member Attendance at CPR and Invasive Procedures Applying Learning to Practice: Patient Care Study Nursing Plan of Care Procedure 44-1: Using a Pulse Oximeter Procedure 44-2: Administering Oxygen by Nasal Cannula Procedure 44-3: Administering Oxygen by Mask Procedure 44-4: Suctioning the Nasopharyngeal and Oropharyngeal Areas Procedure 44-5: Suctioning the Tracheostomy Procedure 44-6: Providing Tracheostomy Care

CHAPTER 45

Fluid, Electrolyte, and Acid–Base Balance

■ Chapter Overview

Chapter 45 provides the learner with basic knowledge of the principles of fluid, electrolyte, and acid–base balance and the etiologies, defining characteristics, and nursing interventions for common disturbances. Sample interview questions for performing a fluid balance nursing history are presented, along with information on specific physical assessment measures and laboratory studies. Numerous examples of nursing diagnoses are offered and expected outcomes and specific nursing strategies for promoting fluid balance are described. The chapter concludes with a patient care study.

■ Teaching–Learning Activities

GROUP ACTIVITIES

1. Have students make a list of common electrolytes found in the body and foods that serve as sources of each electrolyte.

2. Divide the class into three groups. Have students in each group research a screening test for fluid, electrolyte, and acid–base balance and discuss their findings in their group. Have each group report to the class as a whole.

3. Ask the director of a blood bank to discuss blood donations, blood type and cross-matching procedures, and safety measures in blood administration.

4. Demonstrate and have students practice the following procedures:

   • Setting up IV solutions with tubing
   • Starting an IV with an angiocatheter and butterfly needle
   • Practicing timing and regulating IV rates
   • Changing tubing and solutions
   • Adding a solution to "piggyback" onto a main line
   • Assessing an IV site and changing IV site dressing
   • Discontinuing an IV
   • Preparing for blood administration

5. Ask an intensive care nurse to discuss arterial blood gases.

6. Patients with fluid, electrolyte, and acid–base imbalances are often prescribed medications as part of the therapeutic regimen. What blended skills do nurses need to possess to properly administer these medications to their patients?

DISCUSSION QUESTIONS

1. Discuss how the body derives water from ingested liquids, food, and metabolism.

2. What is fluid homeostasis, and what are the primary organs of homeostasis?

3. What goals must nurses meet to be a role model of self-care behaviors that promote fluid, electrolyte, and acid–base balance?

4. What assessments are significant in patients with imbalances of sodium, potassium, calcium, magnesium, chloride, bicarbonate, and phosphate?

5. Discuss the buffer systems of the body that maintain normal acid–base balance.

6. Discuss common assessments and interventions for overhydration and dehydration.

7. What is the role of the nurse in helping a patient: (a) decrease fluids, (b) increase fluids, (c) restrict fluids?

WRITING ACTIVITIES

1. Have students describe the following processes that transport materials to and from intracellular compartments: (a) osmosis, (b) diffusion, (c) active transport, and (d) filtration.

2. Instruct the students to use the following words in a sentence: (a) hyponatremia, (b) hypernatremia, (c) hypokalemia, (d) hyperkalemia, (e) hypocalcemia, (f) hypercalcemia, (g) hypomagnesemia, and (h) hypermagnesemia.

3. Have students describe nursing interventions to maintain or restore fluid and electrolyte balances, including teaching, nutrition, monitoring fluid intake and output, administering medications, and administering IV therapy.

4. Have students summarize a nursing journal article that discusses fluid, electrolyte, or acid–base balance.

5. Instruct students to make a list of the vascular access devices available for delivery of solutions and medications into a vein. Include a brief description of the device, the length of time the infusion therapy is needed, the type of medication or product that will be delivered intravenously, the patient's individualized needs that determine which option is used, and the nursing care involved.

GUIDE TO CRITICAL THINKING AND DEVELOPING BLENDED SKILLS

1. Divide the class into groups and assign to each a particular fluid, electrolyte, and acid–base imbalance. Have the groups describe the imbalance,

identify types of patients who are at greatest risk for these imbalances, and develop related nursing prevention strategies. Guide the class in a discussion of the factors that make it difficult to implement prevention strategies of possible nursing responses.

Using Table 45-8 in the text, discuss the following imbalances:
- Hyponatremia and hypernatremia
- Hypokalemia and hyperkalemia
- Hypocalcemia and hypercalcemia
- Hypomagnesemia and hypermagnesemia
- Hypophosphatemia and hyperphosphatemia
- Respiratory alkalosis
- Respiratory acidosis
- Metabolic acidosis

2. Instruct the class to review the medical record of a patient with a fluid, electrolyte, or acid–base imbalance and to identify all the diagnostic findings that support this diagnosis. Discuss their findings with the class.

TEACHING–LEARNING PLAN: Fluid, Electrolyte, and Acid–Base Balance

Learning Objectives	Content Outline	Resources
Define key terms used in the chapter.		Table 45-1: Water as a Percentage of Body Weight
Describe the location and functions of body fluids and factors that affect variations in fluid compartments.	A. Physiology: body fluids, electrolytes, fluid and electrolyte movement, fluid balance, acid–base balance.	Table 45-2: Homeostatic Mechanisms That Maintain the Composition and Volume of Body Fluid Within Narrow Limits of Normal
Describe the functions, regulation, sources, and mechanisms for loss of the main electrolytes of the body.	B. Disturbances in fluid, electrolytes, and acid–base balance: fluid imbalances, electrolyte imbalances, acid–base imbalances.	Table 45-3: Acid–Base Parameters for Arterial Blood Gas Studies
Explain the principles of osmosis, diffusion, active transport, and filtration.	C. The nurse as role model.	Table 45-4: Imbalances Resulting From Loss of Specific Body Fluid
Describe how thirst and the organs of homeostasis (kidneys, heart and blood vessels, lungs, adrenal glands, pituitary gland, and parathyroid glands) function to maintain fluid homeostasis.	D. Assessing: nursing history, physical assessment. E. Diagnosing. F. Planning: expected outcomes.	Table 45-5: Parameters to be Considered in Clinical Assessment for Fluid, Electrolyte, and Acid–Base Imbalance

(continues)

Learning Objectives	Content Outline	Resources
Describe the role of buffer systems and respiratory and renal mechanisms in achieving acid–base balance.	G. Implementing: preventing fluid imbalances, developing a dietary plan, modifying fluid intake, administering medications, administering intravenous therapy, replacing blood and blood products, giving total parenteral nutrition.	Table 45-6: Acid–Base Disturbances
		Table 45-7: Fluid Volume Disturbances
Identify the etiologies, defining characteristics, and treatment modalities for common fluid, electrolyte, and acid–base disturbances.		Table 45-8: Electrolyte Disturbances
		Table 45-9: Selected IV Solutions
	H. Evaluating.	Table 45-10: Complications Associated With Intravenous Infusions
Perform a fluid, electrolyte, and acid–base balance assessment.	I. Nursing process in clinical practice: the surgical patient, the oncology patient.	Table 45-11: Transfusion Reactions
		Applying Learning to Practice: The Nurse as Role Model: Fluid, Electrolyte, and Acid–Base Balance
Describe the role of dietary modifications, modification of fluid intake, medication administration, intravenous therapy, blood replacement and total parenteral nutrition in resolving fluid, electrolyte, and acid–base imbalances.	J. Patient care study.	Applying Learning to Practice: Promoting Health: Fluid and Electrolyte Balance
		Focused Assessment Guide: Fluid, Electrolyte, and Acid–Base Balance
		Guidelines for Nursing Care: Measuring Fluid Intake and Output
Plan, implement, and evaluate nursing care related to select nursing diagnoses involving fluid, electrolyte, and acid–base imbalances.		Nursing Diagnoses for Common Problems: Fluid and Electrolyte Balance
		Focus on the Older Adult: Nursing Strategies for Ensuring Fluid Balance in Older Adults
		Research in Nursing: Making a Difference: Identifying the Adequacy of Water Intake in an Elderly Population
		Using the Nursing Interventions Classification (NIC): Intravenous (IV) Therapy
		Guidelines for Nursing Care: Caring for a Patient with a PICC
		Guidelines for Nursing Care: Regulating IV Flow Rates
		Applying Learning to Practice: Patient Care Study
		Nursing Plan of Care
		Procedure 45-1: Starting an Intravenous Infusion
		Procedure 45-2: Changing an IV Solution and Tubing
		Procedure 45-3: Monitoring an IV Site and Infusion
		Procedure 45-4: Changing an IV Dressing
		Procedure 45-5: Capping a Primary Line for Intermittent Use
		Procedure 45-6: Administering a Blood Transfusion

INTRODUCTION TO TESTBANK

This testbank consists of over 1,000 multiple choice NCLEX-style questions. All questions are coded by level of difficulty and can be cross-referenced to the page in the textbook where the topic is discussed and the correct answer can be found.

Accompanying each item in this testbank is a set of item descriptors printed below each question. The descriptors contain basic information about an item and are used to determine which items you would like to include on a test. Therefore, you will be able to sort questions based on this criterion. The following key helps to explain descriptors used in this testbank.

<1> 1. Infant mortality is a standard measurement of the quality of healthcare in the country. What does this measure?
    a. The number of babies who die at birth each year.
    b. The number of deaths per 1,000 live births.
<2> c. The number of deaths per 1,000 live births in children under age 12 months each year.*
    d. The number of babies who die of communicable diseases each year.

<3>   **Rationale:** The infant year is birth to 12 months; mortality refers to death.

<4>   Reference: p. 13
    Descriptors:

    <5> 1. 01 **<6>** 2. 03   **<7>** 3. Knowledge
    <8> 4. II-2 **<9>** 5. Documentation **<10>** 6. Easy

Explanation of descriptors:

<1> Question Number

<2> Correct Answer

<3> Question Rationale (or Explanation)
Answer explanations or "rationales" provide brief explanations as to why the answer to the question was chosen.

<4> Referenced Page Number
Indicates the page(s) from the textbook on which the basis for the correct answer may be found. Single pages are indicated as such (e.g., p. 81). Consecutive pages would be indicated by two hyphens (e.g., pp. 31–33; nonconsecutive pages would be indicated by a comma (e.g., pp. 31, 45, 56).

<5> Chapter Number
Indicates the chapter of the textbook on which the item is based.

<6> Chapter Objective
If the textbook chapter has delineated chapter objectives, this item indicates which chapter objective the item relates to by number.

<7> Cognitive Types
Knowledge
Comprehension
Application
Analysis

<8> Patient Needs Step
The framework of *Patient Needs* was selected for the NCLEX-RN examination because it provides a universal structure for defining nursing actions and competencies across all settings for all patients. The four major categories are indicated below.

I. Safe, Effective Care Environment
  1. Management of Care
  2. Safety and Infection Control

II. Health Promotion and Maintenance
  1. Growth and Development Through the Life Span
  2. Prevention and Early Detection of Disease

III. Psychosocial Integrity
  1. Coping and Adaptation
  2. Psychosocial Adaptation

IV. Physiological Integrity
  1. Basic Care and Comfort
  2. Pharmacologic and Parenteral Therapies
  3. Reduction of Risk Potential
  4. Physiologic Adaptation

<9> Patient Needs Concepts and Processes
Integrated within the four categories of *Patient Needs* are **concepts** and **processes**.

Nursing process	Documentation
Caring	Self-care
Communication	Teaching/learning
Cultural awareness	

<10> Difficulty Levels
All items are labeled as either easy, moderate, or difficult. **Easy** items are those you would expect 75% of the students to answer correctly; easy questions are often cognitive ability at the comprehension/recall level. **Moderate** items are those you would expect 50% of the students to answer correctly, and often require cognitive ability at the application level of cognition. **Difficult** items are those you would expect only 25% of the students to answer correctly, and often require cognitive ability at the application or analysis levels.

UNIT I

Foundations of
Nursing Practice

CHAPTER 1

Introduction to Nursing

1. Nursing during the period of the Middle Ages led to
   a. continuity, caring, critical thinking
   b. purpose, direction, leadership*
   c. assessment, rehabilitation, caring
   d. advocacy, rehabilitation, caring

   Reference: p. 7

   Descriptors:

   1. 01   2. 01   3. Knowledge
   4. None   5. None.   6. Moderate

   Rationale: Although the Middle ages ended in chaos, nursing had developed purpose, direction, and leadership.

2. The founder of modern nursing was
   a. Dorothea Dix
   b. Adelaide Nutting
   c. Florence Nightingale*
   d. Sister Jean Jugan

   Reference: p. 7

   Descriptors:

   1. 01   2. 02   3. Knowledge
   4. None   5. None   6. Easy

   Rationale: The founder of professional nursing was Florence Nightingale.

3. The individual who recommended that educational standards for nursing education be established is
   a. Florence Nightingale*
   b. Clara Barton
   c. Louise Schuyler
   d. Jane Adams

   Reference: p. 7

   Descriptors:

   1. 01   2. 06   3. Knowledge
   4. None   5. None   6. Moderate

   Rationale: Florence Nightingale founded modern nursing education.

4. The slow progress to professionalism in nursing throughout the United States following the Civil War was due in part to the
   a. lack of educational standards*
   b. hospital based schools of nursing
   c. lack of influence by Florence Nightingale
   d. independence of religious orders

   Reference: p. 8

   Descriptors:

   1. 01   2. 02   3. Knowledge
   4. None   5. None   6. Moderate

   Rationale: The lack of educational standards, the male dominance in healthcare, and the prevailing Victorian belief that women depended on men contributed to the lack of professionalism.

5. The founder of public health nursing and the Henry Street Settlement is
   a. Lillian Wald*
   b. Adelaide Nutting
   c. Sojurner Truth
   d. Clara Barton

   Reference: p. 9

   Descriptors:

   1. 01   2. 02   3. Knowledge
   4. None   5. None   6. Easy

   Rationale: Lillian Wald established a neighborhood nursing service for the sick poor of the lower East Side of New York City; she was the founder of professional nursing.

6. The essential aspects of nursing as defined by the American Nurses Association include
   a. education, assessment, evaluation
   b. care, cure, coordination*
   c. cure, care, rehabilitation
   d. research, clinical practice, specialization

   Reference: p. 10

   Descriptors:

   1. 01   2. 01   3. Knowledge
   4. None   5. None   6. Easy

   Rationale: The essential components of professional nursing are care, cure, and coordination.

7. Teaching a woman about breast self-examinations is an example of what aspect of professional nursing?
   a. care*
   b. cure
   c. coordination
   d. secondary prevention

   Reference: p. 10

   Descriptors:

1. 01	2. 03	3. Application
4. II-2	5. Teach/Learn	6. Difficult

   Rationale: Nursing is the sharing of responsibility for health and welfare of all those in the community. Breast self-examinations are preventive in nature.

8. Which of the following actions best describes nursing as a profession and a discipline?
   a. university-based education
   b. historical social development and changes
   c. clinically based research for practice*
   d. medical technological advances

   Reference: pp. 10–11

   Descriptors:

1. 01	2. 02	3. Application
4. None	5. None	6. Moderate

   Rationale: Clinically based research for practice is necessary for a group to be classified as a profession and a discipline. Medical technological advances may change the way nurses practice, but it does not influence the profession or the discipline.

9. Providing education about diet and exercise for a healthy diabetic patient is best described as which of the following activities?
   a. promoting wellness
   b. preventing illness*
   c. treating symptoms
   d. restoring wellness

   Reference: p. 10

   Descriptors:

1. 01	2. 03	3. Application
4. II-2	5. Teach/Learn	6. Difficult

   Rationale: Preventive measures such as diet and exercise for a diabetic patient are classified as preventing illness measures.

10. A registered nurse has visited a high school class and presented the topic on nursing as a career. The nurse determines that one of the students needs further instructions when she says that one of the roles of the nurse is to
    a. collaborate with other healthcare professionals
    b. participate in, evaluate, or conduct research
    c. prescribe complex medical and surgical treatments*
    d. assist patients to learn how to conduct self-care activities

    Reference: p. 10

    Descriptors:

1. 01	2. 03	3. Application
4. None	5. None	6. Moderate

    Rationale: Prescription of complex medical and surgical treatments is the responsibility of physicians.

11. Nurses focus on the human response to the
    a. interaction of the environment
    b. impact of disease on the patient
    c. response of the human body to treatment
    d. response to actual or potential health problems*

    Reference: p. 11

    Descriptors:

1. 01	2. 03	3. Comprehension
4. None	5. None	6. Moderate

    Rationale: Nursing focuses on human responses to actual or potential health problems and is increasingly focused on wellness.

12. A faculty member employed by an accredited school of nursing must be prepared at which educational level?
    a. diploma in nursing
    b. vocational certificate in nursing
    c. bachelor's degree in nursing
    d. master's degree in nursing*

    Reference: p. 11

    Descriptors:

1. 01	2. 04	3. Knowledge
4. None	5. None	6. Easy

    Rationale: Master's-prepared nurses have the educational qualifications to teach in an accredited school of nursing.

13. A major rationale for nurses to teach aerobic exercises to groups of senior citizens is to
    a. prevent illness*
    b. allow for socialization
    c. develop diversity in the community
    d. decrease disability

Reference: p. 13

Descriptors:

1. 01	2. 03	3. Comprehension
4. II-2	5. Teach/Learn	6. Difficult

Rationale: Nurses promote health by maximizing the patient's own strengths. Aerobic exercises can promote joint mobility in senior citizens and prevent other illnesses.

14. A nursing student has been assigned to teach a group of expectant parents about car seat safety. This educational presentation is an example of
    a. restoration of health
    b. facilitation of coping
    c. prevention of illness
    d. health promotion*

Reference: p. 13

Descriptors:

1. 01	2. 03	3. Comprehension
4. I-2	5. Teach/Learn	6. Difficult

Rationale: Educational presentations that promote health and prevent illness or injury are emphasized in the objectives of *Healthy People 2000*.

15. Which of the following educational levels describes the LVN (licensed visiting nurse) or LPN (licensed practical nurse)?
    a. 1-year technical degree*
    b. 2-year university degree
    c. 3-year hospital diploma
    d. 4-year health degree

Reference: p. 14

Descriptors:

1. 01	2. 04	3. Knowledge
4. None	5. None	6. Easy

Rationale: Most LVNs or LPNs obtain their license after a 1-year technical degree program.

16. The level of education recommended by the ANA is the
    a. bachelor's degree
    b. master's degree*
    c. specialty certificate
    d. doctorate degree

Reference: p. 14

Descriptors:

1. 01	2. 06	3. Knowledge
4. None	5. None	6. Easy

Rationale: The American Nurses Association has recommended that the entry level for professional practice is the baccalaureate degree.

17. A major difference between nurses prepared with an associate degree and those prepared with a baccalaureate degree is that
    a. only associate degree nurses provide primary care in health settings
    b. baccalaureate degree nurses evaluate research for applicability to practice*
    c. associate degree nurses must delegate care to other healthcare employees
    d. only baccalaureate degree nurses document the nursing process for patients

Reference: pp. 14–15

Descriptors:

1. 01	2. 04	3. Knowledge
4. None	5. None	6. Easy

Rationale: Baccalaureate degree nurses are educated to evaluate research for applicability to practices. All nurses are capable of providing primary care to patients and must also be responsible for delegation of care.

18. A major rationale for the development and continuation of professional nursing organizations for the profession is to
    a. provide socialization and networking for members
    b. regulate members work and career activities
    c. set standards for nursing practice*
    d. provide information to nurses about current practices

Reference: p. 16

Descriptors:

1. 01	2. 05	3. Comprehension
4. None	5. None	6. Moderate

Rationale: Professional organizations have the responsibility to set standards for a specific profession.

19. A nurse wishes to inform a national legislator regarding changes in national healthcare policy. The best action he can take would be to
    a. call the governor of all states in the United States
    b. determine his state legislative representatives
    c. inform the state senators in neighboring states
    d. notify the lobbyist at the American Nurses Association*

    Reference: p. 16

    Descriptors:

1. 01	2. 05	3. Application
4. I-1	5. Communication	6. Difficult

    Rationale: The American Nurses Association is the lobbying body which represents nursing in the state and federal governments.

20. An organization that conducts preentrance testing for nursing is the
    a. American Nurses Association
    b. National League for Nursing*
    c. International Council of Nurses
    d. American Association of Colleges of Nursing

    Reference: p. 16

    Descriptors:

1. 01	2. 05	3. Knowledge
4. None	5. None	6. Easy

    Rationale: The National League for Nursing (NLN) conducts preentrance tests for nursing to measure student progress. The American Nurses Association sets standards for practice.

21. A nursing organization that has established standards of nursing practice is the
    a. National League for Nursing
    b. International Council of Nursing
    c. American Nurses Association*
    d. State Board of Nursing

    Reference: p. 17

    Descriptors:

1. 01	2. 05	3. Knowledge
4. None	5. None	6. Easy

    Rationale: The ANA Standards of Clinical Nursing Practice define the activities of nurses that are specific and unique to nursing.

22. A nurse is moving from Michigan to Ohio. She will be working on a medical/surgical division at Canton Memorial Hospital. The nurse will need to be aware of the
    a. Ohio Nurse Practice Act*
    b. Canton Memorial Hospital policy manual
    c. ANA standards for practice
    d. most recent research on medical/surgical nursing

    Reference: p. 17

    Descriptors:

1. 01	2. 05	3. Comprehension
4. None	5. None	6. Moderate

    Rationale: Nurses must be aware of all aspects of the nurse practice acts in the states they are employed to avoid prosecution or loss of licensure.

23. The nursing administrator at North Dakota Home Health Agency is aware that a nurse in his facility is chemically dependent. It is his responsibility to
    a. confront the nurse regarding the abuse
    b. suspend the nurse for 1 week
    c. make all visits to the patients' homes with the nurse
    d. report the nurse to the state board of nursing*

    Reference: p. 17

    Descriptors:

1. 01	2. 05	3. Application
4. I-1	5. Caring	6. Difficult

    Rationale: The administrator needs to report this to the state board of nursing. The license can be denied, revoked, or suspended because of chemical impairment.

24. To practice nursing in a different state, nurse practice acts must be used because they
    a. provide continuity of care
    b. do not create a regulatory body
    c. define the scope of nursing practice*
    d. determine the educational status for nurses

    Reference: p. 17

    Descriptors:

1. 01	2. 05	3. Comprehension
4. None	5. None	6. Moderate

    Rationale: Each state has a Nurse Practice Act that defines the scope of a nurse's practice in that particular state.

CHAPTER 2

Health of the Individual, Family, and Community

1. The school nurse at the community's junior high school is assisting the teachers in preparing the eighth grade for high school. What must the nurse assess?
   a. cultural factors of the students
   b. students' plans for the future
   c. academic preparation in junior high
   d. psychosocial and physiologic needs*

   Reference: p. 22

   Descriptors:

   1. 02   2. 03   3. Application
   4. II-1   5. Nursing Process 6. Moderate

   Rationale: Through the assessment of psychosocial and physiologic needs of students the nurse can determine interventions that can promote each level of Maslow's Hierarchy of Needs.

2. An 82-year-old patient is being discharged to her home, following a fall in which she sustained a fractured pelvis. The home health nurse plans to assess her home. According to Maslow, the goal of this assessment is
   a. physiologic
   b. social
   c. safety*
   d. anxiety

   Reference: p. 22

   Descriptors:

   1. 02   2. 03   3. Comprehension
   4. I-2   5. Nursing Process 6. Difficult

   Rationale: Physical safety means being protected from physical harm.

3. A 2-year-old patient suffering from asthma is admitted to the hospital. Which of the following is the most immediate patient need for the nurse to address?
   a. ensuring that his favorite toys are nearby
   b. keeping the side rails up at all times
   c. providing oxygen and a clear airway*
   d. providing his favorite snack at bedtime

   Reference: p. 22

   Descriptors:

   1. 02   2. 03   3. Application
   4. IV-1   5. Nursing Process 6. Difficult

   Rationale: Immediate needs for a child with asthma include provision of oxygen and a clear airway. Oxygen needs precede safety needs.

4. The nurse is caring for a 42-year-old male patient. He has just been administered a medication to lower his blood pressure. The nurse must instruct him about
   a. taking a double dose when he misses a scheduled dose of medication
   b. not taking the medication on an empty stomach
   c. exercising on a daily basis and for 45 minutes to 1 hour
   d. taking his medication accurately and watch for adverse reactions*

   Reference: p. 23

   Descriptors:

   1. 02   2. 06   3. Application
   4. IV-2   5. Teach/Learn   6. Moderate

   Rationale: Educating patients about knowledgeable administration of medications promotes safety and security needs. The patient should not be advised to take a double dose of the medication.

5. An adult patient is admitted to the intensive care unit. He will experience
   a. fear of the unknown*
   b. fear of the future
   c. insecurity
   d. sensory depletion

   Reference: p. 23

   Descriptors:

   1. 02   2. 05   3. Application
   4. II-1   5. Caring   6. Moderate

   Rationale: Patients entering the healthcare system often fear the unknown.

6. Consideration and assessment of sexuality in patients is vital to
   a. medical care
   b. holistic care*
   c. evaluative care
   d. respiratory care

   Reference: p. 23

   Descriptors:

1. 02	2. 03	3. Comprehension
4. IV-1	5. Caring	6. Moderate

   Rationale: There is increasing awareness in healthcare that the consideration of sexuality is a vital part of holistic care.

7. To assist a patient to meet self-esteem needs, the nurse should
   a. negate the patient's negative self-perception
   b. compliment the patient about anything to increase self-thought.
   c. determine the patient's goals without any assistance
   d. accept the patient's values and belief systems*

   Reference: p. 24

   Descriptors:

1. 02	2. 03	3. Application
4. III-1	5. Caring	6. Moderate

   Rationale: Acceptance of the patient's values and belief systems by the nurse can help a patient to meet his or her self-esteem needs.

8. A 60-year-old male patient lives alone and has been diagnosed with cancer. His daughter lives in another city. What is the patient at risk for?
   a. physical ailments
   b. death
   c. isolation*
   d. lack of communication

   Reference: p. 25

   Descriptors:

1. 02	2. 04	3. Application
4. III-1	5. Caring	6. Easy

   Rationale: Changes in family structure such as the death of spouse and the mobility of society lead to feelings of loneliness and isolation.

9. The nurse should implement the following nursing intervention for a patient diagnosed with cancer.
   a. referral to a cancer support group*
   b. referral to a cancer survivor
   c. call the physician for a referral to home health
   d. arrange for alternative transportation

   Reference: p. 24

   Descriptors:

1. 02	2. 04	3. Application
4. I-1	5. Nursing Process	6. Difficult

   Rationale: Through the implementation of nursing interventions the patient will feel less isolated and lonely, especially through working with a support group.

10. A 79-year-old woman states, "I am happy with my life and I have my family raised. I've accomplished all my goals." The patient is exhibiting
    a. happiness
    b. trust
    c. problem solving
    d. self-actualization*

    Reference: p. 24

    Descriptors:

1. 02	2. 04	3. Comprehension
4. III-2	5. Communication	6. Moderate

    Rationale: A patient's acceptance of self and others is self-actualization according to Maslow.

11. A nurse is in a food store shopping when another patron complains of chest pain. What is the nurse's immediate concern?
    a. safety
    b. pain
    c. oxygenation*
    d. circulation

    Reference: p. 23

    Descriptors:

1. 02	2. 05	3. Application
4. IV-3	5. Nursing Process	6. Moderate

    Rationale: Oxygen is the most essential of all needs because all body cells require oxygen for survival.

12. To promote a hospitalized patient's love and belonging needs, the nurse should
    a. include significant others in the patient's care*
    b. encourage the patient to set attainable goals
    c. provide the patient with direction and hope
    d. refer the patient to a group therapy session

    Reference: p. 24

    Descriptors:

1. 02	2. 03	3. Application
4. III-2	5. Caring	6. Moderate

    Rationale: Inclusion of the patient's significant others in the physical and emotional care of the patient will help to meet a hospitalized patient's love and belonging needs.

13. A 15-year-old female adolescent is going to live with her mother and her mother's boyfriend. The adolescent begins acting out in the classroom. The school nurse has been asked to assess the adolescent and assist in determining a rationale for her behavior. What question might the nurse ask the adolescent?
    a. "Do you like your new home and you new dad?"
    b. "Who helps you with your homework?"
    c. "Are you able to play outside after school?"
    d. "Who takes care of you and what jobs do they have?"*

    Reference: p. 25

    Descriptors:

1. 02	2. 06	3. Application
4. II-1	5. Communication	6. Difficult

    Rationale: Changes in family structure influence basic human needs. Adolescents may begin acting out due to the stress of the change.

14. A 30-year-old woman has moved in with her parents. She has two young children. What parenting difficulty might she encounter?
    a. separation from familiar rules and regulations
    b. anxiety of fear of the unknown
    c. lack of financial support for her children
    d. changes in role and discipline toward her children*

    Reference: p. 25

    Descriptors:

1. 02	2. 06	3. Application
4. II-1	5. Nursing Process	6. Difficult

    Rationale: Stress can arise when adult children are forced to move back with their parents after they have been established separate. Changes in role and discipline of the children can be a problem.

15. Which of the following societal factors is responsible for helping to change the roles of men and women in traditional families?
    a. decreased educational opportunities for women
    b. increased educational opportunities for men
    c. increased economic standards of living
    d. increased career opportunities for women*

    Reference: p. 26

    Descriptors:

1. 02	2. 04	3. Knowledge
4. II-1	5. Communication	6. Easy

    Rationale: Increased educational and career opportunities for women have helped to change the roles of both men and women in traditional families.

16. Within a family, provision of comfort to family members is an example of
    a. compassion
    b. safety
    c. stress relief
    d. building identity*

    Reference: p. 26

    Descriptors:

1. 02	2. 04	3. Application
4. II-1	5. Caring	6. Difficult

    Rationale: The family provides emotional comfort to family members. It also helps members establish identity and maintain that identity in times of stress.

17. The major effect that a health crisis has on the family structure is
    a. change in family member roles*
    b. adaptation to stress
    c. reevaluation of basic human needs
    d. respect for family identity

    Reference: p. 26

    Descriptors:

1. 02	2. 05	3. Application
4. None	5. None	6. Difficult

    Rationale: During a healthcare crisis certain family members may assume roles they have never performed, such as a daughter may assume the role of the parent.

18. Serving favorite family foods and observing traditional holidays in a prescribed manner accurately describes which family function?
    a. physical
    b. affective
    c. economic
    d. socialization*

    Reference: p. 26

    Descriptors:

1. 02	2. 04	3. Application
4. None	5. None	6. Easy

    Rationale: Rituals such as serving favorite family foods and observing traditional holdiays are part of the soicalization function of the family.

19. Which of the following is considered a risk factor for family development?
    a. support systems readily available
    b. stable economic environment
    c. history of chronic drug abuse*
    d. availability of medical resources

    Reference: p. 28

    Descriptors:

    | 1. 02 | 2. 04 | 3. Application |
    | 4. None | 5. None | 6. Moderate |

    Rationale: Drug abuse, economic instability, frequent moving, and lack of support systems or medical services are all risk factors for family development.

20. To provide nursing care in the community, the community health nurse must be aware of all of the community factors affecting health through the life span *except*
    a. nutritional services
    b. recreational opportunities
    c. healthcare services
    d. educational services*

    Reference: p. 29

    Descriptors:

    | 1. 02 | 2. 04 | 3. Application |
    | 4. None | 5. None | 6. Moderate |

    Rationale: Factors affecting the health of a community include nutritional services, recreational opportunities, and healthcare services.

21. A 2-year-old child was brought to the emergency room by his parents for severe pain in the right shoulder. The parents told the nurse that he accidentally fell down the stairs. Which of the following nursing diagnoses would be appropriate?
    a. Risk for Injury related to age*
    b. Altered Parenting related to the patient's pain
    c. Knowledge Deficit related to injury
    d. Caregiver Role Strain related to emergency room visit

    Reference: p. 28

    Descriptors:

    | 1. 02 | 2. 03 | 3. Comprehensive |
    | 4. II-1 | 5. Nursing Process | 6. Moderate |

    Rationale: Risk for Injury related to age is the appropriate diagnosis. Accidents are one of the leading causes of death in children, particularly toddlers and preschoolers.

CHAPTER 3

Culture and Ethnicity

1. Culture is learned by the younger generation through
   a. ethnic heritage
   b. psychosocial interpretive experience
   c. church involvement
   d. formal and informal experiences*
   Reference: p. 34
   Descriptors:

1. 03	2. 01	3. Knowledge
4. II-1	5. Cultural	6. Moderate

   Rationale: Culture is an integral component of both health and illness. It is learned from our family's beliefs and those of the community.

2. A large group of people who are members of a larger cultural group but have certain ethnic, occupational, or physical characteristics are termed a
   a. culture
   b. subculture*
   c. tribe
   d. heritage
   Reference: p. 35
   Descriptors:

1. 03	2. 02	3. Knowledge
4. II-1	5. Cultural	6. Easy

   Rationale: Subcultures are found in all aspects of society. They are groups within a larger culture.

3. The white middle class people of European ancestry are dominant in the United States. What value is inherent to this group?
   a. blue collar work
   b. thinness*
   c. respect for the elderly
   d. religious affiliation
   Reference: p. 35
   Descriptors:

1. 03	2. 03	3. Comprehensive
4. II-1	5. Cultural	6, Easy

   Rationale: A dominant value in our culture is youth, thinness, and beauty.

4. Which of the following characteristics is a descriptor of one's race in the United States?
   a. language
   b. religion
   c. skin color*
   d. food preferences
   Reference: p. 35
   Descriptors:

1. 03	2. 01	3. Knowledge
4. None	5. None	6. Easy

   Rationale: Racial categories are typically based on specific physical characteristics, such as skin color, body stature, facial features, and hair texture.

5. The statement "Italian Americans are more beautiful than any other cultural group on the planet" is a statement reflecting which cultural misconception?
   a. stereotyping
   b. ethnocentrism*
   c. imposition
   d. conflict
   Reference: p. 35
   Descriptors:

1. 03	2. 02	3. Application
4. None	5. None	6. Moderate

   Rationale: This statement is a misconception termed cultural imposition. Cultural conflict occurs when someone ridicules another's cultural beliefs.

6. A 14-year-old Bosnian refugee is attending a school dance and spending more time with her school friends than her family. She also refuses to speak her native language with her family. She is expressing
   a. cultural blindness
   b. cultural stereotyping
   c. cultural assimilation*
   d. cultural conflict
   Reference: p. 35
   Descriptors:

1. 03	2. 03	3. Application
4. II-1	5. Communication	6. Moderate

Rationale: Assimilation occurs when one's ethnic values are replaced by the values of the dominant culture.

7. A 15-year-old African American girl wears traditional African dress to her high school classes. The students at her school state this is inappropriate. The school nurse understands that the other students are displaying
   a. cultural blindness
   b. cultural stereotyping
   c. cultural assimilation
   d. cultural conflict*

   Reference: p. 35

   Descriptors:

1. 03	2. 03	3. Application
4. II-1	5. Communication	6. Moderate

   Rationale: Cultural conflict occurs when people become aware of cultural differences, feel threatened, and respond by ridiculing beliefs and traditions of others to make themselves feel more secure about their own values.

8. A 40-year-old physician wears her traditional Indian dress. A 50-year-old patient tells the nurse, "They are in America, they should dress like we do." This is an example of
   a. cultural assimilation
   b. cultural imposition*
   c. cultural blindness
   d. cultural conflict

   Reference: p. 35

   Descriptors:

1. 03	2. 03	3. Comprehensive
4. None	5. None	6. Moderate

   Rationale: Cultural imposition is the belief that everyone should conform to the majority belief system.

9. A nurse has begun practicing nursing on an Indian reservation in North Dakota. While on rounds he sees the medicine man using herbs to heal a patient. He tells the medicine man this is inappropriate. This is an example of
   a. cultural assimilation
   b. cultural conflict
   c. cultural blindness*
   d. cultural diversion

   Reference: p. 35

   Descriptors:

1. 03	2. 01	3. Comprehensive
4. None	5. None	6. Moderate

Rationale: Cultural blindness occurs when one ignores differences and proceeds as though they do not exist. This is particularly evident in the healthcare system.

10. While caring for a Hispanic patient, the nurse observes that the patient lowers his eyes while talking to the nurse. The nurse determines that this is a cultural sign of
    a. shame
    b. deference*
    c. modesty
    d. weakness

    Reference: p. 36

    Descriptors:

1. 03	2. 03	3. Application
4. II-1	5. Communication	6. Easy

    Rationale: In some cultures, such as Hispanic, the patient may show deference to the nurse who is sometimes viewed as an authority figure.

11. When completing a cultural assessment, the nurse should consider
    a. that patients may prefer a healthcare provider of a similar cultural background*
    b. knowledge of the particular language a person uses in formal conversation
    c. the type of payment plan the person will use for healthcare needs
    d. that communication will be facilitated by talking in loud, simple phrases of English

    Reference: p. 39

    Descriptors:

1. 03	2. 05	3. Application
4. II-1	5. Nursing Process	6. Moderate

    Rationale: In some cultures, gender and culture of the healthcare provider are important to the patient to establish trust. Some patients prefer someone of the same culture.

12. The home health nurse is visiting a 60-year-old female patient. During the initial visit the patient's husband answered all the questions. The nurse assesses that the
    a. patient does not want the nurse to visit
    b. patient's husband does not trust his wife to answer the questions
    c. patient is an unreliable historian
    d. patient's husband is the dominant member of the family*

Reference: p. 37

Descriptors:

1. 03	2. 05	3. Application
4. II-1	5. Communication	6. Moderate

Rationale: In many cultures, the man is the dominant figure, particularly in traditional households.

13. A 40-year-old man from Vietnam has been admitted to the medical unit after a fall at his home. The nurse should encourage his family to
    a. keep the room cool and open windows
    b. bring in fresh meats and vegetables*
    c. drink fruit beverages and soy milk
    d. pray with the patient and call the priest

Reference: p. 37

Descriptors:

1. 03	2. 05	3. Application
4. II-1	5. Caring	6. Difficult

Rationale: Health promotion activities in the Vietnamese culture include eating large amounts of fresh vegetables, fruit, fish, and meat.

14. When people of other cultures move to North America, those most likely to assimilate to the North American culture are the
    a. children*
    b. stay-at-home mothers
    c. elderly women
    d. unemployed men

Reference: p. 38

Descriptors:

1. 03	2. 05	3. Application
4. II-1	5. Cultural	6. Easy

Rationale: Children assimilate other cultures they are exposed to more readily then adults because they attend school.

15. You are a nurse in New York. You are assigned to care for a Hasidic Jewish man. The patient will be likely to
    a. speak openly about his fears
    b. require family members to hold his hand
    c. understand current healthcare practices
    d. avoid eye contact with the nurses*

Reference: p. 38

Descriptors:

1. 03	2. 04	3. Comprehensive
4. II-1	5. Cultural	6. Moderate

Rationale: Hasidic Jewish men tend to avoid direct eye contact with women.

16. The nurse has learned that Native Americans look down at the floor during conversations with authority figures. The nurse understands that the patient is
    a. listening to the conversation*
    b. uninterested in the information
    c. not understanding what is being said
    d. formulating questions to ask the nurse

Reference: p. 38

Descriptors:

1. 03	2. 04	3. Comprehensive
4. II-1	5. Cultural	6. Moderate

Rationale: Native Americans often stare at the floor during conversations, a behavior that indicates they are carefully listening.

17. The most important factor to consider when caring for patients with limited incomes is
    a. limited access to reliable transportation
    b. basic physiologic needs may go unmet*
    c. limited access to healthcare services
    d. self-actualization needs are left unmet

Reference: p. 40

Descriptors:

1. 03	2. 05	3. Knowledge
4. IV-1	5. Caring	6. Easy

Rationale: Patients with limited incomes may have to choose between food and other necessities versus healthcare. These patients may have basic needs unmet as a result of poverty.

18. Poverty can have a devastating effect on the
    a. image of the family for the future
    b. self-identity of the family with feelings of despair*
    c. self-concept of certain individual family members
    d. increase rate of bonding of family members

Reference: p. 40

Descriptors:

1. 03	2. 05	3. Knowledge
4. IV-1	5. Caring	6. Moderate

Rationale: Poverty cultures have feelings of despair and a decline in self-respect.

19. You are the nursing student caring for a 5-year-old African American patient. She has a laceration over the right eye, which requires sutures. It is important to instruct the mother that her daughter
   a. is more likely to develop an infection then a white child
   b. needs to stay home from school for 1 to 3 days.
   c. will need to be evaluated for damage to the eye
   d. is more likely to develop keloids*

   Reference: p. 41

   Descriptors:

1. 03	2. 06	3. Knowledge
4. IV-1	5. Teach/Learn	6. Moderate

   Rationale: African Americans are most likely to develop keloids; thus, it is important to instruct the patient's caregiver.

20. The transfer of energy from the healer to the patient to stimulates the patient's own healing is termed
   a. holistic health
   b. homeopathy
   c. therapeutic touch*
   d. kinesis

   Reference: p. 43

   Descriptors:

1. 03	2. 06	3. Knowledge
4. IV-1	5. Cultural	6. Easy

   Rationale: Therapeutic touch is an example of alternative therapy, which assists the patient in pain relief.

21. A nurse is caring for a Puerto Rican patient following an automobile accident. The patient is extremely anxious and displays agitated movements resembling seizure activity. The nurse should
   a. ask for a neurologic consult for the patient's abnormal behaviors
   b. stay with the patient to ensure the behaviors are culturally relevant and ensure safety*
   c. allow the patient to have privacy until the behaviors have ceased
   d. ask the patient if he normally reacts this way when he is anxious

   Reference: p. 42

   Descriptors:

1. 03	2. 06	3. Application
4. IV-1	5. Cultural	6. Difficult

   Rationale: Staying with the patient ensures the patient's safety.

22. The nurse is caring for a patient from Taiwan who has undergone abdominal surgery. When assessing a patient's pain, the nurse should
   a. realize that most individuals react to pain in a similar way
   b. use the same criteria for pain assessment for adult patients
   c. encourage a medically prescribed pain regimen
   d. respect a patient's individuality in pain responses*

   Reference: p. 42

   Descriptors:

1. 03	2. 05	3. Application
4. IV-1	5. Cultural	6. Moderate

   Rationale: All patients respond to pain in an individual manner.

23. The nurse enjoys working at the Vietnamese Clinic in the inner city. The nurse
   a. lacks the ability to care for acutely ill individuals
   b. values multicultural healthcare*
   c. is attempting to overcome stereotypes
   d. is attempting to influence patient's beliefs

   Reference: p. 43

   Descriptors:

1. 03	2. 06	3. Application
4. II-1	5. Cultural	6. Difficult

   Rationale: Nurses must value patients' cultural heritage and practices to effectively implement nursing care.

24. A 13-year-old boy has been raised in a home where the individuals are of German descent. He is currently learning health promotion practices regarding nutrition. What might he be experiencing?
   a. an ethnocentric attitude toward health promotion
   b. a cultural attitude toward holistic care
   c. a fear of past nutritional habits
   d. a cultural bind related to upbringing and future beliefs*

   Reference: p. 45

   Descriptors:

1. 03	2. 03	3. Application
4. II-1	5. Teach/Learn	6. Difficult

   Rationale: Culture has a large influence on a patient's eating habits. The ability to implement changes in those habits can be difficult for the patient, leading to conflict.

25. A couple from the Philippines emigrated to the United States a year ago. The couple is expecting their first child. In providing culturally competent care, the nurse should
    a. review his or her own cultural beliefs and biases*
    b. request the couple to use only physicians for healthcare
    c. instruct the couple about new medical practices
    d. determine the male and female gender roles of the couple

Reference: p. 45

Descriptors:

1. 03	2. 06	3. Application
4. II-1	5. Cultural	6. Moderate

Rationale: To provide culturally competent care, the nurse should first review his or her own cultural beliefs and biases.

26. Nursing considerations while caring for African American patients should include
    a. families are generally distant and nonsupportive
    b. special hair and nail care may be necessary*
    c. fad diets are a cultural norm for this group
    d. families are generally future oriented

Reference: p. 46

Descriptors:

1. 03	2. 03	3. Application
4. IV-1	5. Nursing Process	6. Moderate

Rationale: For African American patients, special hair and nail care may be necessary.

27. When caring for a Native American patient and family, the nurse needs to consider which of the following?
    a. Typically the family consists of only the parents and children.
    b. Native Americans tend to be future oriented in time.
    c. Some Native Americans use herbs for treating illnesses.*
    d. Healthcare is usually prescribed by the curandera.

Reference: p. 49

Descriptors:

1. 03	2. 03	3. Application
4. II-1	5. Cultural	6. Moderate

Rationale: Native Americans generally have extended family systems. Some Native Americans use herbal remedies for treating illnesses. The medicine man (shaman) plays an important role in healthcare.

CHAPTER 4

Health and Illness

1. Your patient is diagnosed with diabetes. He is attending classes at the university and works part-time at the university bookstore. This is an example of
   a. debilitating disease
   b. disease with limitations
   c. health not merely the absence of disease*
   d. illness requiring the evaluation of level of activity

   Reference: p. 54

   Descriptors:

   | 1. 04 | 2. 01 | 3. Application |
   | 4. III-1 | 5. Self Care | 6. Moderate |

   Rationale: According to the World Health Organization health is not merely the absence of disease.

2. A family has built a house near an old toxic waste dump. The toxic waste in the soil is an example of a/an
   a. agent*
   b. host
   c. environment
   d. pathogen

   Reference: p. 55

   Descriptors:

   | 1. 04 | 2. 01 | 3. Comprehensive |
   | 4. None | 5. None | 6. Easy |

   Rationale: An agent is an environmental stressor that must be present or absent for illness to occur. The toxic waste dump is the stressor that can cause illness.

3. Deer ticks are a known cause of Lyme disease. Ticks are an example of a/an
   a. agent*
   b. host
   c. environment
   d. risk factor

   Reference: p. 55

   Descriptors:

   | 1. 04 | 2. 01 | 3. Comprehensive |
   | 4. None | 5. None | 6. Easy |

   Rationale: An agent is an environmental stressor that must be present or absent for illness to occur. The tick carries the infection of Lyme disease to the animal or human.

4. A 4-year-old child has been diagnosed with chickenpox. The child is a/an
   a. agent
   b. host*
   c. environment
   d. risk factor

   Reference: p. 55

   Descriptors:

   | 1. 04 | 2. 01 | 3. Comprehensive |
   | 4. None | 5. None | 6. Easy |

   Rationale: The child has been infected with chickenpox. He is a living being capable of being infected by an agent.

5. It is a very hot and humid day in the city. The weather service and health department have classified it as a red day. This means it could be difficult for patients with cardiopulmonary disease. The factor having the most effect on the patients with cardiopulmonary disease is the
   a. agent
   b. host
   c. environment*
   d. disease

   Reference: p. 55

   Descriptors:

   | 1. 04 | 2. 01 | 3. Comprehensive |
   | 4. IV-1 | 5. Nursing Process | 6. Moderate |

   Rationale: All the factors external to the host that make illness more likely must be assessed and interventions implemented.

6. Health is best described as
   a. a noninvasive interaction with the environment
   b. a dynamic, ever-changing state*
   c. constant and developing
   d. static and coexistent status

Reference: p. 56

Descriptors:

1. 04	2. 01	3. Knowledge
4. None	5. None	6. Moderate

Rationale: The person must adapt to changes in the internal and external environments to maintain a state of well-being.

7. One's maximum potential for health is
   a. being part of a whole
   b. a continuum influenced by environments
   c. high-level wellness*
   d. a nonsusceptibility to disease

Reference: p. 56

Descriptors:

1. 04	2. 02	3. Knowledge
4. None	5. None	6. Moderate

Rationale: Halbert Dunn described his model of high-level wellness as functioning to one's maximum potential while maintaining balance and purposeful direction in the environment.

8. Dunn's High-Level Wellness Model encourages the nurse to
   a. place the patient in charge of his or her own care
   b. effect change in one area of the patient's physical being
   c. plan care for the patient in relation to rehabilitation
   d. care for the total person to strive to reach maximum potential*

Reference: p. 56

Descriptors:

1. 04	2. 02	3. Knowledge
4. IV-1	5. Caring	6. Moderate

Rationale: Wellness is a more active state, oriented toward maximizing the potential of the individual, regardless of his state of health.

9. A 16-year-old male patient has been admitted to the hospital following a motor vehicle accident (MVA). He is in traction for a fractured femur. The nurses encourage the patient's family to allow his high school friends to visit. The nurses are meeting the needs of the patient's
   a. emotional dimension
   b. sociocultural dimension*
   c. spiritual dimension
   d. intellectual dimension

Reference: p. 56

Descriptors:

1. 04	2. 03	3. Application
4. II-1	5. Caring	6. Easy

Rationale: Incorporating friends and family into the patient's care satisfies the sociocultural dimension of the patient's recovery.

10. An individual's belief that he or she will contract a disease is related to
    a. Dunn's High-Level Wellness Model
    b. Rosenstoch's Health Belief Model*
    c. Pender's Health Promotion Model
    d. Orem's Self Care Model

Reference: p. 56

Descriptors:

1. 04	2. 03	3. Comprehensive
4. II-1	5. Nursing Process	6. Easy

Rationale: The health belief model by Rosenstoch is concerned with what people perceive, or believe, to be true about themselves in relation to their health.

11. The primary role a nurse can play in health promotion is to
    a. educate the patient in health promotion activities
    b. exercise three times per week
    c. be a role model for health promotion*
    d. implement stress reduction activities

Reference: p. 57

Descriptors:

1. 04	2. 05	3. Application
4. I-1	5. Self Care	6. Difficult

Rationale: Through the implementation of a healthy lifestyle, the nurse can be a more effective role model to educate patients.

12. A 30-year-old patient states that consuming a low-fat diet will help to prevent heart disease. Her statement reflects
    a. an understanding of heart disease as it relates to the diet
    b. a positive outlook on life by consuming a low-fat diet
    c. a belief that there will be a positive outcome to the practice of a healthy diet*
    d. her ability to implement a heart healthy diet is an easy task to accomplish

Reference: p. 57

Descriptors:

1. 04	2. 03	3. Application
4. IV-3	5. Teach/Learn	6. Difficult

Rationale: The health-related behavior that is the outcome is initiated by a commitment to a plan of action, accompanied by the development of associated strategies to perform the valued behavior.

13. A nursing student who practices stress reduction exercises before a test is implementing practices that affect the
    a. intellectual dimension
    b. sociocultural dimension
    c. environmental dimension
    d. emotional dimension*

    Reference: p. 58
    Descriptors:

    1. 04   2. 05   3. Application
    4. IV-3   5. Self Care   6. Moderate

    Rationale: The implementation of stress reduction activities lessens the emotional response associated with a difficult task.

14. When caring for a patient who is a Jehovah's Witness, the nurse must be aware that the patient's religion prohibits the
    a. administration of blood transfusions*
    b. intake of pork products
    c. intake of meat products
    d. administration of medications

    Reference: p. 58
    Descriptors:

    1. 04   2. 05   3. Application
    4. I-1   5. Nursing Process 6. Moderate

    Rationale: The nurse must be respectful of aspects of care that influence the spiritual dimension.

15. A Roman Catholic couple requests communion to be given to them and to their hospitalized child. This is an example of which of the following needs?
    a. environmental
    b. physical
    c. psychological
    d. spiritual*

    Reference: p. 58
    Descriptors:

    1. 04   2. 03   3. Application
    4. III-1   5. Caring   6. Moderate

    Rationale: Taking communion is part of the spiritual dimension for this couple and child who are of the Roman Catholic faith.

16. An appropriate nursing diagnosis for a patient who is overweight and expressing dissatisfaction with her appearance is
    a. ineffective coping
    b. alteration in body image*
    c. spiritual distress
    d. risk for obesity

    Reference: p. 59
    Descriptors:

    1. 04   2. 03   3. Application
    4. III-1   5. Nursing Proces 6. Moderate

    Rationale: An appropriate diagnosis is Alteration in Body Image.

17. Low income families are
    a. more prone to the development of skin cancer
    b. more likely to seek health education
    c. less likely to develop disease
    d. less likely to seek medical advice*

    Reference: p. 58
    Descriptors:

    1. 04   2. 05   3. Knowledge
    4. I-1   5. Caring   6. Moderate

    Rationale: Due to the lack of financial resources patients with low income are less likely to seek medical care.

18. Rapid onset of symptoms that last a short period of time are termed
    a. risk factors
    b. acute illness*
    c. chronic illness
    d. debilitating illness

    Reference: p. 59
    Descriptors:

    1. 04   2. 04   3. Knowledge
    4. None   5. None   6. Easy

    Rationale: An acute illness generally has a rapid onset of symptoms and lasts only a relatively short time.

19. An example of an acute illness is
    a. pneumonia*
    b. hypertension
    c. diabetes mellitus
    d. arthritis

    Reference: p. 59
    Descriptors:

    1. 04   2. 04   3. Knowledge
    4. None   5. None   6. Easy

Rationale: Pneumonia is an acute illness. Hypertension, diabetes mellitus, and arthritis are chronic conditions.

20. When educating teenagers in health promotion activities, it is important to address the
    a. use of immunizations to prevent disease
    b. use of safe sex practices to prevent sexually transmitted diseases*
    c. implementation of safety in the workforce to prevent injury
    d. supplementation of calcium to prevent bone loss

    Reference: p. 59
    Descriptors:

1. 04	2. 05	3. Application
4. IV-3	5. Teach/Learn	6. Moderate

    Rationale: Implementation of health promotion activities that involve teaching must be age specific.

21. A 70-year-old woman has had reconstructive surgery of her left knee. She is unable to bear full weight on the left leg. To assist her in planning for discharge the nurse should
    a. encourage her to only use a wheelchair
    b. prepare her to transfer to a nursing home
    c. encourage her family to assist her*
    d. evaluate her incision site for drainage

    Reference: p. 60
    Descriptors:

1. 04	2. 05	3. Application
4. IV-1	5. Nursing Process	6. Difficult

    Rationale: The family's assistance in care will provide for a smoother transition to discharge and allay anxiety for the patient and family.

22. A patient who calls in to work to follow orders to remain on bedrest is in what stage of illness behavior?
    a. experiencing symptoms
    b. assuming the sick role*
    c. assuming the dependent role
    d. achieving recovery

    Reference: p. 60
    Descriptors:

1. 04	2. 05	3. Application
4. IV-3	5. Nursing Process	6. Moderate

    Rationale: Remaining on bedrest per orders is an example of the patient assuming the sick role.

23. Chronic illness differs from acute illness in that chronic illness
    a. leaves no permanent damage
    b. requires little adaptation for cure
    c. causes irreversible damage or change*
    d. lasts longer than 1 week

    Reference: p. 60
    Descriptors:

1. 04	2. 05	3. Application
4. None	5. None	6. Easy

    Rationale: Chronic illnesses cause irreversible damage or change.

24. A 25-year-old married couple have one child. He is blind in one eye, since birth. They will not allow him to play any sports activities. This is an example of
    a. overreaction
    b. overprotection*
    c. loneliness
    d. caregiving

    Reference: p. 61
    Descriptors:

1. 04	2. 03	3. Application
4. III-2	5. Caring	6. Easy

    Rationale: Parents of a sick child often react with blame, overprotection, and severe anxiety.

25. You are the school nurse at an elementary school. Which of the following is the most appropriate primary prevention program to be presented to the 9-year-old children?
    a. smoking awareness
    b. use of head protection*
    c. low-fat/calorie nutrition
    d. breast self-examination

    Reference: p. 61
    Descriptors:

1. 04	2. 06	3. Comprehensive
4. II-2	5. Teach/Learn	6. Moderate

    Rationale: Primary prevention is directed toward health promotion. Use of head protection and sports injury prevention are appropriate for this age group.

26. When the nurse treats a patient with infection, the administration of antibiotics is an example of
    a. primary prevention
    b. secondary prevention*
    c. tertiary prevention
    d. risk appraisal

    Reference: p. 61

Descriptors:

1. 04	2. 06	3. Comprehensive
4. IV-2	5. Nursing Process	6. Moderate

Rationale: Secondary prevention focuses on prompt treatment of disease, such as administration of medications.

27. A 60-year old patient is receiving physical therapy for her knee reconstruction. What level of prevention is the patient practicing?
    a. primary prevention
    b. secondary prevention
    c. tertiary prevention*
    d. illness prevention

    Reference: p. 61

    Descriptors:

1. 04	2. 06	3. Comprehensive
4. IV-3	5. Nursing Process	6. Moderate

    Rationale: The implementation of physical therapy to restore motion to the knee is an example of tertiary prevention.

28. An 80-year-old man who has difficulty ambulating due to arthritis suffers from a/an
    a. acute disease
    b. debilitating disease
    c. chronic disease*
    d. terminal disease

    Reference: p. 61

    Descriptors:

1. 04	2. 04	3. Comprehensive
4. None	5. None	6. Easy

    Rationale: Chronic illnesses, such as arthritis, have a slow onset with periods of remission and exacerbation.

29. Teaching adolescent girls about monthly breast self-examinations is an example of which type of prevention?
    a. primary*
    b. secondary
    c. tertiary
    d. restorative

    Reference: p. 60

    Descriptors:

1. 04	2. 05	3. Application
4. II-2	5 Teach/Learn	5. Moderate

    Rationale: Teaching monthly self-breast examination is considered primary prevention.

CHAPTER 5

Theoretical Base for Nursing Practice

1. The rationale for nursing actions is the nursing
   a. assessment skills
   b. process and theory
   c. knowledge base*
   d. philosophical base

   Reference: p. 66

   Descriptors:

1. 05	2. 02	3. Knowledge
4. None	5. None	6. Easy

   Rationale: The nursing body of knowledge provides the rationale for nursing actions.

2. A theory is based on
   a. conjecture
   b. proof
   c. unrelated statements
   d. fact*

   Reference: p. 66

   Descriptors:

1. 05	2. 02	3. Knowledge
4. None	5. None	6. Easy

   Rationale: A theory is a group of concepts that describe a pattern of reality.

3. Abstract impressions organized into symbols of reality are termed
   a. theories
   b. concepts*
   c. philosophies
   d. reasoning

   Reference: p. 66

   Descriptors:

1. 05	2. 02	3. Knowledge
4. None	5. None	6. Easy

   Rationale: Concepts are abstract impressions that describe objects, properties, and events and their relations to others.

4. The use of back rubs to enhance pain relief is an example of
   a. philosophy
   b. concept
   c. reasoning
   d. process*

   Reference: p. 66

   Descriptors:

1. 05	2. 02	3. Application
4. IV-1	5. Caring	6. Difficult

   Rationale: Nursing actions are intended to bring about a desired result. Back rubs are an example of a nursing process.

5. The assessment of a patient for pain and the implementation of an appropriate pain relief method is
   a. deductive reasoning*
   b. inductive reasoning
   c. evaluative care
   d. rationale

   Reference: p. 66

   Descriptors:

1. 05	2. 02	3. Application
4. IV-1	5. Nursing Process	6. Difficult

   Rationale: Deductive reasoning examines a general idea then considers specific actions or ideas. Determining the appropriate pain relief measures for the patient requires deductive reasoning.

6. The theory based on psychosocial development on the process of socialization was developed by
   a. Abraham Maslow
   b. Eric Erikson*
   c. Madeleine Leininger
   d. Ludwig von Bertalanffy

   Reference: p. 67

   Descriptors:

1. 05	2. 01	3. Knowledge
4. None	5. None	6. Easy

   Rationale: Erikson's theory emphasizes how individuals learn to interact with the world.

7. The nurse who views the family as an open system that influences and is influenced by the community is using a theoretical framework termed
   a. general systems*
   b. stress/adaptation
   c. developmental
   d. environmental
   Reference: p. 67
   Descriptors:
   1. 05   2. 01   3. Application
   4. None   5. None   6. Moderate
   Rationale: Viewing the family as an open system is an example of general systems theory.

8. Characteristics of nursing theories include
   a. narrow focus and specificity
   b. assumed definitions of concepts
   c. specially formulated technical language
   d. research generation and dissemination*
   Reference: p. 67
   Descriptors:
   1. 05   2. 02   3. Knowledge
   4. None   5. None   6. Easy
   Rationale: Research generation and dissemination are some characteristics of nursing theories.

9. The adjustment a child has to a new school is applicable to
   a. Maslow's hierarchy of needs
   b. moral development theory
   c. general systems theory
   d. adaptation theory*
   Reference: p. 67
   Descriptors:
   1. 05   2. 01   3. Comprehensive
   4. III-1 5. None   6. Moderate
   Rationale: Adaptation theory defines adaptation as the adjustment of living matter to other living thing and to environmental conditions.

10. The factor that differentiates nursing from other disciplines is the
    a. historical development
    b. nursing theory*
    c. assessment and care of the patient
    d. integration of all theories in the provision of care
    Reference: p. 67
    Descriptors:
    1. 05   2. 04   3. Comprehensive
    4. None   5. None   6. Moderate

Rationale: Nursing theory guides nurses in the provision of nursing care.

11. Nursing theory's goal is to influence the
    a. care of the future generations
    b. development of healthcare policy
    c. care of the individual, family, and community*
    d. relationship of the mind and environment
    Reference: p. 67
    Descriptors:
    1. 05   2. 04   3. Knowledge
    4. I-1   5. Nursing Process 6. Moderate
    Rationale: Nursing theories should be simple and general; simple terminology and broadly applicable concepts ensure their usefulness in a wide variety of nursing practice situations.

12. Since the establishment of nursing it has been difficult for nursing to
    a. establish a role in society
    b. establish an identity*
    c. change from care-based to research-based theory
    d. incorporate multiculturalism in care
    Reference: p. 68
    Descriptors:
    1. 05   2. 04   3. Knowledge
    4. None   5. None   6. Moderate
    Rationale: Historically nursing has had difficulty establishing itself as a profession.

13. Nightingale's influence in nursing is still felt in which of the following areas?
    a. Psychomotor skill development
    b. Differentiating nursing practice from medicine*
    c. Promotion of prescriptive privileges for nurses
    d. Promoting "common sense" to nursing care
    Reference: p. 68
    Descriptors:
    1. 05   2. 04   3. Application
    4. None   5. None   6. Moderate
    Rationale: Nightingale's influence can be felt in the area of differentiating nursing practice from medical practice and a promotion of nursing research.

14. The common components of a nursing theory are
    a. evaluation and testability
    b. definition and knowledge*
    c. cure and support
    d. training and rationales

Reference: p. 69

Descriptors:

| 1. 05 | 2. 03 | 3. Application |
| 4. None | 5. None | 6. Difficult |

Rationale: Nursing theory provides a rational knowledge base necessary for acting based on what nursing is and nurses do.

15. The practice of nursing in modern society is based on
    a. research*
    b. clinical practice
    c. evaluation
    d. the women's movement

Reference: p. 69

Descriptors:

| 1. 05 | 2. 04 | 3. Knowledge |
| 4. None | 5. None | 6. Moderate |

Rationale: Beginning in the 1950s, as great advances were made in technology and medical research, nursing leaders realized that research about the practice of nursing was necessary to meet the health needs of modern society.

16. The statement that humans are at the center of nursing's purpose describes
    a. Orem's theory
    b. Henderson's theory
    c. Roy's theory
    d. Rogers' theory*

Reference: p. 70

Descriptors:

| 1. 05 | 2. 05 | 3. Knowledge |
| 4. None | 5. None | 6. Easy |

Rationale: Martha Rogers' theory states that humans are the center of nursing's purpose.

17. A nurse who views patients as being embedded in a sociocultural environment while expressing self within those parameters is using a theory developed by
    a. Johnson
    b. Leininger*
    c. Neuman
    d. Watson

Reference: p. 70

Descriptors:

| 2. 05 | 2. 05 | 3. Knowledge |
| 4. I-1 | 5. Cultural | 6. Easy |

Rationale: Madeleine Leininger is associated with the view that patients are embedded in a

sociocultural environment while they express themselves in those parameters.

18. A nurse is doing private duty on an elderly patient. The nurse cares for the patient in his home and in the acute care setting. This continuity of care is exemplified in which nursing theory?
    a. Johnson's Behavioral Systems Theory*
    b. Imogene King's Theory of Goal Attainment
    c. Myra Levine's Four Conservative Principles Theory of Nursing
    d. Dorothea Orem's Self-Care Deficit Theory of Nursing

Reference: p. 70

Descriptors:

| 1. 05 | 2. 05 | 3.Application |
| 4. I-1 | 5. Caring | 6. Difficult |

Rationale: Dorothy Johnson believes that the care of the whole person facilitates behaviors necessary to prevent illness. Thus the implementation of the continuity of care exemplifies her theory.

19. Assisting an elderly patient in self-actualization prior to death is exemplified by
    a. Virginia Henderson's definition of nursing
    b. Sister Callista Roy's Adaptation Model
    c. Hildegard Peplau's Psychodynamic Nursing Theory
    d. Jean Watson's Philosophy and Science of Caring*

Reference: p. 70

Descriptors:

| 1. 05 | 2. 05 | 3. Application |
| 4. IV-1 | 5. Caring | 6. Moderate |

Rationale: According to Watson, caring is the mechanism by which nurses help individuals and groups reach self-actualization.

20. The nursing theory involved in the interpersonal relationship between a patient and the nursing staff to attain the patient's nursing care goals is
    a. Sister Callista Roy's Adaptation Model
    b. Imogene King's Theory of Goal Attainment*
    c. Myra Levine's Four Conservation Principles Theory of Nursing
    d. Betty Neuman's Healthcare Systems Model

Reference: p. 71

Descriptors:

| 1. 05 | 2. 05 | 3. Comprehensive |
| 4. I-1 | 5. Communication | 6. Moderate |

Rationale: Imogene King's Theory of Goal Attainment is that the focus of nursing should be on the care of humans. The nursing goal is the health of the individual and his or her constant interaction with the environment.

21. A nurse using Watson's theory when caring for a terminally ill patient would
    a. focus on self-care abilities and deficiencies
    b. assist the patient to adapt to biophysical changes
    c. provide pain and comfort measures with optimal hope*
    d. promote a sense of balance between the internal and external environment

Reference: p. 74

Descriptors:

1. 05   2. 05   3. Comprehensive
4. IV-1   5. Caring   6. Moderate

Rationale: Watson's focus is on comfort measures and instilling hope, even if the patient is terminally ill.

22. A 67-year-old patient has hemiparesis of his left side after a stroke. He is unable to perform activities of daily living. The most appropriate nursing diagnosis using Orem's theory is
    a. Knowledge Deficit related to self-care needed
    b. Anxiety related to the stroke and paralysis of his left side
    c. Self-Care Deficit: Bathing, Feeding, Hygiene related to hemiparesis*
    d. Altered Body Image related to age, immobility, and paralysis

Reference: p. 72

Descriptors:

1. 05   2. 05   3. Comprehensive
4. IV-1   5. Nursing Process 6. Moderate

Rationale: The most appropriate diagnosis using Orem's self-care theory is Self-Care Deficit: Bathing, Feeding, Hygiene related to hemiparesis.

CHAPTER 6

Value and Ethics in Nursing

1. A belief about the worth of something is termed a/an
   a. ethic
   b. value*
   c. heritage
   d. moral

   Reference: p. 78

   Descriptors:

1. 06	2. 01	3. Knowledge
4. None	5. None	6. Easy

   Rationale: Values act as a standard guide to one's behavior.

2. In provision of care the nurse must understand the principles of right and wrong. The principles of conduct are termed
   a. ethics*
   b. values
   c. morals
   d. practices

   Reference: p. 78

   Descriptors:

1. 06	2. 01	3. Knowledge
4. I-1	5. None	6. Moderate

   Rationale: Ethics guide professional practice and are principles of right and wrong to guide behavior.

3. The nurse caring for women in an abortion clinic may possess different
   a. values than an obstetrical nurse*
   b. beliefs in a higher being
   c. ethics than other nurses
   d. statutes under which she practices

   Reference: p. 78

   Descriptors:

1. 06	2. 04	3. Application
4. I-1	5. Caring	6. Difficult

   Rationale: A person's values influence beliefs about human needs, health, and illness.

4. Parents who are advancing their education will
   a. cause their children to review their goals
   b. deter their children from advancing their education
   c. model for the children the importance of education*
   d. place too much pressure on their children to advance their education

   Reference: p. 79

   Descriptors:

1. 06	2. 02	3. Application
4. None	5. None	6. Difficult

   Rationale: Children learn values by observing their parents and modeling.

5. A child repeating sayings heard from her parents is an example of what common mode of value transmission?
   a. modeling*
   b. moralizing
   c. laissez-faire
   d. responsibility

   Reference: p. 79

   Descriptors:

1. 06	2. 02	3. Application
4. II-1	5. Communication	6. Easy

   Rationale: Children often will model after their parents. This is an example of modeling.

6. When using the responsible choice mode of value transmission with adolescents, an appropriate nursing intervention would be to instruct the parents to
   a. ground the adolescent when he stays out past curfew
   b. model wearing safety belts in an automobile
   c. provide various viewpoints with discussion*
   d. enroll the adolescent in a religious-sponsored camp

   Reference: p. 79

   Descriptors:

1. 06	2. 02	3. Application
4. II-1	5. Teach/Learn	6. Moderate

Rationale: Providing various viewpoints with discussion is an example of responsible choice mode of transmitting values.

7. A prostitute is a patient on the medical division where the nurse is employed. The nurse is responsible to be
   a. laissez-faire in value transmission
   b. ethically sensitive
   c. value neutral*
   d. moralizing

   Reference: p. 79

   Descriptors:

1. 06	2. 02	3. Application
4. I-1	5. Caring	6. Difficult

   Rationale: Nurses must accept the individuality of patients and be value neutral in providing care.

8. A 50-year-old patient has recently suffered a heart attack. This event has led to him to evaluate his
   a. lifestyle behaviors*
   b. psychosocial behaviors
   c. emotional behaviors
   d. cultural behaviors

   Reference: p. 79

   Descriptors:

1. 06	2. 04	3. Application
4. IV-3	5. Nursing Process	6. Moderate

   Rationale: Values clarification is a process of discovery and allows the person to discover through feelings and analysis of behavior what choices to make when alternatives are presented.

9. Changing behaviors to practice a healthy lifestyle is an example of
   a. values neutrality
   b. ethical implementation
   c. ethical change
   d. values clarification*

   Reference: p. 79

   Descriptors:

2. 06	2. 03	3. Application
4. IV-3	5. Self Care	6. Moderate

   Rationale: Values clarification can lead to changing lifestyle behaviors with a goal toward improving health.

10. A 60-year-old patient states, "I really appreciate your teaching me about a low-fat diet and my future heart healthy lifestyle." This is an example of
    a. choosing
    b. prizing*
    c. acting
    d. evaluating

    Reference: p. 79

    Descriptors:

1. 06	2. 04	3. Application
4. IV-3	5. Teach/Learn	6. Moderate

    Rationale: Prizing is noted when patients appreciate their care and health teaching.

11. A nurse is concerned she will cause pain to her patient with severe burns. The nurse is exhibiting
    a. beneficence
    b. veracity
    c. altruism*
    d. choosing

    Reference: p. 80

    Descriptors:

1. 06	2. 08	3. Application
4. IV-1	5. Caring	6. Difficult

    Rationale: The nurse is concerned about the welfare and well- being of her patient, which is altruism.

12. After careful deliberation, a single patient decides to maintain her pregnancy and keep the baby. This is an example of which step in the value process?
    a. freely choosing from alternatives*
    b. prizing with pride and happiness
    c. acting with consistency
    d. respecting other's beliefs

    Reference: p. 80

    Descriptors:

1. 06	2. 024	3. Application
4. IV-1	5. Caring	6. Moderate

    Rationale: The patient has made a decision and is freely choosing from alternatives.

13. An adult patient with diabetes is compliant in choosing menu items within the prescribed diet plan. The patient is using which step of the values process?
    a. freely choosing from alternatives
    b. understanding the long-term consequences of noncompliance
    c. taking pride in following the diet plan for diabetes
    d. acting consistently on value of diet regimen*

Reference: p. 81

Descriptors:

1. 06	2. 04	3. Application
4. IV-3	5. Teach/Learn	6. Easy

Rationale: When the patient is compliant with the diet regimen for diabetes, the patient is acting consistently on value of diet regimen.

14. A middle-aged man with asthma feels he does not need medical treatment during an episode of symptoms. He is
    a. choosing freely*
    b. prizing with pride
    c. choosing from alternatives
    d. acting without regard to consistency
    Reference: p. 82

Descriptors:

1. 06	2. 08	3. Application
4. II-1	5. Self Care	6. Difficult

Rationale: The patient is choosing freely. It is important that the nurse understand the patient's ability to choose. It should be followed by a teaching session so the patient understands the importance of complying with treatment.

15. An example of a deontologic argument is
    a. abortion is ethically justified
    b. tube feeding a patient is extremely justified
    c. withholding care from a brain dead patient is ethically wrong
    d. abortion is ethically wrong*
    Reference: p. 82

Descriptors:

1. 06	2. 01	3. Comprehensive
4. None	5. None	6. Moderate

Rationale: The deontologic argument is that an action is right or wrong independent of its consequences.

16. A physician has ordered a barium enema for a patient who is terminally ill. The patient does not want the enema and x-ray, but will not tell the physician. The nurse informs the physician of the patient's wishes. This is an example of
    a. autonomy*
    b. fidelity
    c. nonmaleficence
    d. justice
    Reference: p. 84

Descriptors:

1. 06	2. 06	3. Comprehensive
4. IV-1	5. Caring	6. Moderate

Rationale: Autonomy is the nurses' respect for the rights of the patient.

17. The nurse decides not to administer the medication to the patient due to untoward side effects. The nurse notifies the physician. Withholding the medication is an example of
    a. nonmaleficence*
    b. deontologic
    c. justice
    d. morality
    Reference: p. 84

Descriptors:

1. 06	2. 08	3. Application
4. IV-3	5. Nursing Process	6. Moderate

Rationale: Withholding medication from a patient because of untoward side effects is an example of nonmaleficence or doing no harm.

18. When discussing the risks and benefits of a particular procedure with a patient, the nurse is guided by which of the following approaches to ethical conduct?
    a. autonomy*
    b. nonmaleficence
    c. utilitarian
    d. justice
    Reference: p. 84

Descriptors:

1. 06	2. 08	3. Application
4. None	5. None	6. Moderate

Rationale: When the nurse provides information about the risks and benefits of a particular procedure, the nurse is guided by the principle of autonomy, which respects the rights of the patient to make her own decisions related to care.

19. The provision of healthcare to all individuals is termed
    a. autonomy
    b. veracity
    c. justice*
    d. beneficence
    Reference: p. 84

Descriptors:

1. 06	2. 08	3. Comprehensive
4. None	5. None	6. Moderate

Rationale: Justice in nursing is the distribution of nursing care justly.

20. You are the only nurse available to staff the hospital's medical unit. You voice your concerns to supervisor and continue to provide care. This is an act of
    a. fidelity*
    b. justice
    c. nonmaleficence
    d. autonomy

    Reference: p. 84

    Descriptors:

1. 06	2. 08	3. Comprehensive
4. None	5. None	6. Moderate

    Rationale: Fidelity is the act of being faithful to patients entrusted in the nurse's care.

21. An appropriate nursing intervention using a care-based approach for ethical conduct is
    a. focusing care solely on the admission diagnosis
    b. providing care only to assigned patients
    c. distancing self from patients to provide objective care
    d. providing safe, holistic individualized care to each patient*

    Reference: p. 84

    Descriptors:

1. 06	2. 05	3. Application
4. IV-1	5. Caring	6. Moderate

    Rationale: A care-based approach for ethical conduct includes the provision of safe, holistic individualized care to each patient. This approach promotes the dignity and respect of all patients.

22. Which of the following is an example of nurse advocacy?
    a. following hospital rules related to patients' nutritional needs
    b. allowing a patient's underage child to visit the patient*
    c. deferring the patient's rights to medical needs
    d. refusing to relay a patient's request to the physician

    Reference: p. 85

    Descriptors:

1. 06	2. 06	3. Application
4. I-1	5. Caring	6. Moderate

    Rationale: Overlooking a hospital's policy related to visitors who are underage and allowing the child to visit the patient is an example of advocacy.

23. The primary goals and values of the profession are
    a. standards of nursing practice
    b. the patient bill of rights
    c. the state nurse practice acts
    d. nursing code of ethics*

    Reference: p. 85

    Descriptors:

1. 06	2. 09	3. Knowledge
4. None	5. None	6. Easy

    Rationale: A professional code of ethics provides a framework for making ethical decisions and sets forth professional expectations.

24. When a nurse participates in the profession's efforts to maintain high-quality nursing care, he is
    a. collaborating with other professions
    b. practicing within the code of ethics*
    c. implementing competence
    d. evaluating the care provided

    Reference: p. 86

    Descriptors:

1. 06	2. 09	3.Comprehensive
4. I-1	5. Nursing Process	6. Difficult

    Rationale: Nursing codes of ethics inform both nurses and society of the primary goals and values of the profession.

25. A nursing student leaves the patient's home with the patient's name on her school papers. The student is violating
    a. informed consent
    b. accountability
    c. confidentiality*
    d. mission statements

    Reference: p. 87

    Descriptors:

1. 06	2. 09	3. Comprehensive
4. I-1	5. Communication	6. Easy

    Rationale: When the student leaves papers around that have a patient's name on them, the student is violating confidentiality.

26. Which of the following statements reflects an ethical action by the nurse as described in the nursing code of ethics?
    a. "Did you hear about the patient's husband in room 27D?"
    b. "It's not my job to get permission for your baby to visit."
    c. "Let me see if I find a way for you to see your new grandchild."*
    d. "You know that those kind of people always act like that."

Reference: p. 87

Descriptors:

1. 06	2. 07	3. Comprehensive
4. I-1	5. Communication	6. Easy

Rationale: When the nurse says "Let me see if I find a way for you to see your new grandchild," the nurse is acting as a patient advocate, which is part of the nursing code of ethics.

27. Which of the following is an example of paternalistic behavior?
    a. telling a patient that a painful procedure will not hurt
    b. deciding to close an intensive care unit when no beds are available
    c. intercepting a visitor's gift of candy to a diabetic patient*
    d. discussing the status of a patient with the patient's roommate

Reference: pp. 87–89

Descriptors:

1. 06	2. 07	3. Comprehensive
4. I-1	5. Caring	6. Easy

Rationale: Paternalistic behavior assumes that the healthcare provider knows more about what should occur with the patient than the patient. Intercepting candy from a visitor to a diabetic patient is an example of paternalistic behavior.

28. An illiterate patient is awaiting gallbladder surgery. The nurse obtains the patient's signature on the surgical permit without verbal discussion of the risks and benefits of the procedure. This is an ethical dilemma involving
    a. confidentiality
    b. informed consent*
    c. deception
    d. nurse–patient conflict

Reference: p. 90

Descriptors:

1. 06	2. 07	3. Application
4. I-1	5. Documentation	6. Easy

Rationale: When the nurse obtains a signature from an illiterate patient without verbal discussion, the nurse is involved in an ethical dilemma related to informed consent.

29. A physician writes an order for a patient that states "Do not resuscitate." The nurse determines that this is in opposition to the patient's living will and notifies the physician who refuses to rescind the order. This is an example of
    a. deception over proposed medical regimen
    b. physician incompetence or malpractice
    c. conflict regarding the scope of nursing practice
    d. disagreement over proposed medical regimen*

Reference: p. 90

Descriptors:

1. 06	2. 07	3. Comprehensive
4. I-1	5. Caring	6. Easy

Rationale: When the physician refuses to rescind a medical order that conflicts with the patient's wishes, this is an example of disagreement over proposed medical regimen.

30. A common ethical dilemma between nurse practitioners and physicians involves conflict related to
    a. patient deception
    b. use of resources
    c. scope of nursing practice*
    d. patient confidentiality

Reference: p. 90

Descriptors:

1. 06	2. 08	3. Application
4. I-1	5. Nursing Process	6. Easy

Rationale: Nurse practitioners practice under the state's nurse practice act, yet there is often conflict related to their scope of nursing practice.

31. A nurse manager notes a discrepancy in the narcotic count at the end of the shift. The manager finds a staff nurse with the narcotic and syringe in the dressing room. The nurse asks the manager not to tell anyone about her addiction to morphine. This is an example of an ethical dilemma related to
    a. nurse malpractice on a unit
    b. claims of loyalty among colleagues*
    c. moral convictions versus practice demands
    d. professional fraud and lying

Reference: p. 91

Descriptors:

1. 06	2. 08	3. Application
4. I-1	5. Caring	6. Easy

Rationale: When the nurse asks the manager not to tell anyone of her addiction, this is an ethical dilemma related to claims of loyalty among colleagues.

32. You are the nurse who is working on a medical unit that is understaffed and you feel safe patient care is in jeopardy. After notifying your supervisor about your concerns, nothing has changed. You decide to go public with your concerns. Which of the following tactics would be appropriate?
    a. healthcare rationing
    b. patient advocacy
    c. whistle blowing*
    d. personal moral convictions

    Reference: p. 91

    Descriptors:

    1. 06   2. 09   3. Comprehensive

    4. I-1   5. Communication   6. Easy

    Rationale: Short staffing and whistle blowing are used to notify the public of the problem related to unsafe patient care.

33. The primary function of a healthcare institution's ethics committee is to
    a. enforce regulations set forth by the institution
    b. provide staff development related to ethical decisions*
    c. revoke professional licensure as appropriate by law
    d. provide legal services to staff members when needed

    Reference: p. 92

    Descriptors:

    1. 06   2. 10   3. Knowledge

    4. None   5. None   6. Moderate

    Rationale: Chief functions of ethics committees include education, policy making, case review, and consultation. Legal services are not part of the functions.

CHAPTER 7

Legal Implications of Nursing

1. To reduce the risk of a lawsuit within a nursing facility, the nurse should
   a. call the family daily with a report on the patient
   b. only have licensed staff caring for the patient
   c. develop a trusting relationship with the patient and family*
   d. answer the patient's call light immediately

   Reference: p. 96

   Descriptors:

1. 07	2. 10	3. Application
4. I-1	5. Caring	6. Easy

   Rationale: Nurses who wish to avoid legal conflicts need to develop trusting nurse–patient relationships and maintain competent practice.

2. State nurse practice acts are designed to protect the
   a. patient*
   b. nurse
   c. healthcare agency
   d. educational institution

   Reference: p. 96

   Descriptors:

1. 07	2. 04	3. Knowledge
4. None	5. None	6. Easy

   Rationale: Each state has a nurse practice act that protects the public by broadly defining the legal scope of nursing practice.

3. A nurse employed in the intensive care unit has been arrested for possession of narcotics. He is in violation of
   a. criminal law*
   b. civil law
   c. administrative law
   d. common law

   Reference: p. 96

   Descriptors:

1. 07	2. 05	3. Comprehensive
4. I-1	5. None	6. Easy

Rationale: Criminal law concerns state and federal criminal statutes, which define criminal actions such as illegal possession of drugs.

4. Nurse practice acts are an example of which type of law?
   a. constitutional
   b. statutory*
   c. administrative
   d. common

   Reference: p. 96

   Descriptors:

1. 07	2. 01	3. Knowledge
4. None	5. None	6. Easy

   Rationale: Nurse practice acts are an example of statutory law.

5. Laws governing the practice of nursing and medicine are termed
   a. public
   b. civil*
   c. constitutional
   d. statutory

   Reference: p. 96

   Descriptors:

1. 07	2. 01	3. Knowledge
4. None	5. None	6. Easy

   Rationale: Laws governing the practice of nursing and medicine are termed civil laws.

6. An example of a voluntary standard for nursing is
   a. licensure
   b. nurse practice acts
   c. state boards of nursing
   d. NLN accreditation*

   Reference: p. 98

   Descriptors:

1. 07	2. 03	3. Knowledge
4. None	5. None	6. Easy

   Rationale: An example of a voluntary standard for nursing is NLN accreditation.

7. Which of the following is necessary for a nurse to practice nursing?
   a. accreditation
   b. certification
   c. credentials
   d. licensure*

   Reference: p. 98–99

   Descriptors:

1. 07	2. 04	3. Knowledge
4. None	5. None	6. Easy

   Rationale: Licensure is required to practice nursing.

8. The most frequently seen violation of the state nurse practice acts is
   a. substance abuse*
   b. abandonment
   c. negligence
   d. assault

   Reference: p. 98

   Descriptors:

1. 07	2. 05	3. Knowledge
4. None	5. None	6. Moderate

   Rationale: Substance abuse by nurses is the most frequently noted violation of nurse practice acts.

9. A nurse was employed at a clinic in rural Montana. While working in the capacity of a staff nurse she was taking practitioner classes at the local university. Her lab jacket listed her title as nurse practitioner. The nurse is
   a. allowed to be addressed as practitioner since she is in school
   b. in violation of the Montana Nurse Practice Act*
   c. not practicing in the capacity of nurse practitioner, thus it is acceptable to wear the title
   d. allowed to wear the jacket and title until she becomes licensed

   Reference: p. 98

   Descriptors:

1. 07	2. 04	3. Application
4. None	5. None	6. Difficult

   Rationale: If a nurse does not possess the proper credentialing she is in violation of the nurse practice act.

10. Accreditation of schools of nursing is
    a. voluntary from the state governments
    b. voluntary from the National League for Nursing Accrediting Commission
    c. required by the NLNAC in order that graduates practice nursing
    d. an evaluation of the nursing program and that the program has met certain standards*

    Reference: p. 98

    Descriptors:

1.07	2. 04	3. Knowledge
4. None	5. None	6. Moderate

    Rationale: Nursing is one of the groups operating under state laws that promote the general welfare by determining minimum standards of education through accreditation of educational programs in nursing.

11. A nurse is being sued by a patient for negligence. The plaintiff in the case is the
    a. judge
    b. nurse
    c. patient*
    d. attorney

    Reference: p. 98

    Descriptors:

1. 07	2. 08	3. Knowledge
4. None	5. None	6. Easy

    Rationale: In a court of law the individual who is suing is the plaintiff.

12. Striking an out-of-control hospitalized patient is a/an
    a. intentional tort*
    b. unintentional tort
    c. act of fraud
    d. common law

    Reference: p. 99

    Descriptors:

1. 07	2. 05	3. Application
4. None	5. None	6. Moderate

    Rationale: Intentional torts for which the nurse may be held liable include assault and battery, defamation of character, invasion of privacy, false imprisonment, and fraud.

13. A signed consent form is not required for
    a. outpatient surgery
    b. blood transfusion
    c. admission to the hospital

d. an emergency that threatens life*

Reference: p. 100

Descriptors:

1. 07   2. 10   3. Knowledge

4. None   5. None   6. Moderate

Rationale: A signed consent is not needed in an emergency if there is an immediate threat to life.

14. The nurse is caring for a hospitalized patient when the nurse gives an injection to the patient after he has refused the medication. This may be considered a type of crime termed
    a. defamation
    b. negligence
    c. battery*
    d. assault

Reference: p. 100

Descriptors:

1. 07   2. 06   3. Application

4. None   5. None   6. Moderate

Rationale: When a nurse administers a medication against the patient's wishes, this may be considered battery.

15. A nurse is caring for a 45-year-old male patient. The patient is scheduled to have coronary bypass surgery in the morning. The nurse's responsibility is to
    a. explain the surgery to the patient
    b. have the patient's wife sign his operative permit
    c. witness the patient's signature when he signs the permit*
    d. explain anesthesia procedures to the patient

Reference: p. 101

Descriptors:

2. 07   2. 10   3. Application

4. I-1   5. Nursing Process   6. Moderate

Rationale: The nurse's responsibility is to witness the patient's signature on the operative permit.

16. The nurse caring for an elderly patient. Another nurse on the unit states, "She is a chronic complainer and she is addicted to morphine." The nurse could be sued for
    a. libel
    b. battery
    c. negligence
    d. slander*

Reference: p. 100

Descriptors:

1. 07   2. 07   3. Comprehensive

4. None   5. None   6. Moderate

Rationale: The nurse's statements constitute an oral defamation of character and slander.

17. A written defamation of character is termed
    a. libel*
    b. slander
    c. assault
    d. felony

Reference: p. 100

Descriptors:

1. 07   2. 07   3. Knowledge

4. None   5. None   6. Easy

Rationale: The nurse's written statements can constitute a written defamation of character.

18. An elderly patient is confused and verbally abusive. The nursing staff is fearful he will fall so they place him in restraints for 10 hours per day. This nursing action can be
    a. false imprisonment*
    b. justified for the patient's condition
    c. an applicable use of restraints
    d. deemed appropriate by the state board of nursing

Reference: p. 101

Descriptors:

1. 07   2. 06   3. Application

4. None   5. None   6. Difficult

Rationale: Unjustified retention or prevention of the movement of another person without proper consent can constitute the act of false imprisonment.

19. An appropriate nursing intervention to prevent possible invasion of a patient's privacy is for the nurse to
    a. assess the patient's verbal and written communication skills
    b. request only necessary information to provide care*
    c. promote a stress-free environment for decision making
    d. chart only objective information that has been discussed

Reference: p. 101

Descriptors:

1. 07   2. 06   3. Application

4. I-1   5. Nursing Process   6. Difficult

Rationale: The nurse should request only the necessary information to provide safe care as a way of ensuring against the patient's invasion of privacy.

20. To prevent being sued for negligence the nurse should
    a. care for patients only if adequately staffed
    b. care for patients he is most familiar with
    c. refuse to be assigned to a division he has no expertise in caring for patients
    d. accurately assess the patients assigned to his care*

    Reference: p. 102

    Descriptors:

1. 07	2. 10	3. Comprehensive
4. I-1	5. Nursing Process	6. Difficult

    Rationale: Accurate assessment of the patient is the nurse's responsibility according to the standards for nursing practice.

21. A nurse works full-time on a rehabilitation unit. He is pulled to telemetry where he does not have the advanced skills that the nurses possess on this unit. The nurse should
    a. refuse to be pulled to telemetry and go home
    b. ask to be paired with one of the experienced nurses on telemetry*
    c. ask for another assignment on a less technical floor
    d. quit and call the Joint Commission on Accreditation of Healthcare Organizations

    Reference: p. 102

    Descriptors:

1. 07	2. 10	3. Application
4. I-1	5. Caring	6. Difficult

    Rationale: It is the responsibility of the nurse to work on the unit needing help. To safeguard himself, the nurse should use help from experienced staff members.

22. Of the following examples, which possesses the most liability for nurses?
    a. An infant is left unattended with the side rail down, but no injury occurs.
    b. A mother's labor is progressing, and the nurse informs the physician of possible signs of fetal distress.
    c. Tylenol elixir is ingested by a mentally challenged patient; however, no injury is sustained.
    d. An elderly woman falls out of bed with the side rails down and fractures her left hip.*

    Reference: p. 102

    Descriptors:

1. 07	2. 07	3. Application
4. I-1	5. Nursing Process	6. Difficult

    Rationale: Malpractice exists when failure to use appropriate safety measures can be proved. This failure causes the patient to fall while attempting to get out of bed, resulting in a fractured hip.

23. When the nurse fails to raise the side rails of a crib of a toddler who is hospitalized, this could be considered what type of crime?
    a. battery
    b. fraud
    c. false imprisonment
    d. negligence*

    Reference: p. 102

    Descriptors:

1. 07	2. 06. 07	3. Application
4. I-1	5. Nursing Process	6. Easy

    Rationale: The nurse's failure to raise the side rails could be considered negligence.

24. A hospitalized patient fell and sustained injuries while the hospital bed was in the highest elevated position. The most difficult aspect of liability to prove is
    a. duty
    b. breach of duty
    c. causation*
    d. standard of care

    Reference: p. 102

    Descriptors:

1. 07	2. 06	3. Application
4. I-1	5. Nursing Process	6. Easy

    Rationale: Causation of the injury is the most difficult to prove.

25. A nurse was at the doorway of a patient and another nurse was in the room. The nurse observed the other nurse and patient fall onto the floor. Later, the nurse who was observing the event is called to testify about the events. In this situation the nurse is serving as a/an
    a. defendant
    b. fact witness*
    c. expert witness
    d. plaintiff

    Reference: p. 104

    Descriptors:

1. 07	2. 09	3. Comprehensive
4. None	5. None	6. Easy

    Rationale: The nurse who observed the incident is termed a fact witness.

26. Failure of the nurse to teach a patient information required for his care is
    a. to be documented by the next nurse caring for the patient
    b. in violation of the state nurse practice act
    c. in violation of local statute*
    d. the responsibility of the physician

    Reference: p. 105

    Descriptors:

    1. 07   2. 12   3. Comprehensive
    4. IV-3   5. Teach/Learn   6. Easy

    Rationale: Educating a patient on all aspects of the patient's care is a statute in all nurse practice acts.

27. An example of potential liability in nursing is a failure to
    a. detect a change in the patient's condition*
    b. formulate a correct nursing diagnosis
    c. be sensitive to the patient's perceived needs
    d. implement supplementary interventions

    Reference: p. 106

    Descriptors:

    1. 07   2. 07   3. Comprehensive
    4. I-1   5. Nursing Process   6. Moderate

    Rationale: Failure to detect and report a change in a patient's condition is a potential liability. Formulating a correct diagnosis, being sensitive to the patient's perceived needs, and implementing supplementary interventions are not conditions of liability.

28. Which of the following statements is legally required by a nurse who has provided patient care education?
    a. using a variety of audiovisual equipment
    b. teaching a family member along with the patient
    c. not documenting the teaching provided*
    d. using only a family member as an interpreter for the patient

    Reference: p. 105

    Descriptors:

    1. 07   2. 07   3. Comprehensive
    4. I-1   5. Documentation   6. Moderate

    Rationale: Legally, nurses are required to document any patient education provided. The nurse can use a hospital's interpreter and is not limited to the family members.

29. Verbal or telephone orders given by a physician are
    a. required to be countersigned in 24 hours*
    b. illegal in some institutions
    c. contraindicated when narcotics are ordered
    d. only appropriate when two nurses listen to the order

    Reference: p. 107

    Descriptors:

    1. 07   2. 12   3. Knowledge
    4. I-1   5. Documentation   6. Easy

    Rationale: Verbal or telephone orders should be countersigned by the physician within 24 hours.

30. The primary aim of risk management programs is to
    a. provide marginal healthcare required by law
    b. protect the family in case of early discharge
    c. provide advice to healthcare staff regarding patient care
    d. protect the patient in regard to safety and quality healthcare*

    Reference: p. 108

    Descriptors:

    1. 07   2. 10   3. Knowledge
    4. I-2   5. Nursing Process   6. Moderate

    Rationale: Elements of a risk management program are patient safety, product safety, and quality assurance.

31. A nursing student is caring for a 2-year-old child. He has just administered the wrong medication to the child. The student is
    a. not responsible; however, his nursing instructor is liable
    b. responsible for his action and is held to the same standard as a registered nurse*
    c. responsible for his action and is not held to the same standard as a registered nurse
    d. liable only if the action causes medication causes harm to the child

    Reference: p. 110

    Descriptors:

    1. 07   2. 07   3. Application
    4. IV-2   5. Nursing Process   6. Difficult

    Rationale: Nursing students are responsible for their own acts of negligence if these result in patient injury. Moreover, they are held to the same standard of care that would be used to evaluate the actions of a registered nurse.

32. A nurse practitioner is driving to work when she comes across a serious accident. According to the Good Samaritan law the nurse
    a. is liable for all her actions
    b. can be sued if the patient dies
    c. may be able to provide care without fear of being sued*
    d. is protected by the law to provide care without fear of reprisal

    Reference: p. 110

    Descriptors:

1. 07	2. 12	3. Application
4. I-2	5. Nursing Process	5. Moderate

    Rationale: Good Samaritan laws are designed to protect health practitioners when they give aid to people in emergency situations.

33. As a student nurse, you are held to the same standard of care as a/an
    a. registered nurse*
    b. staff member
    c. nursing assistant
    d. medical student

    Reference: p. 110

    Descriptors:

1. 07	2. 12	3. Knowledge
4. I-1	5. Nursing Process	6. Easy

    Rationale: Student nurses are held to the same standard of care as registered nurses; for this reason, they should carry liability insurance.

UNIT II

Promoting Health Across the Life Span

CHAPTER 8

Developmental Concepts

1. A normal phase of development involves
   a. a period of spirituality
   b. a period of disequilibrium*
   c. a state of constant adaptation
   d. major difficulties in development

   Reference: p. 118

   Descriptors:

1. 08	2. 02	3. Knowledge
4. II-1	5. Nursing Process	6. Easy

   Rationale: Each phase of development involves a time for adjustment. In phases with difficult internal and external demands, a period of disequilibrium will exist.

2. The first trend of growth and development occurs
   a. from head to toe*
   b. slowly in infancy
   c. rapidly at school age
   d. from side to side

   Reference: p. 119

   Descriptors:

1. 08	2. 02	3. Knowledge
4. II-1	5. Nursing Process	6. Easy

   Rationale: Growth and development follow regular trends. The first trend is cephalocaudal (proceeding from head to tail).

3. The public health department in the inner city has specific concerns about mental retardation in children. This concern comes from the
   a. crime in the inner city
   b. single-parent households
   c. lack of psychosocial development
   d. lead-based paint in older homes*

   Reference: p. 119

   Descriptors:

1. 08	2. 06	3. Comprehensive
4. II-4	5. Teach/Learn	6. Difficult

   Rationale: Growth and development are influenced by the environment.

4. Which of the following is not a general principle of growth and development?
   a. Children learn to walk before learning to run.
   b. Genetics determines the level of developmental maturity.*
   c. Head control occurs before hand clapping.
   d. An ill child may experience delayed puberty.

   Reference: p. 119

   Descriptors:

1. 08	2. 01, 02	3. Application
4. II-1	5. Nursing Process	6. Easy

   Rationale: Genetics does not determine the level of developmental maturity.

5. To prevent increasing rates of mental retardation in older neighborhoods it is important for the public health nurse to
   a. educate the families on signs and symptoms of mental retardation
   b. assess the children in school for disability
   c. instruct families on interventions to prevent child abuse
   d. educate family members on lead-based paint abatement*

   Reference: p. 119

   Descriptors:

1. 08	2. 06	3. Application
4. II-1	5. Teach/Learn	6. Difficult

   Rationale: Environmental changes such as lead-based paint abatement will decrease the rate of lead poisoning in areas that are at risk. Lead poisoning can lead to retardation.

6. According to Freud the pleasure-seeking instincts are defined as the
   a. id
   b. ego
   c. superego
   d. libido*

   Reference: p. 120

   Descriptors:

1. 08	2. 03	3. Knowledge
4. None	5. None	6. Easy

Rationale: Freud defined libido as the general pleasure-seeking instincts rather than purely gratification.

7. An adolescent who is actively maintaining her virginity until marriage is considered to be in which of Freud's stages of psychosocial development?
   a. conscious mind, latent stage
   b. id, latent stage
   c. ego, genital stage
   d. superego, genital stage*

   Reference: p. 120

   Descriptors:

   1. 08   2. 03   3. Comprehensive
   4. None   5. None   6. Moderate

   Rationale: An adolescent who is actively maintaining her virginity until marriage is considered to be in Freud's stage of psychosocial development termed superego, genital stage.

8. According to Freud's theory, viewing oneself as separate from others occurs at age
   a. 3 years
   b. 2 years
   c. 1 year
   d. 6 months*

   Reference: p. 120

   Descriptors:

   1. 08   2. 02   3. Knowledge
   4. II-1   5. Nursing Process   6. Easy

   Rationale: Development of the ego in the first year of life allows the infant, by 6 months of age, to view self as separate from others, according to Freud.

9. A 3-year-old child understands rules coupled with right and wrong. According to Freud, this activity is developed in the
   a. id
   b. ego
   c. superego*
   d. unconscious mind

   Reference: p. 120

   Descriptors:

   1. 08   2. 03   3. Application
   4. II-1   5. Nursing Process   6. Moderate

   Rationale: The superego represents the internalization of rules and values so that socially acceptable behavior is practiced.

10. According to Freud, gratification from sucking occurs in the
    a. oral stage (0–18 months)*
    b. anal stage (8 months–4 years)
    c. phallic stage (3–7 years)
    d. latency stage (7–12 years)

    Reference: p. 120

    Descriptors:

    1. 08   2. 03   3. Knowledge
    4. II-1   5. Nursing Process   6. Easy

    Rationale: The infant's pleasures center on gratification by using the mouth for sucking and satisfying hunger.

11. Teaching parents to interact with their children through their schoolwork and athletic games is best to assist them in what stage of development?
    a. initiative versus guilt
    b. industry versus inferiority*
    c. identity versus role confusion
    d. intimacy versus isolation

    Reference: p. 122

    Descriptors:

    1. 08   2. 03   3. Comprehensive
    4. II-1   5. Teach/Learn   6. Moderate

    Rationale: Focusing on the end result of achievements, the school-aged child gains pleasure from finishing projects and receiving recognition for accomplishments.

12. When discussing life goals a patient voices his desire to advance his standing in his church. To accomplish this goal he must devote time through hours of school and church work. He states, "I want to do this to be a role model to my children." According to Erikson, this is seen in
    a. intimacy versus isolation
    b. generativity versus stagnation*
    c. ego integrity versus despair
    d. cognitive development

    Reference: pp. 122–123

    Descriptors:

    1. 08   2. 03   3. Application
    4. II-1   5. Self Care   6. Moderate

    Rationale: The middle adult has a desire to make a contribution to the world.

13. According to Robert J. Havinghurst the development of a conscience, morality, and scale of values occurs in
    a. early childhood
    b. middle childhood*
    c. adolescence
    d. young adulthood

    Reference: p. 123

    Descriptors:

    | 1. 08 | 2. 03 | 3. Knowledge |
    | 4. II-1 | 5. Nursing Process | 6. Moderate |

    Rationale: Developing a conscience, morality, and a scale of values occurs at middle childhood.

14. The ability to apply the nursing process and critically think through patient care situations requires the nurse to be at which stage of development according to Piaget?
    a. Sensorimotor
    b. Preoperational
    c. Concrete operational
    d. Formal operational*

    Reference: p. 123

    Descriptors:

    | 1. 08 | 2. 03 | 3. Application |
    | 4. II-1 | 5. Nursing Process | 6. Moderate |

    Rationale: The ability to apply the nursing process and critically think through patient care situations requires the nurse to be at Piaget's formal operational stage of development.

15. The patient visiting the clinic has a son with a mental disability that stems back to the Vietnam War. He states, "I don't understand why he won't work. I went to the war and I always supported my family and was proud of being in the military." This statement reflects
    a. civic responsibility
    b. accommodation
    c. despair*
    d. integrity

    Reference: p. 123

    Descriptors:

    | 1. 08 | 2. 03 | 3. Application |
    | 4. II-1 | 5. Nursing Process | 6. Difficult |

    Rationale: If one believes that one's life has been a series of failures or missed directions, a sense of despair may prevail.

16. According to Piaget, the process of integrating new experiences into existing schema is termed
    a. assimilation*
    b. accommodation
    c. integrity
    d. developmental tasks

    Reference: p. 123

    Descriptors:

    | 1. 08 | 2. 03 | 3. Knowledge |
    | 4. II-1 | 5. Nursing Process | 6. Easy |

    Rationale: Assimilation is the process of integrating new experiences into existing schemata.

17. A perception of goodness or badness occurs at which stage of Kohlberg's moral development theory?
    a. preconventional level*
    b. instrumental relativist orientation
    c. conventional level
    d. postconventional level

    Reference: p. 124

    Descriptors:

    | 1. 08 | 2. 03 | 3. Knowledge |
    | 4. II-1 | 5. Nursing Process | 6. Moderate |

    Rationale: The motivation for choices of action is fear of physical consequences of authority's disapproval. As a result of the consequences, a perception of goodness or badness develops.

18. Nursing's code of ethics requires nurses to provide holistic healthcare for all patients. This is an example of which of the following stages of Kohlberg and Gilligan's moral development theory?
    a. social contract, utilitarian
    b. universal ethical principle*
    c. law and order
    d. instrumental relativist

    Reference: p. 124

    Descriptors:

    | 1. 08 | 2. 03 | 3. Application |
    | 4. II-1 | 5. Caring | 6. Moderate |

    Rationale: Providing holistic care is an example of Kohlberg and Gilligan's universal ethical principle.

19. Adults who think abstractly and feel as though they are contributors to society, have entered Kohlberg's
    a. stage 3: good boy–good girl orientation
    b. stage 4: law and order*
    c. stage 5: social contract–utilitarian orientation
    d. stage 6: universal ethical principle orientation

    Reference: p. 124

    Descriptors:

    1. 08   2. 03   3. Knowledge
    4. II-1   5. Nursing Process 6. Moderate

    Rationale: Behavior follows social or religious rules from a respect for authority. Adults at this stage think abstractly and view themselves as members of society.

20. Gilligan's feminist theory of moral development is in agreement with nursing philosophy because it provides for
    a. creation of equal rights for all
    b. promotion of social norms
    c. an ethic of care*
    d. internal sense of justice for society

    Reference: p. 125

    Descriptors:

    1. 08   2. 03   3. Knowledge
    4. II-1   5. Nursing Process 6. Moderate

    Rationale: Gilligan's feminist theory provides for an ethic of care that is basic to nursing's philosophy.

21. A theory that states females are more likely to see moral requirements emerging from needs of others is
    a. Kohlberg's Moral Development Theory
    b. James Fowler's Faith Development Theory
    c. Carol Gilligan's Moral Development Theory*
    d. Jean Piaget's Cognitive Development Theory

    Reference: p. 125

    Descriptors:

    1. 08   2. 03   3. Knowledge
    4. II-1   5. Caring   6. Easy

    Rationale: Gilligan's theory views females as developing a morality of response and care and males as developing a morality of justice.

22. A young woman tells the school nurse, "I am a loner. I prefer to be by myself." This statement reflects
    a. Kohlberg's instrumental relativist orientation
    b. Kohlberg's social contract, Utilitarian orientation
    c. Gilligan's level 1: selfishness*
    d. Gilligan's level 3: nonviolence

    Reference: p. 125

    Descriptors:

    1. 08   2. 03   3. Comprehensive
    4. II-1   5. Self Care   6. Moderate

    Rationale: Level 1 is selfishness. The focus is on one's own needs. Relationships are often disappointing, and as a result, a woman may isolate herself to avoid getting hurt.

23. A 14-year-old girl has written an eloquent essay against abortion. According to James Fowler's theory, she is in which stage of faith development?
    a. intuitive-projective faith
    b. mystical-literal faith
    c. synthetic-conventional faith
    d. individuative-reflective faith*

    Reference: p. 125

    Descriptors:

    1. 08   2. 03   3. Comprehensive
    4. II-1   5. Nursing Process 6. Difficult

    Rationale: Individuative-reflective faith is a crucial time for older adolescents and young adults because they become responsible for their own commitments, beliefs, and attitudes.

24. To promote health in the adolescent population the most appropriate education program for all adolescents would be
    a. safe sex practices*
    b. stress reduction
    c. prevention of osteoporosis
    d. iron-rich foods

    Reference: p. 126

    Descriptors:

    1. 08   2. 04   3. Application
    4. II-1   5. Teach/Learn 6. Moderate

    Rationale: Pregnancy and parenthood in adolescent girls continues to be a concern. Adolescents must be educated on the risk of unsafe sex practices.

25. Two preadolescent boys are best friends. One is 6 feet, 4 inches tall and weighs 142 pounds. The other is 4 feet, 10 inches tall and weighs 90 pounds. The smaller of the two boys feels "scrawny" next to his friend. Which developmental crisis needs to be mastered by the smaller boy?
   a. mistrust
   b. isolation
   c. role confusion
   d. inferiority*

Reference: p. 122
Descriptors:
1. 08   2. 03   3. Application
4. II-1   5. Nursing Process   6. Moderate
Rationale: The smaller boy must master feelings of inferiority.

CHAPTER 9

Conception Through Young Adult

1. A patient has been admitted to the emergency room following a motor vehicle accident. The patient is 6 months pregnant with her first child. She states, "I have had one drink per day, usually beer." The most appropriate question to ask her is
   a. "Did you drink before you became pregnant?"
   b. "Has anyone ever told you what effect alcoholic beverages have on your unborn baby?"*
   c. "Do you experience emotional problems that cause you to drink while you are pregnant?"
   d. "Do you drink any other alcoholic beverage or just beer?"

   Reference: p. 132

   Descriptors:

1. 09	2. 02	3. Application
4. II-1	5. Caring	6. Difficult

   Rationale: Human growth and development begins at the moment of fertilization. Environment and nutrition influence all stages of development.

2. During which prenatal time period is the unborn at greatest risk for anomalies due to teratogenic exposure?
   a. conception
   b. preembryonic*
   c. embryonic
   d. zygote

   Reference: p. 133

   Descriptors:

1. 09	2. 02	3. Knowledge
4. II-1	5. Nursing Process	6. Easy

   Rationale: The prenatal time period when the unborn is at greatest risk for anomalies due to teratogenic exposure is the preembryonic stage.

3. When caring for a pregnant woman it is important to teach her to increase her consumption of calcium-containing products during the
   a. preembryonic stage
   b. ectoderm stage
   c. embyronic stage
   d. fetal stage*

   Reference: p. 133

   Descriptors:

1. 09	2. 02	3. Application
4. II-1	5. Teach/Learn	6. Difficult

   Rationale: Fetal stage lasts from 9 weeks to birth. All body organs and systems continue to grow and develop.

4. Assessment of an infant at birth is made with the use of
   a. Denver Developmental Screening Test
   b. Apgar Rating Scale*
   c. Glasgow Scale
   d. Reflex Rating Scale

   Reference: p. 133

   Descriptors:

1. 09	2. 01	3. Knowledge
4. II-1	5. Nursing Process	6. Easy

   Rationale: At birth the infant is assessed and assigned an Apgar score. This score indicates the baby's physical condition with 10 being the highest score.

5. The neonate inherits
   a. no immunity from the mother
   b. active immunity from the mother
   c. transient immunity from the mother*
   d. humoral immunity from the mother

   Reference: p. 133

   Descriptors:

1. 09	2. 01	3. Knowledge
4. II-1	5. Nursing Process	6. Easy

   Rationale: The neonate inherits a transient immunity from infections as a result of immunoglobulins that cross the placenta.

6. The nurse caring for a newborn infant following delivery by cesarean section should assess the newborn for
   a. decreased heart rate
   b. excessive crying
   c. excessive sleeping
   d. increased secretions*

   Reference: p. 134

Descriptors:

1. 09	2. 04	3. Application
4. II-1	5. Nursing Process	6. Moderate

Rationale: Neonates delivered by cesarean birth are at risk for respiratory difficulties because of excess mucus in the lungs, often requiring frequent suctioning.

7. Following delivery an infant has edema of the scalp. This is referred to as
   a. a brain injury
   b. subchondral edema
   c. hydrocephalus
   d. caput succedaneum*

Reference: p. 134

Descriptors:

1. 09	2. 03	3. Comprehensive
4. II-1	5. Nursing Process	6. Easy

Rationale: Caput succedaneum is a birth trauma that causes temporary symptoms and parents need to be reassured.

8. The home health nurse visiting a newborn and his family must assess for a common condition that is seen a few days after birth. This condition is
   a. colic
   b. jaundice*
   c. hypospadias
   d. cleft palate

Reference: p. 134

Descriptors:

1. 09	2. 03	3. Comprehensive
4. II-1	5. Nursing Process	6. Moderate

Rationale: The nonthreatening nature of physiologic jaundice, which commonly occurs in the neonate's first days, should be explained to parents.

9. Which of the following is most immediately life-threatening to a neonate?
   a. Apgar score of 3*
   b. physiologic jaundice
   c. molding of the skull
   d. cyanosis of the hands

Reference: pp. 133–134

Descriptors:

1. 09	2. 03	3. Comprehensive
4. II-1	5. Nursing Process	6. Moderate

Rationale: An Apgar score of 3 indicates severe neonatal distress and can be life-threatening if treatment is not instituted.

10. A infant's mother asks the home health nurse, "Why he is so yellow?" The nurse's best response is
    a. "That is a normal occurrence in newborns due to the bilirubin in the blood."*
    b. "This condition is indicative of increased red blood cells due to incompatibility."
    c. "Liver damage is very rare, but could be a serious condition so that he will need to be hospitalized."
    d. "Your baby cannot breakdown bilirubin so the liver is atrophying."

Reference: p. 134

Descriptors:

1. 09	2. 03	3. Application
4. II-1	5. Teach/Learn	6. Difficult

Rationale: The nonthreatening nature of physiologic jaundice, which commonly occurs in the neonate's first days because of excess bilirubin, should be explained to parents.

11. Long-term growth and development effects are most likely to occur in a neonate affected with
    a. caput succedaneum
    b. subconjunctival hemorrhage
    c. physiologic jaundice
    d. fetal alcohol syndrome*

Reference: p. 134

Descriptors:

1. 09	2. 03	3. Knowledge
4. II-1	5. Nursing Process	6. Moderate

Rationale: Fetal alcohol syndrome causes long-term detrimental effects in the newborn.

12. A patient is 3 months pregnant and smokes cigarettes. What will the nurse teach her about cigarette smoking?
    a. Cigarette smoking can be fatal to the baby.
    b. Cigarette smoking causes low birthweight.*
    c. Cigarette smoking causes fetal lung cancer.
    d. Cigarette smoking increases fetal blood flow.

Reference: p. 134

Descriptors:

1. 09	2. 03	3. Knowledge
4. II-1	5. Teach/Learn	6. Moderate

Rationale: Cigarette smoking causes low-birthweight infants; thus, expectant mothers should be informed.

13. On delivery of a 6 pound 3 ounce baby girl, the nurse assesses jittering of the baby's body. The nurse suspects
    a. she has a birth defect
    b. she is cold and clammy
    c. she is a crack cocaine baby*
    d. her mother abused alcohol

    Reference: p. 134

    Descriptors:

1. 09	2. 03	3. Application
4. II-1	5. Nursing Process	6. Difficult

    Rationale: Crack cocaine babies are jittery, hypersensitive to noise, and intolerant of cuddling, and feed poorly.

14. At birth an infant is 6 pounds 3 ounces. The baby should weigh
    a. 12 pounds, 6 ounces by her first birthday
    b. 14 pounds by her first birthday
    c. 18 pounds, 9 ounces by her first birthday*
    d. 24 pounds, 4 ounces by her first birthday

    Reference: p. 135

    Descriptors:

1. 09	2. 02	3. Comprehensive
4. II-1	5. Nursing Process	6. Moderate

    Rationale: Infants triple their birthweight by the first birthday.

15. A mother's or father's emotional linkage to their baby is called
    a. attachment
    b. relationship
    c. bonding*
    d. love

    Reference: p. 136

    Descriptors:

1. 09	2. 01	3. Knowledge
4. II-1	5. Caring	6. Moderate

    Rationale: Bonding occurs after birth and is necessary for attachment.

16. An expensive way to assess an infant's or child's development is with the
    a. Denver Developmental Screening Test*
    b. Apgar Rating Scale
    c. Glasgow Scale
    d. Reflex Rating Scale

    Reference: p. 135

    Descriptors:

1. 09	2. 03	3. Knowledge
4. II-1	5. Nursing Process	6. Moderate

Rationale: The Denver Developmental Screening Test is commonly used to determine quickly and inexpensively atypical developmental patterns in infants and children.

17. A mother brings her 2-month-old infant into the clinic for a checkup. She asks, "Why is my baby a restless sleeper and she only takes 3 to 4 ounces of formula every 2 hours?" The nurse's best explanation is
    a. "All babies' temperaments are different and she will probably change soon."
    b. "Some babies are easier to deal with in regards to eating, but others require additional time."
    c. "Your child may have an uneasy temperament and be sensitive to noise."*
    d. "Your child is probably passive and distant and will be difficult to raise."

    Reference: p. 136

    Descriptors:

1. 09	2. 03	3. Application
4. II-1	5. Teach/Learn	6. Difficult

    Rationale: The difficult infant has a volatile and labile response. They are restless sleepers, eat poorly, and are sensitive to noise.

18. To prevent sudden infant death syndrome (SIDS), nurses should teach parents to position the infant
    a. in a pumpkin seat to sleep
    b. on her back to sleep*
    c. in a bassinet to age 6 months
    c. on her abdomen to sleep

    Reference: p. 137

    Descriptors:

1. 09	2. 04	3. Knowledge
4. II-1	5. Teach/Learn	6. Easy

    Rationale: Because sleep habits have been implicated with SIDS, it is recommended that infants up to the age of 6 months sleep on their side or back.

19. A 2-month-old infant is diagnosed with colic. His mother is concerned about his development. The most appropriate response to her concern is
    a. babies often gain weight more slowly with colic
    b. babies gain weight appropriately for their age*
    c. babies with colic are prone to failure to thrive
    d. babies with colic often develop with delays

    Reference: p. 136

    Descriptors:

1. 09	2. 03	3. Application
4. II-1	5.Teach/Learn	6. Moderate

Rationale: Despite the symptoms of colic, babies develop normally.

20. The home health nurse is visiting a patient. During the visit the nurse suspects another family member is abusing a baby in the home. The nurse's legal responsibility is to
    a. report it to the authorities*
    b. call the nursing supervisor
    c. report it to the physician
    d. educate on parenting skills

    Reference: p. 137

    Descriptors:

    1. 09   2. 04   3. Comprehensive
    4. II-1   5. Caring 6. Moderate

    Rationale: Healthcare workers have a legal obligation to report suspected maltreatment.

21. Parents who have infants in day-care centers can anticipate behaviors such as
    a. withdrawal without difficulty in early infancy
    b. crying with separation in early infancy
    c. crying with separation in late infancy*
    d. fear as a result of the day-care center

    Reference: p. 137

    Descriptors:

    1. 09   2. 02   3. Application
    4. II-1   5. Nursing Process 6. Moderate

    Rationale: In late infancy behaviors of separation anxiety are common.

22. Teaching a mother parenting skills that help to deter child abuse is an example of
    a. illness prevention
    b. primary prevention*
    c. secondary prevention
    d. tertiary prevention

    Reference: p. 137

    Descriptors:

    1. 09   2. 04   3. Comprehensive
    4. II-1   5. Teach/Learn 6. Moderate

    Rationale: Education provided to the patient is primary prevention.

23. Appropriate toys for toddlers typically include
    a. pull toys and tricycles*
    b. drinking glasses and party items
    c. car seats and bicycles
    d. hard candies and board games

    Reference: p. 138

    Descriptors:

    1. 09   2. 04   3. Application
    4. II-1   5. Nursing Process 6. Easy

    Rationale: Pull toys and tricycles are appropriate toys for toddlers.

24. A 3-year-old boy has been toilet trained for 2 months. Last week his newborn brother came home from the hospital. He now has been wetting the bed and having elimination accidents. The best explanation for this is that he is
    a. saying "no" through negativism
    b. expressing stress through regression*
    c. having anxiety attacks over the new baby
    d. experiencing a medical abnormality

    Reference: p. 139

    Descriptors:

    1. 09   2. 03   3. Application
    4. II-1   5. Nursing Process 6. Moderate

    Rationale: Regression, or behavior that is more characteristic of a younger age, can occur at any time in response to stressful circumstances.

25. When interviewing a child's mother the nurse determines that she is putting the child to bed with a bottle. What intervention would be most appropriate?
    a. The nurse should instruct the mother to change formula due to possible gastrointestinal upset.
    b. The nurse should give the mother new angled bottles.
    c. The nurse should instruct the mother on the development of dental caries.*
    d. The nurse should provide the mother information on dietary sugar.

    Reference: p. 139

    Descriptors:

    1. 09   2. 04   3. Application
    4. II-1   5. Teach/Learn 6. Difficult

    Rationale: Dental problems occur when children are sucking on sweetened milk.

26. Appropriate teaching principles to discuss with parents of toddlers include
    a. providing rationale to a toddler when discipline is needed
    b. discipline is necessary when the toddler cries at bedtime
    c. safe placement of household cleaning agents*
    d. hard candies and sweets will calm a crying child

    Reference: p. 139

    Descriptors:

1. 09	2. 03, 04	3. Application
4. II-1	5. Teach/Learn	6. Moderate

    Rationale: Accidents including poisonings are a major cause of death in toddlers.

27. When educating parents of preschoolers on development the nurse should inform them that
    a. play is more related to fantasy and is not related to fact
    b. the preschooler is very fearful of activities and people
    c. the preschooler thinks logically with a concept of weight
    d. the preschooler increases socialization with other children*

    Reference: p. 140

    Descriptors:

1. 09	2. 02	3. Knowledge
4. II-1	5. Teach/Learn	6. Moderate

    Rationale: Socialization increases with preschoolers.

28. Preschoolers learn sex differences and modesty. This factor is described in
    a. Freud's theory
    b. Erikson's theory
    c. Piaget's theory
    d. Havinghurst's theory*

    Reference: p. 141

    Descriptors:

1. 09	2. 02	3. Knowledge
4. II-1	5. Nursing Process	6. Easy

    Rationale: Havinghurst's theory states preschoolers learn sex differences and modesty.

29. The nursing education director at the outpatient surgical center is developing a program for preschoolers. What would be the best education program for preschoolers?
    a. a video series of the operating room experience
    b. pamphlets and books that describe the experience
    c. the use of puppets with the surgical equipment*
    d. education for the parents to teach the children

    Reference: p. 142

    Descriptors:

1. 09	2. 04	3. Application
4. II-1	5. Teach/Learn	6. Difficult

    Rationale: A hands-on education experience is more easily understood for preschoolers.

30. A father is concerned about his preschooler's inability to fall asleep. It is important to explain to the father about the
    a. limitation of fluids after 7:00 PM
    b. importance of bedtime rituals*
    c. use of a pacifier as security
    d. practice of sleeping with the parent is important

    Reference: p. 143

    Descriptors:

1. 09	2. 04	3. Comprehensive
4. II-1	5. Teach/Learn	6. Easy

    Rationale: The implementation of bedtime rituals with children enhances sleep.

31. The brain of a school-aged child is
    a. growing rapidly
    b. 50% of adult size
    c. 90% of adult size*
    d. the same as an adult

    Reference: p. 143

    Descriptors:

1. 09	2. 02	3. Knowledge
4. None	5. None	6. Easy

    Rationale: The brain of the school-aged child is 90% of adult size.

32. A school-aged child frequently voices
    a. anxiety over independence
    b. positive self-esteem regarding useful skills*
    c. understanding of being separate from others
    d. ability to express self verbally

    Reference: p. 144

    Descriptors:

1. 09	2. 02	3. Comprehensive
4. II-1	5. Nursing Process	6. Moderate

Rationale: The school-aged child is focused on learning new skills and developing a positive self-esteem.

33. A 7-year-old boy is having trouble listening in school and moves around the room indiscriminately. The school nurse and teacher suspect that he is
    a. under pressure from the parents and acting out
    b. bored with school and he knows the material
    c. displaying symptoms of attention deficit/hyperactivity disorder (ADHD)*
    d. presenting with an anxiety disorder

    Reference: p. 145

    Descriptors:

    1. 09   2. 03   3. Application
    4. II-1   5. Nursing Process   6. Moderate

    Rationale: ADHD is a developmentally inappropriate degree of inattention, impulsiveness, and hyperactivity.

34. The adolescent is in the stage of
    a. protest and despair
    b. egocentrism
    c. emotional maturity
    d. formal operation*

    Reference: p. 146

    Descriptors:

    1. 09   2. 02   3. Knowledge
    4. II-1   5. Nursing Process   6. Easy

    Rationale: According to Piaget, adolescence is the stage when the cognitive development of formal operations is developed.

35. The school nurse observes that one group of teenage girls has rejected the permissive behavior of another group of girls. This is noted in adolescence as
    a. development of moral values*
    b. jealous among adolescent girls
    c. each group's lack of self-esteem
    d. emotional instability of girls

    Reference: p. 146

    Descriptors:

    1. 09   2. 02   3. Comprehensive
    4. II-1   5. Nursing Process   6. Moderate

    Rationale: Self-concept is being stabilized, with peer group acting as the greatest influence.

36. Adolescents begin to determine
    a. care of parents
    b. emotional stability
    c. choice of profession*
    d. relationship with same sex

    Reference: p. 147

    Descriptors:

    1. 09   2. 02   3. Knowledge
    4. II-1   5. Nursing Process   6. Easy

    Rationale: Adolescence is the time when career choices are being considered.

37. Educating adolescents on safe sex is an example of
    a. primary prevention*
    b. secondary prevention
    c. tertiary prevention
    d. risk assessment

    Reference: p. 148

    Descriptors:

    1. 09   2. 04   3. Comprehensive
    4. II-1   5. Teach/Learn   6. Easy

    Rationale: Health education is primary prevention.

38. What is the most appropriate nursing diagnosis for a young woman who has fear and obsession over being overweight?
    a. Risk of Injury related to purging.
    b. Anxiety related to fear of obesity.*
    c. Altered Nutrition: More than Body Requirements related to overeating.
    d. Social Isolation related to inability to be popular.

    Reference: p. 149

    Descriptors:

    1. 09   2. 03   3. Application
    4. II-1   5. Nursing Process   6. Difficult

    Rationale: The fear she has indicated is an actual health problem, which produces anxiety.

39. In the United States suicide is the third leading cause of death for adolescents. Of the following which is true regarding suicide in the adolescent population?
    a. The occurrence of suicide is the same for men and women.
    b. The occurrence of suicide is more likely in women.
    c. The occurrence of suicide attempts is greater in women.*
    d. The suicide rates are higher in women than men.

Reference: p. 150

Descriptors:

| 1. 09 | 2. 03 | 3. Knowledge |
| 4. II-4 | 5. Nursing Process | 6. Moderate |

Rationale: The occurrence of suicide attempts is greater in women. The understanding of this phenomenon can assist nurses in their assessment of women for injury.

40. The school nurse and high school counselor are planning a program to promote psychosocial health and build relationships in adolescents. It is important that the program include
    a. nutritional health
    b. communication techniques*
    c. therapeutic touch
    d. study skills

Reference: p. 150

Descriptors:

| 1. 09 | 2. 04 | 3. Comprehensive |
| 4. III-1 | 5. Communication | 6. Moderate |

Rationale: Education on communication builds psychosocial development and strengthens relationships.

41. By teaching parents to communicate with their teenagers the nurse will help parents build
    a. school performance in teens
    b. self-esteem in teens*
    c. role development in teens
    d. psychosexual development

Reference: p. 151

Descriptors:

| 1. 09 | 2. 04 | 3. Comprehensive |
| 4. II-1 | 5. Teach/Learn | 6. Difficult |

Rationale: Teaching communication techniques with parents will help to build the self-esteem of the teen.

CHAPTER 10

The Aging Adult

1. The development of osteoarthritis and its effect on joints can be described by the
   a. genetic theory
   b. wear-and-tear theory*
   c. immunity theory
   d. free radical theory

   Reference: p. 154

   Descriptors:

   1. 10   2. 03   3. Application

   4. None   5. None   6. Moderate

   Rationale: According to the wear-and-tear theory, organisms wear out. The development of osteoarthritis occurs due to the wear and tear on the joints.

2. The development of cancer in older individuals can be associated with information in the
   a. genetic theory
   b. wear-and-tear theory
   c. immunity theory*
   d. free radical theory

   Reference: p. 154

   Descriptors:

   1. 10   2. 03   3. Application

   4. None   5. None   6. Moderate

   Rationale: The immune system declines steadily after young adulthood, and rates of cancer increases in adults.

3. Middle-aged adults are known to
   a. plan goals in their lives
   b. evaluate goal achievement*
   c. review their life's accomplishments
   d. change their long-term relationships

   Reference: p. 154

   Descriptors:

   1. 10   2. 02   3. Application

   4. II-1   5. Nursing Process   6. Moderate

   Rationale: The aging of parents causes the middle adult to evaluate one's achievements.

4. A gradual decrease in ovarian function in adult women is
   a. prepuce
   b. prepubescent
   c. andropause
   d. menopause*

   Reference: p. 155

   Descriptors:

   1. 10   2. 02   3. Knowledge

   4. II-1   5. Nursing Process   6. Easy

   Rationale: Nurses need to be aware of the physiologic process of menopause and its effect on the care provided.

5. A patient's family member states, "Well, when I get older I hope I am able to care for myself. If I have to die, I hope I just have a heart attack and be gone." This statement reflects
   a. Piaget's Theory of Development
   b. Erikson's Theory of Development*
   c. Fowler's Faith Development Theory
   d. Gilligan's Theory of Development

   Reference: p. 155

   Descriptors:

   1. 10   2. 02   3. Comprehensive

   4. II-1   5. Nursing Process   6. Moderate

   Rationale: According to Erikson, adults who do not achieve the tasks of middle adulthood will focus on themselves, becoming overly concerned about their own emotional and physical health needs (integrity vs. despair).

6. A 42-year-old male patient states to you, "I am so confused. I don't know how to balance care of my children and my ill parents." The patient is experiencing
   a. the empty nest syndrome
   b. a midlife crisis
   c. dissemination syndrome
   d. the sandwich generation*

Reference: p. 155

Descriptors:

1. 10   2. 02   3. Comprehensive

4. II-1   5. Nursing Process   6. Moderate

Rationale: Caring for aging parents and growing children is described as the sandwich generation. Middle adults faced with this situation often express feelings of powerlessness.

7. The loss of a spouse during middle adulthood is a threat to
   a. self-concept*
   b. body image
   c. role overload
   d. goal achievement

Reference: p. 156

Descriptors:

1. 10   2. 02   3. Comprehensive

4. II-1   5. Nursing Process   6. Moderate

Rationale: The loss of a spouse is a major crisis and threat to one's self-concept.

8. Weight gain during middle adulthood is a result of
   a. increased caloric intake
   b. less physical activity*
   c. increased time alone
   d. decreased hormone function

Reference: p. 157

Descriptors:

1. 10   2. 04   3. Comprehensive

4. II-1   5. Nursing Process   6. Easy

Rationale: Middle adults tend to maintain previous eating habits and caloric intake while being less physically active.

9. By age 40 it is recommended that individuals have a/an
   a. digital examination for rectal cancer
   b. prostate-specific antigen test for prostate cancer
   c. colonoscopy for polyps
   d. eye examination for glaucoma*

Reference: p. 157

Descriptors:

1. 10   2. 06   3. Knowledge

4. II-2   5. Nursing Process   6. Moderate

Rationale: Middle adults should have an eye examination every 1 to 2 years with a test for glaucoma.

10. A developmental task for a 45-year-old patient is the
    a. development of a sense of independence
    b. acceptance of wrinkles and gray hair*
    c. establishment of a personal philosophy
    d. establishment of peer and intimate relationships

Reference: p. 155

Descriptors:

1. 10   2. 02   3. Knowledge

4. II-1   5. Nursing Process   6. Moderate

Rationale: For a 45-year-old patient, a developmental task is the acceptance of aging, which includes wrinkles and gray hair.

11. A moderately obese 48-year-old patient is seen in the ambulatory care clinic complaining of chest pain. He states, "My father died at age 50 of a heart attack." There is no evidence of the patient suffering a heart attack. Prior to discharge, the nurse should instruct the patient that he should
    a. change occupations
    b. attend psychotherapy sessions
    c. switch to a low-fat diet*
    d. practice hyperventilation

Reference: p. 157

Descriptors:

1. 10   2. 06   3. Application

4. II-2   5. Teach/Learn   6. Moderate

Rationale: Due to the genetic factors the patient should be educated on a low-fat diet to prevent heart disease.

12. The scientific and behavioral study of all aspects of aging is termed
    a. gynecology
    b. oncology
    c. gerontology*
    d. radiology

Reference: p. 158

Descriptors:

1. 10   2. 01   3. Knowledge

4. None   5. None   6. Easy

Rationale: Gerontology is the study of aging.

13. Truth about the aging process includes which statement?
    a. Older men outnumber older women.
    b. Aging is an individual experience.*
    c. Few "old-old" require healthcare assistance.
    d. Over 50% of those over 60 live in assisted housing.

Reference: p. 158

Descriptors:

| 1. 10 | 2. 02 | 3. Knowledge |
| 4. None | 5. None | 6. Moderate |

Rationale: Women outnumber men in old age. Aging is an individual experience and health status and functioning depend on many factors.

14. Many elderly feel isolated. This is usually related to
    a. death of loved ones*
    b. lack of faith in God
    c. societal changes
    d. decreased income

Reference: p. 159

Descriptors:

| 1. 10 | 2. 02 | 3. Comprehensive |
| 4. II-1 | 5. Nursing Process | 6. Moderate |

Rationale: Loneliness results from death of loved ones or other losses.

15. A 78-year-old patient complains of shortness of breath, rapid heart rate, and swelling of his feet. These physiologic symptoms are related to aging
    a. blood vessels
    b. liver metabolism
    c. heart muscles*
    d. lung tissue

Reference: p. 159

Descriptors:

| 1. 10 | 2. 04 | 3. Application |
| 4. II-1 | 5. Nursing Process | 6. Moderate |

Rationale: Aging heart muscles cause fluid retention and shortness of breath.

16. The skin in the elderly is very fragile. This is due to
    a. loss of elasticity*
    b. edema of tissues
    c. decreased blood flow
    d. lack of vitamin E

Reference: p. 160

Descriptors:

| 1. 10 | 2. 04 | 3. Application |
| 4. II-1 | 5. Nursing Process | 6. Easy |

Rationale: Wrinkling and sagging of skin occur with decreased skin elasticity; dryness and scaling are common. Loss of elasticity leads to skin tears and ulcerations.

17. Musculoskeletal changes noted in the older adult include
    a. increased activity
    b. night pain
    c. moderate strength
    d. stiff joints*

Reference: p. 160

Descriptors:

| 1. 10 | 2. 04 | 3. Knowledge |
| 4. II-1 | 5. Nursing Process | 6. Easy |

Rationale: Joints in elderly patients stiffen and lose flexibility and motion.

18. Older individuals often experience presbycusis. The nurse should
    a. communicate with the patient by writing
    b. speak to the patient in a high-pitched tone
    c. speak to the patient in a low-pitched tone*
    d. refer the patient to speech pathologist

Reference: p. 160

Descriptors:

| 1. 10 | 2. 06 | 3. Application |
| 4. II-1 | 5. Nursing Process | 6. Moderate |

Rationale: Older patients experience decreased hearing ability (presbycusis) and should be spoken to in a low-pitched tone.

19. An 80-year-old patient has fallen in his home, fracturing his right hip. Following surgery he is most prone to
    a. edema
    b. heart attack
    c. pneumonia*
    d. stroke

Reference: p. 161

Descriptors:

| 1. 1 | 2. 07 | 3. Comprehensive |
| 4. IV-3 | 5. Nursing Process | 6. Easy |

Rationale: An older patient with a hip fracture is at high risk for pneumonia.

20. An elderly patient who experiences patterns of forgetfulness and progressive confusion with the inability to perform activities of daily living is most likely experiencing
    a. Lou Gehrig's disease
    b. Alzheimer's disease*
    c. hypothyroidism
    d. heart disease

Reference: p. 161

Descriptors:

| 1. 10 | 2. 03 | 3. Knowledge |
| 4. IV-4 | 5. Nursing Process | 6. Easy |

Rationale: Alzheimer's disease is the leading cause of cognitive impairment in old age. It is progressive confusion and disorientation to physical surroundings.

21. Which of the following is true of the relationship between the physiologic and functional status in aging?
    a. There is little correlation between the two concepts.
    b. Adaptation to abilities varies among individuals.*
    c. Usually only one functional status is affected.
    d. Lifestyle factors have little influence on functional status.

Reference: p. 161

Descriptors:

| 1. 10 | 2. 05 | 3. Knowledge |
| 4. IV-4 | 5. Nursing Process | 6. Moderate |

Rationale: Adaptation to abilities varies among individuals and depends on many factors.

22. To assist patients diagnosed with Alzheimer's disease to identify their rooms in a nursing home, it is important to
    a. have their names written on the door
    b. have a memory box outside the room*
    c. decorate the room differently for patients
    d. have a tag on the room with their name

Reference: p. 162

Descriptors:

| 1. 10 | 2. 07 | 3. Application |
| 4. IV-4 | 5. Nursing Process | 6. Difficult |

Rationale: Alzheimer's patients have the ability to identify their rooms more easily if they can identify photographs or knick knacks from their homes.

23. An 80-year-old woman rarely leaves her home and has become more introspective. This describes
    a. isolation theory
    b. disengagement theory*
    c. reality theory
    d. moral development theory

Reference: p. 162

Descriptors:

| 1. 10 | 2. 02 | 3. Comprehensive |
| 4. III-1 | 5. Nursing Process | 6. Easy |

Rationale: Older adults often withdraw from usual roles and become introspective.

24. Older women and men at the local Catholic church talk that life was better years ago. They state the church is just not the same as it was in the past. This is an example of
    a. life review*
    b. verbal expression
    c. moral adjustment
    d. value change

Reference: p. 163

Descriptors:

| 1. 10 | 2. 02 | 3. Comprehensive |
| 4. III-2 | 5. Nursing Process | 6. Easy |

Rationale: Older adults often like to tell stories of past events or life review.

25. Reminiscence can assist the older adult in accomplishing which of the Erikson's developmental tasks?
    a. resolution of future failures and disappointments
    b. restructuring of achieved and yet to be achieved accomplishments*
    c. maintaining a sense of right and wrong behaviors
    d. an opportunity to view life as a series of unresolved problems

Reference: p. 163

Descriptors:

| 1. 10 | 2. 06 | 3. Knowledge |
| 4. III-1 | 5. Nursing Process | 6. Moderate |

Rationale: Reminiscence can assist the older adult to achieve ego integrity and helps by the restructuring of the achieved and yet-to-be-achieved accomplishments.

26. Sexuality in the older patient
    a. increases
    b. decreases
    c. is the same*
    d. is nonexistent

Reference: p. 164

Descriptors:

| 1. 10 | 2. 05 | 3. Knowledge |
| 4. III-3 | 5. Nursing Process | 5. Easy |

Rationale: Libido remains the same in older patients unless there is a physiologic reason associated with a change or medications.

27. An elderly patient will not go to sleep at night until she says her prayers. The term that describes the importance of prayers is
    a. self-transcendence*
    b. moral development
    c. individuative-reflective
    d. atonement for sins

    Reference: p. 165

    Descriptors:

1. 10	2. 02	3. Comprehensive
4. III-2	5. Nursing Process	6. Moderate

    Rationale: Self-transcendence is a characteristic of later life that helps one expand beyond personal limits to reach out to others. It is a greater awareness of one's beliefs and values.

28. While caring for a hospitalized 91-year-old patient, the nurse should consider that
    a. there is a decreased capacity in the elderly to adapt to illness*
    b. senility is a common problem for older adults who are ill
    c. medication dosages may need to be increased for the elderly
    d. learning capacities are generally quite diminished

    Reference: p. 166

    Descriptors:

1. 10	2. 06	3. Knowledge
4. IV-4	5. Nursing Process	6. Moderate

    Rationale: Elderly patients often have a decreased ability to adapt to illness for a variety of reasons. Senility is not common in the elderly.

29. An elderly patient is hospitalized for treatment of an infection. The nurse should be aware that the patient is
    a. likely to be isolated in a separate unit
    b. often confused by the strange surroundings*
    c. frequently malnourished because of loneliness
    d. prone to chronic fatigue from exertion

    Reference: p. 167

    Descriptors:

1. 10	2. 07	3. Application
4. III-1	5. Nursing Process	6. Difficult

    Rationale: Elderly patients who are hospitalized are prone to the development of confusion due to unfamiliar surroundings.

30. Nursing actions to promote wellness or prevent illness in the elderly population include
    a. administering antidepressants for unresolved grief
    b. teaching the importance of healthy diets and exercise*
    c. advising patients to eliminate strenuous activity due to injuries
    d. promoting frequent naps throughout the day to reduce fatigue

    Reference: p. 167

    Descriptors:

1. 10	2. 06	3. Knowledge
4. II-1	5. Nursing Process	6. Moderate

    Rationale: Healthy diets and exercise for the elderly population can reduce or prevent illness.

UNIT III

Community-Based
Settings for Patient Care

CHAPTER 11

Community-Based Healthcare

1. Care provided to people who live within a defined geographic region or have common needs requires
   a. collaborative care
   b. community-based healthcare*
   c. home-based healthcare
   d. occupational nursing care

   Reference: p. 174

   Descriptors:

1. 11	2. 01	3. Knowledge
4. None	5. None	6. Easy

   Rationale: Community-based healthcare is centered on individual and family healthcare needs for a defined geographic region.

2. The 1996 Health Insurance Portability and Accountability Act has
   a. provided healthcare to the underprivileged
   b. extended COBRA benefits to the unemployed
   c. prohibited denial of coverage for preexisting illness*
   d. allowed for the establishment of community clinics

   Reference: p. 174

   Descriptors:

1. 11	2. 06	3. Knowledge
4. None	5. None	6. Easy

   Rationale: Federal legislation up through the 1996 Health Insurance Portability and Accountability Act has improved access to insurance for employed persons and prohibits denial of coverage for an existing illness.

3. The focus on health and care, not on illness, is the main theme of
   a. Americans With Disabilities Act
   b. Social Security of Act of 1935
   c. Nursing's Agenda for Healthcare Reform*
   d. Hill-Burton Act for Healthcare Construction

   Reference: p. 175

   Descriptors:

1. 11	2. 07	3. Knowledge
4. None	5. None	6. Easy

   Rationale: Nursing's Agenda for Healthcare Reform recommends that the focus be on health and care, not on illness and cure.

4. Patients who enter a hospital for more than 24 hours are considered
   a. inpatients*
   b. outpatients
   c. terminal patients
   d. ambulatory patients

   Reference: p. 176

   Descriptors:

1. 11	2. 01	3. Knowledge
4. None	5. None	6. Easy

   Rationale: People who enter a healthcare facility such as a hospital and stay more than 24 hours are said to be inpatients.

5. According to the DRG (diagnosis-related group) system of Medicare, shorter hospital stays have become the norm. Following discharge patients are most often referred to the
   a. physician's office
   b. occupational nurse
   c. clinical nurse specialist
   d. home health nurse*

   Reference: p. 176

   Descriptors:

1. 11	2. 01	3. Knowledge
4. None	5. None	6. Moderate

   Rationale: Home healthcare's importance is evidenced by the prospective payment system of reimbursement (DRG), which encourages early discharge from the hospital.

6. A community health nurse is planning a presentation to a group of high school students on nursing as a profession. Which of the following should be included in the teaching plan?
   a. Home-based care is one of the most rapidly growing areas of the healthcare system.*
   b. Advanced practice nurses are declining in their numbers.
   c. The scope of nursing practice has been narrowed due to the number of other healthcare workers.
   d. Patients admitted to the hospital are usually severely ill and remain hospitalized for lengthy periods.

   Reference: p. 176

   Descriptors:

1. 11	2. 02	3. Knowledge
4. I-1	5. None	6. Easy

   Rationale: Home healthcare or home-based care is one of the most rapidly growing areas of the healthcare system due to decreased hospital stays.

7. Public hospitals are financed by
   a. charitable contributions
   b. insurance payments
   c. for profit corporations
   d. government agencies*

   Reference: p. 177

   Descriptors:

1. 11	2. 01	3. Knowledge
4. None	None	6. Easy

   Rationale: Public hospitals, which are nonprofit institutions, are financed and operated by local, state, or national agencies.

8. An adult without health insurance will most likely receive care in a hospital that is termed
   a. rehabilitative
   b. private, for profit
   c. private, not for profit
   d. public, not for profit*

   Reference: p. 177

   Descriptors:

1. 11	2. 01	3. Knowledge
4. None	5. None	6. Easy

   Rationale: Public not-for-profit hospitals provide care for patients without insurance.

9. Certified nurse practitioners in private practice implement their nursing skills in
   a. primary care centers*
   b. acute care centers
   c. home health agencies
   d. outpatient clinics

   Reference: p. 177

   Descriptors:

1. 11	2. 03	3. Knowledge
4. None	5. None	6. Easy

   Rationale: Primary healthcare services are provided by physicians and advanced practice nurses in offices and clinics offering the diagnosis and treatment of minor illnesses, minor surgical procedures, obstetrical care, well-child care, counseling, and referrals.

10. A 76-year-old male patient is unable to care for himself while his family is at work and school. The nurse should suggest to the family that they explore using a/an
    a. extended care facility
    b. adult day-care center*
    c. skilled nursing facility
    d. respite care center

    Reference: p. 177

    Descriptors:

1. 11	2. 03	3. Comprehensive
4. IV-1	5. Self Care	6. Moderate

    Rationale: An adult day-care center might be an appropriate facility for the family to explore for daytime use.

11. A patient's family would like to take a cruise, but they are unsure of who will care for the patient in their absence. The home health nurse should suggest that the family place the patient in a/an
    a. acute care facility
    b. skilled nursing facility
    c. respite care center*
    d. long-term care center

    Reference: p. 178

    Descriptors:

1. 11	2. 03	3. Application
4. IV-1	5. Self Care	6. Moderate

    Rationale: The primary purpose of a respite care center is to enable the primary caregiver some time away from the responsibilities of day-to-day care.

12. One of the major sources of emergency care and health education for children in the United States are nurses employed in
    a. ambulatory care centers
    b. ambulatory surgery centers
    c. hospital-based emergency rooms
    d. elementary and high schools*

    Reference: p. 178

    Descriptors:

1. 11	2. 04	3. Knowledge
4. None	5. None	6. Easy

    Rationale: School nurses in both elementary and secondary schools provide both emergency care and health education to this population.

13. The nurse has presented a class on healthy lifestyles to a group of adults ages 65 and older. The nurse determines that one of the participants needs further instruction when he says that long-term care facilities have increased due to the
    a. increased number of older adults with long-term care insurance*
    b. number of older adults who are living longer
    c. lack of caregivers within the person's family
    d. decreased length of hospital stays

    Reference: pp. 178–179

    Descriptors:

1. 11	2. 03	3. Application
4. I-1	5. Teach/Learn	6. Moderate

    Rationale: The increase in long-term care facilities is related to the number of older adults who are living longer, lack of caregivers in a family, and decreased length of hospital stays.

14. The nursing staff of an occupational health center will assist with patients from
    a. work-related injuries*
    b. home infusion services
    c. rehabilitation of disabilities
    d. chemotherapy administration

    Reference: p. 178

    Descriptors:

1. 11	2. 03	3. Knowledge
4. None	5. None	6. Moderate

    Rationale: Occupational health nurses practicing in industrial clinics focus on preventing work-related injury and illness. They also care for minor accidents and illnesses and make referrals for more serious health problems.

15. A 72-year-old patient has terminal cancer. He has less than 6 months to live. You are the home health nurse caring for the patient. The nurse should refer the patient to
    a. respite care
    b. hospice care*
    c. skilled care
    d. extended care

    Reference: p. 179

    Descriptors:

1. 11	2. 03	3. Comprehensive
4. I-1	5. Self Care	6. Moderate

    Rationale: Hospices are special services for terminally ill patients and their families.

16. A 77-year-old man has recently been disabled from a stroke and experienced the death of a spouse. He is a deeply religious man and prays often. Based on this information, he would benefit from the care provided by the
    a. parish nurse*
    b. physician's assistant
    c. social worker
    d. home health aid

    Reference: p. 179

    Descriptors:

1. 11	2. 05	3. Comprehensive
4. I-1	5. Self Care	6. Easy

    Rationale: Parish nurses reach out to those who are suffering from losses.

17. The nurse is employed in a healthcare facility in which the cost-effective care of the patient is carefully monitored from initial contact to discharge. This type of system is termed
    a. case management
    b. primary healthcare
    c. collaborative care
    d. managed care*

    Reference: p. 182

    Descriptors:

1. 11	2. 05	3. Knowledge
4. None	5. None	6. Easy

    Rationale: This type of system is termed managed care.

18. Military hospitals are operated by
    a. state governments
    b. Veterans Administration
    c. for profit companies
    d. the armed forces*

    Reference: p. 180

    Descriptors:

1. 11	2. 06	3. Knowledge
4. None	5. None	6. Easy

    Rationale: Military hospitals provide care to active members of the armed forces and their immediate families.

19. The rate of pneumonia after severe flooding is often investigated by the
    a. US Air Force Hospital.
    b. Centers for Disease Control and Prevention*
    c. National Institutes of Health
    d. US Department of Justice

    Reference: p. 180

    Descriptors:

1. 11	2. 07	3. Application
4. None	5. None	6. Difficult

    Rationale: The Centers for Disease Control and Prevention focuses on the epidemiology, prevention, control, and treatment of communicable diseases.

20. A 46-year-old woman has fallen and believes she fractured her wrist. Under her managed care system, she may need to be referred by the
    a. orthopedic surgeon
    b. insurance company
    c. primary care physician*
    d. orthopedic doctor of choice

    Reference: p. 180

    Descriptors:

1. 11	2. 05	3. Comprehensive
4. None	5. None	6. Difficult

    Rationale: Under a managed care system, the patient may need to be referred by her primary care physician if an orthopedic surgeon is needed.

21. Monitoring of care provided and determining the healthcare needs and referrals fall under the auspices of the
    a. physical therapist
    b. nurse practitioner
    c. case manager*
    d. social worker

    Reference: p. 180

    Descriptors:

1. 11	2. 04	3. Comprehensive
4. None	5. None	6. Moderate

    Rationale: The RN case manager monitors the care provided and ensures that appropriate referrals are made and that the plan of care follows established standards.

22. When nurses are working with physician assistants they are
    a. legally bound to follow only the guidelines of the physician
    b. in some states, not bound to follow the physician assistant's orders*
    c. able to provide the same level of care as physician assistants
    d. able to receive orders including narcotics from physician assistants

    Reference: p. 181

    Descriptors:

1. 11	2. 07	3. Comprehensive
4. None	5. None	6. Moderate

    Rationale: In most states, nurses are not legally bound to follow a physician assistant's orders unless they are cosigned by a physician.

23. The nurse is caring for a pregnant woman in the community clinic, who has decided to put her baby up for adoption. The nurse should refer the patient to a
    a. social worker*
    b. family planner
    c. physician assistant
    d. chaplain

    Reference: p. 182

    Descriptors:

1. 11	2. 06	3. Application
4. I-1	5. Nursing Process	6. Easy

    Rationale: A social worker can assist the patient with the process of adoption.

24. Nurses must keep in mind that the consumer of healthcare is
    a. legally responsible to follow the healthcare team orders
    b. unable to sue if they cannot pay for healthcare
    c. more educated about healthcare than previously*
    d. required by law to report practitioner misconduct

    Reference: p. 184

    Descriptors:

1. 11	2. 07	3. Knowledge
4. None	5. None	6. Moderate

    Rationale: Consumers of healthcare are more educated about healthcare and treatments than ever before.

25. A professional trained in techniques that improve pulmonary function is termed a
    a. respiratory therapist*
    b. physician assistant
    c. speech therapist
    d. social worker

    Reference: p. 182

    Descriptors:

1. 11	2. 05	3. Knowledge
4. None	5. None	6. Easy

Rationale: Respiratory therapists are trained in techniques that improve pulmonary function.

26. Prepaid group managed care plans that allow subscribers to receive all medical services through affiliated providers are called
    a. private insurance plans
    b. health maintenance organizations*
    c. preferred provider organizations
    d. self-care insurance plans

    Reference: p. 183

    Descriptors:

1. 11	2. 06	3. Knowledge
4. None	5. None	6. Moderate

    Rationale: Health maintenance organizations are prepaid plans that allow members to receive all medical services through specific providers.

CHAPTER 12

Continuity of Care

1. When the home health nurse notifies the acute care setting with a report on the status and condition of the patient, this activity constitutes the provision of
   a. coordination of care
   b. fluidity of care
   c. continuity of care*
   d. management of care
   Reference: p. 188
   Descriptors:

1. 12	2. 01	3. Comprehensive
4. I-1	5. Nursing Process	6. Moderate

   Rationale: The nurse is the primary person responsible for communicating the patient's needs in the continuity of care.

2. Through the home health nurse's activity of informing the acute care setting of the status of the patient, the patient will experience
   a. a smoother transition to the acute care setting*
   b. health promotion activities at the acute setting
   c. anxiety with the change of healthcare staff
   d. care and attention to his physical needs only
   Reference: p. 188
   Descriptors:

1. 12	2. 02	3. Application
4. I-1	5. Nursing Process	6. Difficult

   Rationale: Through communication the patient's needs are consistently met as the patient moves from one level of care to another.

3. A 3-year-old child is discharged following the diagnosis of leukemia. He will be receiving chemotherapy at home. What are the most important referrals the nurse must make?
   a. speech therapy, occupational therapy, durable medical equipment
   b. home health nurse, pharmacy, durable medical equipment*
   c. home health nurse, social worker, parish nurse
   d. perfusionist, physician assistant, registered nurse

   Reference: p. 190
   Descriptors:

1. 12	2. 02	3. Application
4. I-1	5. Nursing Process	6. Difficult

   Rationale: This child will require the services of the home health nurse to administer and teach the family about the chemotherapy. The pharmacy will provide the chemotherapy and the durable medical equipment company will provide the needed intravenous equipment.

4. The nurse has discussed continuity of care with a group of beginning nursing students. The nurse determines that one of the students needs further instruction when she says that continuity of care includes
   a. collaborating with other members of the healthcare team
   b. discharge planning for any patient who enters the healthcare system
   c. involving the patient and family in decisions related to care
   d. documenting the patient's physical assessment findings*
   Reference: p. 188
   Descriptors:

1. 12	2. 01	3. Application
4. I-1	5. Caring	6. Moderate

   Rationale: Documenting the patient's physical assessment findings is not part of the continuity of care process.

5. A patient is scheduled to have surgery on his feet in an ambulatory surgery facility. Before the surgery is performed, the nurse should determine if the patient
   a. has had appropriate screening tests*
   b. has assistance from a family member at home
   c. needs a bath or shower with betadine soap
   d. should be admitted to the hospital following surgery

Reference: p. 190

Descriptors:

| 1. 12 | 2. 04 | 3. Application |
| 4. IV-3 | 5. Nursing Process | 6. Moderate |

Rationale: Most patients who are scheduled for ambulatory surgery have various screening tests (eg, electrocardiogram) before the surgery date.

6. A 5-year-old boy is admitted to the pediatric unit for the treatment of acute asthma. Prior to administering a breathing treatment and while the child watches, the nurse should demonstrate the procedure
   a. to the parents
   b. to the student nurse
   c. on a stuffed animal*
   d. on another nurse

Reference: p. 189

Descriptors:

| 1. 12 | 2. 03 | 3. Application |
| 3. II-1 | 5. Nursing Process | 6. Difficult |

Rationale: The best intervention is to demonstrate the procedure on the stuffed animal. This will allow the child time to understand the procedure and allay anxiety.

7. Adequate teaching to a patient prior to surgery will
   a. help to alleviate anxiety*
   b. provide an improved response
   c. allow payment from the insurance
   d. have limited effect on care

Reference: p. 189

Descriptors:

| 1. 12 | 2. 06 | 3. Comprehensive |
| 4. IV-3 | 5. Nursing Process | 6. Moderate |

Rationale: Thorough and adequate patient teaching will assist the patient in the alleviation of anxiety.

8. When a patient is admitted to the acute care setting, the nurse must first
   a. perform a physical assessment*
   b. have pastoral care visit
   c. orient the patient to the floor
   d. provide for the patient's nutrition

Reference: p. 190

Descriptors:

| 1. 12 | 2. 04 | 3. Application |
| 4. IV-3 | 5. Nursing Process | 6. Easy |

Rationale: The physical assessment provides a database for the development of the plan of care and should be done first.

9. A 48-year-old woman is being transferred to the surgical unit following surgery. Before the patient's arrival, the nurse should
   a. have the nursing assistant prepare the room
   b. raise the bed to the high position*
   c. lower the bed to the lowest position
   d. place the bed in high Fowler's position

Reference: p. 190

Descriptors:

| 1. 12 | 2. 04 | 3. Application |
| 4. IV-3 | 5. Nursing Process | 6. Easy |

Rationale: Placing the bed in the high position allows for the ease of patient transfer from the stretcher to the bed.

10. To ensure that the patient is discharged with all her belongings, during the admission process the nurse should
    a. send the belongings home with the family
    b. notify security of the patient's belongings
    c. inventory all of the patient's belongings*
    d. place the patient's belongings in a closet

Reference: p. 191

Descriptors:

| 1. 12 | 2. 04 | 3. Knowledge |
| 4. I-1 | 5. Nursing Process | 6. Easy |

Rationale: An inventory of the patient's personal belongings is completed to ensure that the belongings are returned to the patient on discharge.

11. Information documented on the admission form will
    a. assist the nurse in the evaluation of care
    b. provide the patient with discharge information
    c. assist in the development of the care plan*
    d. be used only by the nursing staff

Reference: p. 191

Descriptors:

| 1. 12 | 2. 04 | 3. Knowledge |
| 4. I-1 | 5. Documentation | 6. Moderate |

Rationale: The information gathered on the admission form is used to develop the nursing care plan for the patient and is used as a database for discharge planning and home care.

12. A 55-year-old man is transferred from the medical division to the intensive care unit. He will most likely be
    a. experiencing unfamiliar sounds*
    b. heavily sedated and unresponsive
    c. unable to communicate with family
    d. experiencing severe discomfort

Reference: p. 191

Descriptors:

| 1. 12 | 2. 05 | 3. Comprehensive |
| 4. III-2 | 5. Nursing Process | 6. Moderate |

Rationale: The patient needs to be oriented to the intensive care unit and taught the unfamiliar sights and sounds he will experience.

13. A homeless man who is a patient in the public hospital leaves against medical advice (AMA). The next day you hear that he is found dead in an abandoned building. Which of the following statements is true?
    a. His family will probably file suit you for negligence.
    b. The family can sue because you witnessed the signature.
    c. The physician failed to provide adequate medical care.
    d. The institution and physician are released from liability.*

Reference: p. 194

Descriptors:

| 1. 12 | 2. 06 | 3. Comprehensive |
| 4. I-1 | 5. Documentation | 6. Moderate |

Rationale: A patient who leaves a healthcare facility against medical advice signs a form releasing the physician and institution from legal responsibility.

14. The nurse has assisted with the transfer of an adult patient to a different unit in the hospital setting. Following the transfer, the nurse should
    a. provide the receiving nurse with a verbal report*
    b. be certain the patient's personal belongings have been sent home
    c. ask the patient to review the advance directives
    d. provide the receiving nurse with the patient's prescriptions

Reference: p. 194

Descriptors:

| 1. 12 | 2. 05 | 3. Application |
| 4. I-1 | 5. Nursing Process | 6. Moderate |

Rationale: The transferring nurse needs to provide a verbal report.

15. A 33-year-old patient is newly diagnosed with diabetes mellitus. She is insulin dependent. Prior to discharge the nurse must instruct the patient on her insulin. It is important to teach the insulin action, side effects, and
    a. administration*
    b. cost
    c. exercise
    d. diet

Reference: p. 195

Descriptors:

| 1. 12 | 2. 06 | 3. Application |
| 4. IV-3 | 5. Teach/Learn | 6. Moderate |

Rationale: Discharge planning should include all the patient teaching necessary for self-care.

16. A systematic process for preparing the patient to leave the healthcare setting and maintain continuity of care is
    a. transfer of service
    b. case management
    c. discharge planning*
    d. needs assessment

Reference: p. 194

Descriptors:

| 1. 12 | 2. 06 | 3. Knowledge |
| 4. I-1 | 5. Communication | 6. Moderate |

Rationale: Planning for discharge begins on admission and is a systematic process to prepare the patient to leave the facility and maintain continuity of care.

17. To ensure continuity of care of a newly hospitalized patient, the nurse initiates discharge planning for the patient
    a. as soon as possible after admission*
    b. within 48 hours after admission
    c. the day before dismissal
    d. on the day of dismissal

Reference: p. 194

Descriptors:

1. 12	2. 06	3. Application
4. I-1	5. Communication	6. Easy

Rationale: Discharge planning should begin as soon as possible after admission.

18. An adult patient hospitalized for abdominal surgery will be dismissed to home in the morning. The nurse has instructed the patient how to perform necessary dressing changes at home. Before the patient is released the nurse should
    a. ask the patient to verbalize the procedure
    b. provide the patient with a short quiz about the procedure
    c. determine if the patient has any questions about his treatment plan
    d. ask the patient to perform a demonstration of the dressing change*

Reference: p. 195

Descriptors:

1. 12	2. 06	3. Application
4. IV-3	5. Teach/Learn	6. Moderate

Rationale: A demonstration of the procedure by the patient is the best way for the nurse to determine that the patient can perform the procedure.

19. The nurse is preparing to discharge an adult patient who will be using a wheelchair at home. A priority assessment for the nurse to make is
    a. who the caregiver will be when the patient is home
    b. how often the patient needs to have home care
    c. whether the patient's dwelling can accommodate a wheelchair*
    d. whether or not the patient has adequate insurance coverage

Reference: p. 196

Descriptors:

1. 12	2. 06	3. Application
4. I-1	5. Nursing Process	6. Moderate

Rationale: An important assessment for a patient who is being discharged in a wheelchair is whether or not the patient's dwelling can accommodate a wheelchair.

20. A frail 86-year-old patient will be dismissed from the hospital to home following a total knee replacement. For the patient's home care referral to be reimbursed, the nurse should
    a. have a written order by the physician*
    b. ask the social worker to document the patient's needs
    c. have the patient give her permission for home care
    d. document the patient's home care needs in the medical record

Reference: p. 197

Descriptors:

1. 12	2. 06	3. Application
4. I-1	5. Nursing Process	6. Moderate

Rationale: A written order by the physician is required for reimbursement.

21. An 80-year-old patient is being discharged with a Foley catheter. Prior to discharge the nurse should
    a. instruct the patient on safe and appropriate transfers
    b. assess whether the patient has physical limitations
    c. instruct the patient and family on catheter care*
    d. arrange for the patient's transfer to a nursing home

Reference: p. 197

Descriptors:

1. 12	2. 06	3. Application
4. IV-3	5. Teach/Learn	6. Difficult

Rationale: All aspects of patient care including patient education must be provided before discharge.

22. An 85-year-old patient is being discharged from the hospital after suffering a stroke. The family is very anxious that they will be unable to care for her. The most appropriate referral for the patient is a/an
    a. extended care facility
    b. home health agency*
    c. in-home hospice
    d. respite care center

Reference: 195

Descriptors:

1. 12	2. 05	3. Application
4. III-1	5. Teach/Learn	6. Moderate

Rationale: The nurse must assess the proper agency to refer a patient so that continuity of care is maintained.

23. An adult patient who has been hospitalized decides to leave the hospital against medical advice (AMA) and refuses to sign the release form. The nurse should
    a. try to convince the patient to remain hospitalized
    b. notify the hospital security department
    c. contact the hospital's legal department
    d. document the explanation to the patient in the medical record*

Reference: p. 194

Descriptors:

1. 12	2. 05	3. Application
4. I-1	5. Documentation	6. Moderate

Rationale: If a patient decides to leave the hospital against medical advice (AMA), and refuses to sign the release, the nurse should document this in the patient's chart or record.

CHAPTER 13

Home Healthcare

1. One of the most important aspects to consider in the care of the patient and family in the home is the
   a. setting
   b. climate
   c. culture*
   d. finances

   Reference: p. 200

   Descriptors:

1. 13	2. 03	3. Comprehensive
4. IV-1	5. Culture	6. Moderate

   Rationale: When providing home healthcare, nurses integrate community health principles, focusing on cultural and personal habits.

2. A major purpose of home healthcare is to
   a. care for acutely ill patients
   b. promote self-care within the family
   c. rehabilitate patients who have had injuries
   d. minimize the effects of illness and disability*

   Reference: p. 200

   Descriptors:

1. 13	2. 01	3. Knowledge
4. IV-3	5. Nursing Process	6. Easy

   Rationale: A major purpose of home healthcare is to minimize the effects of illness and disability.

3. The founders of the Henry Street Settlement, which was eventually known as the Visiting Nurses Association, were
   a. Lillian Wald and Mary Brewster*
   b. Adelaid Nutting and Sojourner Truth
   c. Mary Brewster and Dorothea Dix
   d. Elizabeth Blackwell and Lillian Wald

   Reference: p. 200

   Descriptors:

1. 13	2. 02	3. Knowledge
4. None	5. None	6. Easy

   Rationale: Lillian Wald and Mary Brewster founded the Henry Street Settlement in 1893. They provided nursing care for poor residents living in tenements.

4. What makes home healthcare different from hospital-based nursing?
   a. The nurse is more skilled in the hospital than home care.
   b. The home health nurse is more skilled in assessments.
   c. A hospital-based nurse is only employed in hospitals.
   d. The home health nurse conforms to patient's schedule.*

   Reference: p. 200

   Descriptors:

1. 13	2. 03	3. Comprehensive
4. IV-1	5. Nursing Process	6. Moderate

   Rationale: Home care nursing is unique because when the nurse crosses the threshold of the patient's home, care must be adapted to the patient's home and to the patient's schedule.

5. The role of the home health nurse is to
   a. work independently of the physician
   b. work under the prescribed plan*
   c. develop a plan of care by the nurse
   d. collaborate with family only

   Reference: p. 201

   Descriptors:

1. 13	2. 03	3. Knowledge
4. IV-1	5. Nursing Process	6. Moderate

   Rationale: The physician certifies that the patient has a health problem to receive home healthcare. The physician prescribes a plan of care treatment for the patient receiving home healthcare.

6. The rise in home healthcare in the last 15 years is primarily due to
   a. an increase rate of illness
   b. early discharge from hospitals*
   c. a greater need for continuity
   d. the advancement of technology

Reference: p. 201

Descriptors:

| 1. 13 | 2. 04 | 3. Knowledge |
| 4. II-2 | 5. Nursing Process | 6. Moderate |

Rationale: The introduction of diagnosis-related groups in hospitals led to an earlier discharge from the hospital than in the past.

7. Home care for the patient with a colostomy will most often be by a/an
   a. enterostomal therapist*
   b. nurse practitioner
   c. licensed practical nurse
   d. nurse anesthetist

Reference: p. 201

Descriptors:

| 1. 13 | 2. 03 | 3. Knowledge |
| 4. IV-1 | 5. Nursing Process | 6. Moderate |

Rationale: Nursing care administered by enterostomal therapists is appropriate for patients with ostomies or severe skin breakdown.

8. One of the most positive aspects of home care is that it is
   a. less expensive than other facilities
   b. staffed with greater stability than hospitals
   c. more comfortable for the patient*
   d. a better place to teach patients

Reference: p. 201

Descriptors:

| 1. 13 | 2. 05 | 3. Application |
| 4. IV-1 | 5. Caring | 6. Moderate |

Rationale: The home is a place of security, having meaning and given value because of ownership, family relationships and memories, independence, and protection.

9. Home care nurses must be knowledgeable and skilled. They must use
   a. effective transfer techniques
   b. effective communication skills*
   c. an understanding of catheters
   d. an understanding of dietetics

Reference: p. 202

Descriptors:

| 1. 13 | 2. 03 | 3. Application |
| 4. IV-1 | 5. Communication | 6. Easy |

Rationale: Nurses who provide care in the home must be knowledgeable and skilled with effective communication techniques as the most important aspect of their care.

10. A major difference between nurses who work in an acute care setting and those employed in a home care agency is the nurse's
    a. rapport skills
    b. independence*
    c. technical skills
    d. reimbursement for services

Reference: p. 202

Descriptors:

| 1. 13 | 2. 03 | 3. Knowledge |
| 4. IV-1 | 5. Nursing Process | 6. Easy |

Rationale: A major difference for nurses in acute care settings and home healthcare is the nurse's independence.

11. Home health nurses must be able to
    a. provide care autonomously*
    b. reach the patient's family members at all times
    c. provide care without an order
    d. use all medical equipment

Reference: p. 202

Descriptors:

| 1. 13 | 2. 03 | 3. Knowledge |
| 4. IV-1 | 5. Nursing Process | 6. Moderate |

Rationale: Home health nurses must make independent decisions and assume responsibility for decision making. Consultation with other professionals is not as easily available.

12. There are 21 inches of snow on the ground and the roads are impassable. An 82-year-old patient is unable to give her own insulin. How will the home health nurse administer the insulin to the patient? The nurse should
    a. see the patient no matter how difficult it is to get to the home
    b. have the patient call 911 and go to the emergency room
    c. call emergency transportation for herself and to go to the home*
    d. explain the insulin administration to the neighbor over the phone

Reference: p. 203

Descriptors:

| 1. 13 | 2. 03 | 3. Application |
| 4. IV-3 | 5. Caring | 6. Difficult |

Rationale: The nurse is accountable to the patient and must be a coordinator of the care. During extreme weather emergencies, volunteer and emergency personnel will assist with transportation.

13. The home care nurse visiting an 83-year-old patient is trying to assist him in understanding his medical bills. The nurse has also communicated with the insurance company. However, after several attempts the nurse is unable to ascertain the amount of insurance coverage for the patient. The most appropriate referral he can make is to call the
a. patient's lawyer
b. insurance company president
c. patient's power of attorney
d. agency's social worker*
Reference: p. 203
Descriptors:
1. 13　　　2. 03　　　3. Application
4. I-1　　　5. Caring　　6. Difficult
Rationale: When the patient requires assistance with billing and knowledge of community resources, it is most appropriate to refer the patient to the social worker.

14. An appropriate goal for a 40-year-old newly diagnosed insulin-dependent diabetic is to be able to
a. attend diabetic classes at the local hospital
b. be independent in nursing care in 1 week
c. administer his insulin in 3 days*
d. be knowledgeable about hypoglycemia today
Reference: p. 203
Descriptors:
1. 13　　　2. 05　　　3. Application
4. IV-4　　　5. Teach/Learn　　6. Difficult
Rationale: It is important for the nurse to develop with the patient goals that are easily attainable.

15. The preentry phase of the home visit is
a. a visit to the patient in the hospital
b. the time the referral is received*
c. the date of the first visit
d. the period of goal development
Reference: p. 203
Descriptors:
1. 13　　　2. 04　　　3. Knowledge
4. IV-1　　　5. Nursing Process　　6. Easy
Rationale: The preentry phase is the time when the nurse reviews the information and calls the patient to set up the first visit.

16. During the preentry phase of the home visit, the nurse assigned to the patient should plan to
a. negotiate the times of the visits
b. develop detailed nursing care plans
c. establish rapport with the patient
d. gather information about the patient*
Reference: p. 203
Descriptors:
1. 13　　　2. 04　　　3. Application
4. IV-1　　　5. Nursing Process　　6. Moderate
Rationale: During the preentry phase, the nurse should gather information about the patient.

17. The most important aspect for the nurse to consider when making a home care visit is
a. time
b. safety*
c. activities
d. skills
Reference: p. 204
Descriptors:
1. 13　　　2. 03　　　3. Knowledge
4. I-2　　　5. Nursing Process　　6. Easy
Rationale: The nurse must evaluate safety issues before making the first home visit.

18. The nurse caring for the home care patient must be aware of the fact that she
a. is a guest in the patient's home*
b. is the leader of the health team
c. needs to focus more heavily on the family
d. needs to be attentive to the community
Reference: p. 205
Descriptors:
1. 13　　　2. 04　　　3. Comprehensive
4. IV-1　　　5. Nursing Process　　6. Moderate
Rationale: The nurse must remember that she is a guest in the patient's home and is offering services that the patient may or may not accept.

19. During the entry phase of the home visit the nurse should
a. determine desired outcomes with the patient*
b. determine past surgical experiences
c. gather necessary supplies for the patient
d. obtain a doctor's order for the visits

Reference: p. 203

Descriptors:

1. 13   2. 04   3. Application

4. IV-1   5. Nursing Process 6. Moderate

Rationale: During the entry phase of the home visit, the nurse should determine desired outcomes with the patient.

20. Home health nursing requires that the nurse implement good nursing bag technique. This includes
    a. leaving the nursing bag in the car
    b. keeping items concealed in the bag
    c. place protection under the bag*
    d. wear latex gloves at all times

Reference: p. 207

Descriptors:

1. 13   2. 04   3. Knowledge

4. I-2   5. Nursing Process 6. Moderate

Rationale: There is risk for infection in homes that are not clean. It is important that the nurse place a barrier between the nursing bag and the table or floor.

21. To implement total care to the patient the home care nurse must be most familiar with
    a. the educational level of the patient and family
    b. the holidays the patient and family celebrate
    c. the nutritional content of the patient's diet
    d. the spiritual practices of the patient and family*

Reference: p. 207

Descriptors:

1. 13   2. 05   3. Application

4. IV-1   5. Nursing Process 6. Difficult

Rationale: Spirituality is often an important aspect of the patient's life. It is important that the nurse be aware of these practices and implement them in the patient's care.

22. The home health nurse is caring for a patient who is on a soft diet and immobilized due to partial paralysis. The patient has several family members to care for her. A primary nursing diagnosis for this patient is
    a. Impaired Social Interaction related to injuries
    b. Risk for Trauma related to immobility
    c. Risk for Constipation related to lack of dietary bulk*
    d. Altered Coping: Individual, related to partial paralysis

Reference: p. 207

Descriptors:

1. 13   2. 03   3. Application

4. IV-3   5. Nursing Process 6. Moderate

Rationale: Because of the immobility and soft diet, a priority diagnosis is Risk for Constipation related to lack of dietary fiber.

23. Care of the family after the death of a loved one is termed
    a. grief counseling
    b. bereavement care*
    c. hospice care
    d. psychological counseling

Reference: p. 208

Descriptors:

1. 13   2. 05   3. Knowledge

4. III-1   5. Caring   6. Easy

Rationale: The continuation of care after the death of the patient is bereavement care.

24. Nursing that provides care to patients who are dying is
    a. grief counseling
    b. bereavement care
    c. hospice care*
    d. psychological counseling

Reference: p. 208

Descriptors:

1. 13   2. 06   3. Knowledge

4. III-1   5. Caring   6. Easy

Rationale: Hospice nursing provides care to patients who are dying from a terminal illness.

25. The nurse is preparing to discharge an adult patient from the hospital to home where the patient's wife will be the major care provider for the patient. One of the primary differences for family members between acute care and home care is that for patients in acute care settings, the family member
    a. may not be competent to provide care
    b. has limited knowledge of the patient's needs
    c. usually has limited skills for providing care
    d. may become overwhelmed by the provision of care*

Reference: p. 208

Descriptors:

1. 13	2. 05	3. Application
4. IV-1	5. Caring	6. Moderate

Rationale: Family members may become overwhelmed by providing care.

26. The nurse has explained hospice care to a family member of a patient dying from cancer. The nurse determines that the family member understands the nurse's instructions when she says that hospice care
    a. is most often provided in a hospice center
    b. begins when the patient has 1 year to live
    c. ends with the family 1 year after the death*
    d. is not reimbursed by Medicare insurance

Reference: p. 208

Descriptors:

1. 13	2. 06	3. Application
4. IV-1	5. Caring	6. Moderate

Rationale: Hospice care ends with the family 1 year after the death.

27. If current trends in the United States continue, home healthcare will
    a. require more specialized nurses*
    b. provide greater emphasis on illness care
    c. depend on nurses who are more generalized
    d. care for patients with less acuity than in the past

Reference: p. 209

Descriptors:

1. 13	2. 02	3. Knowledge
4. None	5. None	6. Easy

Rationale: With the advent of newer technological advances, and people living longer, it is highly likely that home healthcare will require more specialized nurses, for example, cardiac care nurses.

UNIT IV

The Nursing Process

Blended Skills and Critical Thinking Throughout the Nursing Process

1. Nurses are responsible for the
   a. prescribing of medications
   b. diagnosis of medical diseases
   c. diagnosis of human responses*
   d. ordering of treatments

   Reference: p. 214

   Descriptors:

1. 14	2. 02	3. Knowledge
4. IV-1	5. Nursing Process	6. Easy

   Rationale: Nurse are responsible for the diagnosis and treatment of human responses actual or potential.

2. The nursing process was first introduced by
   a. Jean Watson
   b. Lydia Hall*
   c. Nell Watts
   d. Faye Abdellah

   Reference: p. 214

   Descriptors:

1. 14	2. 02	3. Knowledge
4. None	5. Nursing Process	5. Easy

   Rationale: The nursing process was first introduced by Lydia Hall in 1955.

3. The National League for Nursing recommended that
   a. all care is based on the nursing process
   b. the nursing process is the guideline for care
   c. education programs incorporate nursing process*
   d. the nursing process is the standard for care

   Reference: p. 215

   Descriptors:

1. 14	2. 02	3. Knowledge
4. None	5. Nursing Process	6. Easy

   Rationale: The National League for Nursing has recommended that educational programs incorporate the nursing process as their intellectual process.

4. The nurse reviews a patient's blood pressure recordings for the last 24 hours. What part of the nursing process is this action?
   a. assessment*
   b. diagnosis
   c. evaluation
   d. implementation

   Reference: p. 215

   Descriptors:

1. 14	2. 03	3. Application
4. IV-1	5. Nursing Process	6. Moderate

   Rationale: Through the assessment of the patient the nurse can determine an appropriate plan of care.

5. In the five steps of the nursing process, the goal is for the
   a. patient's family and patient to work together
   b. physician and the patient to work together
   c. patient and the nurse to work together*
   d. nurse and the patient's family to work together

   Reference: p. 215

   Descriptors:

1. 14	2. 03	3. Knowledge
4. IV-1	5. Nursing Process	6. Moderate

   Rationale: In the nursing process the nurse and patient are partners.

6. When a nurse is caring for an infant, who becomes the partner in the infant's care? The
   a. parent*
   b. social worker
   c. physical therapist
   d. other nurses

   Reference: p. 215

   Descriptors:

1. 14	2. 03	3. Comprehensive
4. IV-1	5. Nursing Process	6. Moderate

   Rationale: A parent or significant support person should assist in the nursing process.

7. The state board examination for nurse licensure
reflects the view that nursing has evolved to a
   a. more disease-based perspective
   b. holistic approach using the nursing process*
   c. general systems approach
   d. technologically based profession

Reference: p. 215

Descriptors:

| 1. 14 | 2. 02 | 3. Knowledge |
| 4. None | 5. Nursing Process | 6. Easy |

Rationale: Since changes were made in 1982, the
state board licensure examination has been
developed around the steps of the nursing process.

8. The steps of the nursing process include all of the
following *except*
   a. assessing patients, communities, and families
   b. deriving a medical diagnosis for curing disease*
   c. planning care for mutual goal setting
   d. evaluating the planned care responses

Reference: p. 216

Descriptors:

| 1. 14 | 2. 03 | 3. Application |
| 4. None | 5. Nursing Process | 6. Moderate |

Rationale: Nursing process focuses on human
responses, not medical diagnosis for curing
disease.

9. A major benefit for patients and nurses when the
nursing process is used includes care that is
provided in which of the following ways?
   a. ritualistic
   b. standardized
   c. individualized*
   d. technical

Reference: p. 216

Descriptors:

| 1. 14 | 2. 05 | 3. Knowledge |
| 4. I-1 | 5. Nursing Process | 6. Easy |

Rationale: When the nursing process is used,
patients and nurses benefit from individualized
care.

10. The assessment phase of the nursing process is
    a. the documented problem
    b. the database*
    c. the physician's order
    d. the evaluation

Reference: p. 216

Descriptors:

| 1. 14 | 2. 03 | 3. Knowledge |
| 4. None | 5. Nursing Process | 6. Moderate |

Rationale: The base contains all assessment data
collected and should be continuously updated.

11. In developing a nursing care plan the nurse
describes a decubitus ulcer in regard to location,
size, shape, color, drainage, and odor. This is an
example of the contribution to
    a. a one-time nursing phenomenon
    b. a complete and accurate database*
    c. a patient's understanding of wounds
    d. a rationale for care in implementation

Reference: p. 217

Descriptors:

| 1. 14 | 2. 04 | 3. Application |
| 4. IV-3 | 5. Nursing Process | 6. Difficult |

Rationale: Without a complete and accurate
database, the nurse cannot identify the patient's
strengths and weaknesses.

12. A 52-year-old patient is recovering from a bicycle
accident in which she sustained a brain injury. The
nurse and patient identify goals to be attained.
This is an example of
    a. health promotion
    b. disease prevention
    c. risk identification
    d. health restoration*

Reference: p. 218

Descriptors:

| 1. 14 | 2. 04 | 3. Application |
| 4. IV-3 | 5. Nursing Process | 6. Moderate |

Rationale: The nursing process offers a means for
nurses and patients to work together to identify
specific goals related to restoration of health.

13. An elderly patient has an inability to swallow. The
patient is being fed through a tube. Assessment of
the patient's response to the tube feeding helps to
determine whether the
    a. family can provide care
    b. nursing action achieves goals*
    c. future of the patient's condition
    d. speech therapist is needed

Reference: p. 218

Descriptors:

1. 14	2. 04	3. Application
4. IV-1	5. Nursing Process	6. Moderate

Rationale: The nursing process offers direction for all the activities carried out by the nurse during the patient's care.

14. A nurse administers a sleeping medication to a patient; however, she does not document her intervention. Based on the information the
    a. medication was never given*
    b. medication should be repeated
    c. nurse should obtain a new order
    d. nurse should assess for side effects

Reference: p. 218

Descriptors:

1. 14	2. 10	3. Application
4. IV-2	5. Documentation	6. Moderate

Rationale: Legally speaking, a nursing action not documented is a nursing action not met.

15. A patient develops a grayish color of his skin, but no change in vital signs. The nurse notifies the attending physician. Within minutes the patient becomes diaphoretic and complains of chest pain. This scenario describes
    a. trial-and-error problem solving
    b. scientific problem solving
    c. goal-oriented problem solving
    d. intuitive problem solving*

Reference: p. 218

Descriptors:

1. 14	2. 01	3. Comprehensive
4. IV-3	5. Nursing Process	6. Moderate

Rationale: Intuitive problem solving is a skill developed through years of experience. Intuitive problem solving comes with years of practice and observation.

16. Following a patient's assessment and the development of the database the nurse should develop a/an
    a. nursing diagnosis*
    b. nursing intervention
    c. patient goal
    d. evaluation of care

Reference: p. 219

Descriptors:

1. 14	2. 03	3. Comprehensive
4. IV-1	5. Nursing Process	6. Moderate

Rationale: A nursing diagnosis is formulated after the data collection.

17. A systematic way to form and shape one's thinking defines
    a. technical skills
    b. cognitive skills
    c. critical thinking*
    d. purposeful thinking

Reference: p. 221

Descriptors:

1. 14	2. 07	3. Knowledge
4. None	5. None	6. Easy

Rationale: Critical thinking is a systematic way to form and shape one's thinking. It is disciplined, comprehensive, based on intellectual standards, and well reasoned.

18. A nurse who is skilled in interpersonal relationships is able to accomplish which of the following? The nurse will
    a. interact with patients and families*
    b. use equipment competently
    c. mediate ethical conflict with others
    d. advance the interests of patients

Reference: p. 221

Descriptors:

1. 14	2. 09	3. Comprehensive
4. I-1	5. Communication	6. Moderate

Rationale: Interactions with patients, families, significant others, and colleagues affirms the individual's self-worth.

19. Critical thinking allows the nurse to determine the
    a. best outcome of care
    b. best intervention*
    c. evaluation of care
    d. diagnosis of care

Reference: p. 221

Descriptors:

1. 14	2. 07	3. Comprehensive
4. None	5. None	6. Difficult

Rationale: The purpose of critical thinking is to make a judgment about a particular patient or situation and determine how best to intervene.

20. A patient has complained about pain at her incision site hourly since surgery 3 days ago. She has been named the "great complainer." At 8:30 PM she complains of chest pain. However, the nurse refuses to assess her. The nurse is exhibiting
    a. good faith and integrity
    b. use of the nursing process
    c. ability to think independently
    d. judgmental behavior*

    Reference: p. 233

    Descriptors:

1. 14	2. 10	3. Application
4. IV-3	5. Nursing Process	6. Difficult

    Rationale: Nurses who are independent thinkers are careful not to allow the status quo or persuasive individuals control behaviors.

21. A nurse who is employed by an agency is working on a medical unit at a local hospital. The nurse is unfamiliar with the infusion pump at this institution. What would be the nurse's best plan? The nurse should
    a. implement the trial-and-error approach
    b. ask for assistance from an experienced nurse*
    c. set the machine and then check its operation
    d. infuse the medication without a pump

    Reference: p. 225

    Descriptors:

1. 14	2. 10	3. Application
4. IV-2	5. Nursing Process	6. Difficult

    Rationale: The nurse should identify nurses who are technical experts, and ask for help. The patient's life may depend on the nurse's technical competence.

22. Visiting with a patient for 60 seconds at eye level and with a close touch indicates to the patient that the nurse
    a. cares for the patient as a person*
    b. is limited in time with the patient
    c. has too much work to accomplish
    d. requires extra help to provide care

    Reference: p. 225

    Descriptors:

1. 14	2. 11	3. Application
4. IV-1	5. Caring	6. Difficult

    Rationale: A 60-second nurse—patient interaction can enhance the patient's well-being.

23. Employees who report their employer's violation of the law to the appropriate state authorities are called
    a. patient advocates
    b. whistle blowers*
    c. unethical nurses
    d. critical thinkers

    Reference: p. 230

    Descriptors:

1. 14	2. 01	3. Comprehensive
4. I-1	5. Caring	6. Easy

    Rationale: Reporting an employer's violations may not be protected by the state or federal government. These employees are termed "whistle blowers."

CHAPTER 15

Assessing

1. The ability to safely and effectively use an electronic intravenous pump is an example of a skill termed
   a. cognitive
   b. technical*
   c. interpersonal
   d. legal

   Reference: p. 236

   Descriptors:

1. 15	2. 02	3. Knowledge
4. IV-1	5. Nursing Process	6. Easy

   Rationale: Using an electronic intravenous pump in a safe manner is a technical skill.

2. Maintaining a trusting and accountable relationship with patients and other health professionals is an example of a skill termed
   a. cognitive
   b. ethical/legal*
   c. introspective
   d. technical

   Reference: p. 236

   Descriptors:

1. 15	2. 01	3. Application
4. I-1	5. Nursing Process	6. Easy

   Rationale: Maintaining a trusting and accountable relationship with patients and other health professionals is an example of a skill termed ethical/legal. Ethical/legal skills involve maintaining a trusting relationship.

3. The collection of the patient's assessment information is termed the
   a. plan
   b. database*
   c. evaluation
   d. chart

   Reference: p. 236

   Descriptors:

3. 15	2. 01	3. Knowledge
4. I-1	5. Nursing Process	6. Easy

   Rationale: A database includes all pertinent patient information collected by the nurse and other healthcare professionals.

4. Nursing assessments differ from medical assessments in that
   a. medical assessments target community health issues
   b. nursing assessments focus on patient responses*
   c. medical assessments focus on health promotion
   d. nursing assessments diagnose pathological illness

   Reference: p. 236

   Descriptors:

1. 15	2. 03	3. Knowledge
4. I-1	5. Nursing Process	6. Moderate

   Rationale: Medical assessments target data pointing to pathologic conditions. Nursing assessments focus on the patient's responses to health problems.

5. Which of the following is *not* a source of information for the database?
   a. patient
   b. family
   c. Medicare*
   d. physician

   Reference: p. 236

   Descriptors:

1. 15	2. 03	3. Knowledge
4. I-1	5. Nursing Process	6. Easy

   Rationale: The sources of patient information are the patient, the patient's support people, the patient record, the patient's healthcare professionals, and other nurses, not Medicare.

6. The unique focus of nursing assessments is the
   a. patient's response to actual or potential health problems*
   b. family's needs and the provision of wellness information
   c. reason for treatments and medications to treat disease process
   d. rationale for the appropriate levels of prevention and healthcare

Reference: p. 236

Descriptors:

1. 15	2. 03	3. Knowledge
4. I-1	5. Nursing Process	6. Moderate

Rationale: The unique focus of nursing assessment is on the patient's response to actual or potential health problems.

7. Information about the patient, in the patient's own words, is
   a. objective data
   b. subjective data*
   c. recorded data
   d. historical data

   Reference: p. 236

   Descriptors:

1. 15	2. 01	3. Knowledge
4. I-1	5. Nursing Process	6. Easy

   Rationale: Subjective data is information that only the patient can validate.

8. The nurse assesses the patient's blood pressure and records it at 148/90. This is an example of
   a. objective data*
   b. subjective data
   c. recorded data
   d. historical data

   Reference: p. 237

   Descriptors:

1. 15	2. 01	3. Comprehensive
4. IV-1	5. Nursing Process	6. Moderate

   Rationale: Objective data are observable and measurable data that can be seen, heard, or felt by someone other than the person experiencing them.

9. A nurse is assessing an anorectic teenager. The patient states, "I don't want to eat. I don't feel well." Following this statement the patient vomits and displays flulike symptoms. The nurse charts that the patient refused to eat and vomited, indicating that she displays acute anorectic symptoms. These data indicate that
   a. the patient is lying and the nurse confirms the anorectic symptoms
   b. based on the information the nurse should isolate the patient
   c. the nurse has not documented the patient's factual information*
   d. the physician should be notified of the patient's behavior

Reference: p. 237

Descriptors:

1. 15	2. 02	3. Application
4. III-2	5. Documentation	6. Difficult

Rationale: The patient's condition must be represented and documented accurately.

10. The home health nurse has received a referral on an 88-year-old man who had a craniotomy 2 weeks ago. On the initial visit the patient states, "I haven't had any surgery, I need new medicine." The nurse assesses a healed incision on the skull. This information indicates that the
    a. patient's record is inadequate
    b. patient's medicines were changed
    c. patient is poor historian*
    d. patient wasn't hospitalized

    Reference: p. 238

    Descriptors:

1. 15	2. 05	3. Application
4. IV-1	5. Nursing Process	6. Difficult

    Rationale: Patients with decreased mental capacity should respond as accurately as possible. During the interview the nurse may validate the patient's inability to answer accurately.

11. The home health nurse reviews the patient's record and information from the hospital. This is an example of the phase termed
    a. introduction
    b. preparatory*
    c. working
    d. termination

    Reference: p. 239

    Descriptors:

1. 15	2. 05	3. Comprehensive
4. I-1	5. Nursing Process	6. Moderate

    Rationale: The preparatory phase involves a review of the patient's record.

12. A patient's blood sugar is 195. What source of data does this represent?
    a. consultation
    b. medical history
    c. progress notes
    d. laboratory data*

Reference: p. 238

Descriptors:

| 1. 15 | 2. 07 | 3. Comprehensive |
| 4. IV-3 | 5. Nursing Process | 6. Easy |

Rationale: Results of diagnostic studies are helpful to physicians for establishing diagnosis and monitoring treatment. The results of these same studies may also be helpful to nurses in evaluating the success of nursing interventions.

13. During the patient interview, the patient's significant other is answering all the questions. The nurse observes the patient attempting to answer but seems unable to do so. The nurse's most appropriate statement would be
    a. "Please let the patient answer her questions. I am sure she is able to answer."
    b. "Let me show you the sitting room, and I'll call you when we are finished."*
    c. "I understand your concern, but I really need to hear what she has to say."
    d. "I don't think you are capable of answering questions about her health."

Reference: p. 239

Descriptors:

| 1. 15 | 2. 08 | 3. Application |
| 4. IV-1 | 5. Nursing Process | 6. Difficult |

Rationale: The nurse should interview the patient alone, either in the patient's room or in a quiet office.

14. The nurse introduces himself to the patient, and informs the patient of the length of the interview. This occurs in the phase termed
    a. introduction*
    b. preparatory
    c. working
    d. termination

Reference: p. 240

Descriptors:

| 1. 15 | 2. 05 | 3. Comprehensive |
| 4. IV-1 | 5. Nursing Process | 6. Easy |

Rationale: The introduction to the interview sets the tone for the interview.

15. During the interview, the patient states, "I have pain in my right knee." To clarify the information the nurse states, "Your pain is in your right knee." This is an example of what communication technique?
    a. silence
    b. blocking
    c. paraphrase*
    d. pause

Reference: p. 240

Descriptors:

| 1. 15 | 2. 08 | 3. Comprehensive |
| 4. IV-1 | 5. Communication | 6. Easy |

Rationale: It is best to use reflection and paraphrase to communicate to the patient that you understand him.

16. The nurse thanks the patient for his cooperation during the interview and highlights the key points. This occurs during the phase termed
    a. introductory
    b. preentry
    c. postinterview
    d. termination*

Reference: p. 241

Descriptors:

| 1. 15 | 2. 08 | 3. Comprehensive |
| 4. I-1 | 5. Communication | 6. Easy |

Rationale: The nurse should thank the patient during the termination phase.

17. The physical assessment performed by the nurse focuses on the patient's
    a. neurologic deficits
    b. medical history
    c. functional abilities*
    d. pathologic conditions

Reference: p. 242

Descriptors:

| 1. 15 | 2. 08 | 3. Knowledge |
| 4. IV-1 | 5. Nursing Process | 6. Easy |

Rationale: The nursing physical assessment focuses primarily on the patient's functional abilities.

18. The nurse gathers data about the patient's left arm pain. This is an example of a/an
    a. initial assessment
    b. focused assessment*
    c. emergency assessment
    d. evaluative assessment

Reference: p. 243

Descriptors:

| 1. 15 | 2. 12 | 3. Application |
| 4. IV-1 | 5. Nursing Process | 6. Moderate |

Rationale: In a focused assessment, the nurse gathers data about a specific problem that has already been identified.

19. A 5-month-old infant is admitted with lethargy and failure to thrive. The most important assessment to make is the baby's
a. length
b. pupil reaction
c. weight*
d. fontanelle size

Reference: p. 244

Descriptors:

| 1. 15 | 2. 11 | 3. Application |
| 4. IV-3 | 5. Nursing Process | 6. Difficult |

Rationale: If failure to thrive is suspected, it is most important to assess the weight accurately. Nursing assessments are modified according to the developmental needs of the patient.

20. Structuring the assessment data allows for
a. comprehensive data collection*
b. limitation of data collected
c. nursing care development
d. evaluation of interventions

Reference: p. 246

Descriptors:

| 1. 15 | 2. 11 | 3. Knowledge |
| 4. I-1 | 5. Nursing Process | 6. Moderate |

Rationale: Structuring assessment data systematically ensures that comprehensive holistic data are collected for each patient and lead to the formulation of nursing diagnosis.

21. Data that may need validation include
a. confirmed reports when data are retrieved
b. suspicious findings or observations*
c. supporting data from previous findings
d. patient or family member reports of findings

Reference: p. 249

Descriptors:

| 1. 15 | 2. 10 | 3. Application |
| 4. None | 5. Nursing Process | 6. Easy |

Rationale: Suspicious findings or observations need validation.

22. Which of the following findings is significant and requires immediate communication to the patient's physician?
a. weight loss of 3 ounces in an 8-pound infant at 24 hours of age
b. diminished breath sounds in a patient diagnosed with pneumonia*
c. patient response to a newly ordered pain medication
d. patient's request for husband to stay with her in the room

Reference: p. 250

Descriptors:

| 1. 15 | 2. 12 | 3. Application |
| 4. IV-3 | 5. Communication | 6. Moderate |

Rationale: Diminished breath sounds in a patient diagnosed with pneumonia is an important finding because the patient could experience respiratory arrest.

CHAPTER 16

Diagnosing

1. Based on the information collected in the database, the nurse identifies the patient's
   a. correct medical diagnosis to plan care
   b. actual or potential health problems*
   c. health promotion diagnoses only
   d. interventions to assist the patient

   Reference: p. 254

   Descriptors:

1. 16	2. 02	3. Knowledge
4. I-1	5. Nursing Process	6. Easy

   Rationale: After the nurse has collected and recorded the patient data, the work of diagnosing begins with the identification of actual or potential health problems.

2. A condition that necessitates intervening to prevent or resolve disease/illness or to promote coping and wellness is termed a
   a. health problem*
   b. disease process
   c. communicable illness
   d. infectious disease

   Reference: p. 254

   Descriptors:

1. 16	2. 01	3. Knowledge
4. I-1	5. Nursing Process	6. Easy

   Rationale: A health problem is a condition that necessitates intervening to prevent or resolve disease or illness or to promote coping or wellness.

3. Nursing diagnoses are written to describe patient problems that nurses can treat
   a. dependently
   b. interdependently
   c. independently*
   d. collaboratively

   Reference: p. 255

   Descriptors:

1. 16	2. 02	3. Knowledge
4. I-1	5. Nursing Process	6. Easy

   Rationale: Nursing diagnoses are written to describe patient problems that nurses can treat independently.

4. Medical diagnoses identify
   a. disease*
   b. promotion
   c. prevention
   d. prescription

   Reference: p. 255

   Descriptors:

1. 16	2. 02	3. Knowledge
4. None	5. None	6. Easy

   Rationale: Physicians diagnose disease processes; nurses describe patient problems that are treated by nurses.

5. Physiologic complications that nurses monitor to detect onset or changes in status are defined as
   a. medical diagnoses
   b. nursing diagnoses
   c. problem interventions
   d. collaborative problems*

   Reference: p. 255

   Descriptors:

1. 16	2. 01	3. Knowledge
4. IV-3	5. Nursing Process	6. Moderate

   Rationale: Nurses manage collaborative problems using physician-prescribed and nursing-prescribed interventions to minimize complications.

6. A 68-year-old woman has loss of elasticity of the skin, edema, redness, and an open wound measuring 2.5 cm. According to data interpretation, what do these symptoms indicate?
   a. cues to the nurse*
   b. no significance at this time
   c. a physician is required
   d. a dermatologist should be called

   Reference: p. 256

   Descriptors:

1. 16	2. 03	3. Application
4. IV-1	5. Nursing Process	6. Moderate

   Rationale: The term "cue" is often used to denote significant data or data that influence this analysis.

7. The grouping of data that point to the existence of a significant health problem is termed
   a. diagnosis
   b. clustering*
   c. cue
   d. analysis

   Reference: p. 257

   Descriptors:

1. 16	2. 03	3. Knowledge
4. I-1	5. Nursing Process	6. Moderate

   Rationale: A data cluster is a grouping of patient data or cues that points to the existence of a patient problem.

8. The purpose of the problem statement is the
   a. diagnosis of a medical condition
   b. evaluation of the care provided
   c. implementation of nursing care
   d. description of patient health problems*

   Reference: p. 259

   Descriptors:

1. 16	2. 04	3. Knowledge
4. I-1	5. Nursing Process	6. Moderate

   Rationale: The problem statement identifies what is unhealthy about the patient. The problem statement describes the health state or health problem clearly and concisely.

9. Advantages to using the NANDA-approved list of nursing diagnoses include
   a. promoting the use of an exclusive nursing language
   b. allowing nurses to use computer-based programs
   c. facilitating and disseminating research findings*
   d. assisting in the organized nursing care of patients

   Reference: p. 259

   Descriptors:

1. 16	2. 05	3. Application
4. I-1	5. Nursing Process	6. Moderate

   Rationale: One of the advantages to using NANDA-approved nursing diagnoses is the facilitation and dissemination of nursing research findings.

10. The component of the nursing diagnosis that directs the nursing interventions is termed the
    a. problem
    b. characteristics
    c. etiology*
    d. rationale

    Reference: p. 260

    Descriptors:

1. 16	2. 05	3. Knowledge
4. I-1	5. Nursing Process	6. Easy

    Rationale: The etiology is the cause or contributing factor. The interventions will be developed and directed at the etiology.

11. Defining characteristics that are included in the nursing diagnosis should
    a. precede the problem statement
    b. include treatment plans
    c. follow the etiology statement*
    d. indicate unhealthy symptoms

    Reference: p. 260

    Descriptors:

1. 16	2. 05	3. Knowledge
4. I-1	5. Nursing Process	6. Moderate

    Rationale: Defining characteristics, when included in the nursing diagnosis, should follow the etiology statement and be linked by the phrase "as manifested by" or "as evidenced by."

12. Of the following nursing diagnoses, which is worded incorrectly?
    a. Fluid Volume Excess related to edema of the lower extremities
    b. Constipation related to reduced fiber intake
    c. Stress Incontinence related to cancer of the bladder*
    d. Impaired Skin Integrity related to pressure on coccyx

Reference: p. 260

Descriptors:

1. 16	2. 05	3. Application
4. I-1	5. Nursing Process	6. Difficult

Rationale: Stress Incontinence related to cancer of the bladder contains a medical diagnosis at the etiology of the problem. The use of medical diagnosis is improper in the development of the nursing diagnosis.

13. Which of the following is considered a NANDA-approved nursing diagnosis?
    a. Powerlessness*
    b. Congestive heart failure
    c. Skin breakdown
    d. Dermatitis

Reference: p. 261

Descriptors:

1. 16	2. 01, 02	3. Knowledge
4. I-1	5. Nursing Process	6. Moderate

Rationale: A NANDA-approved diagnosis is a problem that nurses can treat. Powerlessness is a NANDA-approved diagnosis. The others are medical diagnoses.

14. A clinical judgment that the individual, family, or community is more vulnerable to develop a problem is a/an
    a. possible problem
    b. diagnosed need
    c. potential problem*
    d. actual problem

Reference: p. 263

Descriptors:

1. 16	2. 05	3. Knowledge
4. IV-3	5. Nursing Process	6. Moderate

Rationale: A risk nursing diagnosis is a clinical judgment that an individual, family, or community is more vulnerable to develop the problem than others in the same situation.

15. A clinical judgment about an individual, family, or community in transition from a specific level of wellness to a higher level of wellness is termed the
    a. actual problem
    b. potential diagnosis
    c. possible problem
    d. wellness diagnosis*

Reference: p. 265

Descriptors:

1. 16	2. 05	3. Knowledge
4. I-1	5. Nursing Process	6. Easy

Rationale: The inclusion of a wellness diagnosis acknowledges the importance of the use of nursing diagnoses for healthy patients.

16. Validation of derived nursing diagnoses can be done by
    a. noting when a pattern emerges from the database*
    b. determining that a review is not consistent with the defining characteristics
    c. ascertaining if the diagnosis is amenable to medical treatment
    d. asking other nurses to verify the data about the patient

Reference: p. 265

Descriptors:

1. 16	2. 05	3. Application
4. I-1	5. Nursing Process	6. Easy

Rationale: Noting when a pattern emerges from the database validates the diagnosis.

17. The major advantage of the nursing diagnosis is the
    a. ability to individualize each plan of care*
    b. lack of an acceptable patient taxonomy
    c. ability to apply care plans to all patients
    d. lack of input from patients in development

Reference: pp. 265–266

Descriptors:

1. 16	2. 06	3. Comprehensive
4. I-1	5. Nursing Process	6. Difficult

Rationale: The nursing diagnosis allows for every patient an individualized plan of care.

18. A young woman is crying after an encounter with a coworker. The occupational health nurse sees the patient and assumes she has "Defensive Coping." This is an example of
    a. negligence
    b. misdiagnosis*
    c. incompetence
    d. inexperience

Reference: p. 266

Descriptors:

1. 16	2. 06	3. Comprehensive
4. IV-1	5. Nursing Process	6. Difficult

Rationale: Nurses must implement adequate assessments to avoid misdiagnosing patients' health problems.

19. Ways to lessen the limitations of NANDA-approved nursing diagnoses include
    a. ensuring that the patient and family are not aware of the diagnoses
    b. using the nursing diagnoses in conjunction with the medical plan of care
    c. identifying patients who fit under the same level of diagnoses
    d. instituting great care in decreasing cultural misinterpretations of the diagnoses*

Reference: p. 267

Descriptors:

1. 16	2. 07	3. Application
4. I-1	5. Culture	6. Moderate

Rationale: Ways to lessen the limitations of NANDA-approved nursing diagnoses include instituting great care in decreasing cultural misinterpretations of the diagnoses. There is some criticism that cultural aspects of a patient are not considered when nurses formulate nursing diagnoses.

CHAPTER 17

Planning

1. The expected patient outcome in the nursing care plan is the
   a. goal*
   b. diagnosis
   c. intervention
   d. evaluation

   Reference: p. 270

   Descriptors:

1. 17	2. 01	3. Knowledge
4. I-1	5. Nursing Process	6. Easy

   Rationale: The patient goal is the expected outcome of care.

2. After 3 weeks of rehabilitation a 48-year-old patient is able to ambulate 50 feet without assistance. This is an example of a/an
   a. nursing diagnosis
   b. patient intervention
   c. expected outcome*
   d. nursing assessment

   Reference: p. 270

   Descriptors:

1. 17	2. 01	3. Application
4. IV-1	5. Nursing Process	6. Difficult

   Rationale: An expected outcome is the measurable criterion used to evaluate the extent to which the goal is met.

3. A nurse is giving a bath to a patient when she is notified that a postoperative patient is vomiting. She quickly makes the first patient comfortable and attends to the postoperative patient. The action by the nurse is considered
   a. formal planning
   b. nursing evaluation
   c. database establishment
   d. informal planning*

   Reference: p. 270

   Descriptors:

1. 17	2. 02	3. Application
4. I-1	5. Nursing Process	6. Moderate

   Rationale: This action by the nurse is considered informal planning because the nurse had to quickly determine what nursing actions were necessary for the patient who was vomiting.

4. The most important purpose of planning care with the patient and other family members is to
   a. individualize patient care*
   b. ensure continuity of care
   c. follow standardized plans of care
   d. provide similar staff for each patient

   Reference: p. 270

   Descriptors:

1. 17	2. 02	3. Application
4. IV-1	5. Nursing Process	6. Moderate

   Rationale: Not all patients are the same, even if they have the same nursing diagnoses. Planning care with the patient and family helps to individualize nursing care.

5. The school nurse instructs junior high school students on smoking prevention. During high school, two-thirds of the students are noted not to smoke. In the planning step of the nursing process this is considered
   a. resolution of health problems
   b. prevention of health problems*
   c. reduction of health problems
   d. negative goal attainment

   Reference: p. 271

   Descriptors:

1. 17	2. 08	3. Application
4. II-1	5. Teach/Learn	6. Difficult

   Rationale: The primary purpose in planning is a positive patient outcome.

6. A hospice nurse caring for a terminally ill patient will provide
   a. ongoing problem-oriented planning*
   b. initial problem-oriented planning
   c. assessment problem-oriented planning
   d. discharge problem-oriented planning

   Reference: p. 271

   Descriptors:

1. 17	2. 03	3. Application
4. III-1	5. Caring	6. Moderate

   Rationale: Hospice nurses use ongoing problem-oriented planning.

7. A local hospital has developed standardized care plans. It is important that the nurse providing care
   a. assess the need for the nursing care plan
   b. evaluate the effectiveness of the nursing plan
   c. individualize the plan to meet patient needs*
   d. reject the standardized plan and develop a new one

   Reference: p. 272

   Descriptors:

1. 17	2. 01	3. Comprehensive
4. IV-1	5. Nursing Process	6. Easy

   Rationale: Standardized care plans provide an excellent basis for the initial plan if the nurse individualizes them.

8. The nurse who uses Maslow's hierarchy of needs would indicate which of the following nursing diagnoses is a priority?
   a. Ineffective Coping
   b. Ineffective Breathing Pattern*
   c. Risk for Grief
   d. Alteration in Comfort

   Reference: p. 272

   Descriptors:

1. 17	2. 06	3. Application
4. IV-1	5. Nursing Process	6. Easy

   Rationale: Using Maslow's hierarchy, physiologic needs such as Ineffective Breathing Pattern take priority over other needs.

9. A 43-year-old mother of two has been hospitalized for vertigo and dehydration. The nurse notes that the woman's 14-year-old daughter is anxious about her mother's condition. After caring for the woman she speaks to the daughter and provides reassurance. This is an example of a/an
   a. initial plan
   b. ongoing plan*
   c. assessment plan
   d. discharge plan

   Reference: p. 272

   Descriptors:

1. 17	2. 03	3. Application
4. III-2	5. Nursing Process	6. Difficult

   Rationale: Ongoing planning is problem oriented and is carried out by any nurse who interacts with the patient.

10. A 48-year-old business man is required to travel because of his job. He complains of constipation and anxiety over the separation from his family. In planning his nursing care, the nurse's priority is to address the patient's
    a. physiologic needs*
    b. safety needs
    c. love and belonging needs
    d. self-esteem needs

    Reference: p. 272

    Descriptors:

1. 17	2. 04	3. Application
4. III-1	5. Nursing Process	6. Moderate

    Rationale: In the establishment of the nursing care plan and inherent goal development the nurse must apply Maslow's hierarchy of human needs.

11. Of the following nursing actions, which would have the highest priority?
    a. offering the patient 30 mL of juice between meals
    b. suctioning when signs of dyspnea appear*
    c. ambulating the patient in the hallway 3 times per day
    d. performing active range of motion exercises twice a day

    Reference: p. 272

    Descriptors:

1. 17	2. 04	3. Comprehensive
4. IV-3	5. Nursing Process	6. Moderate

    Rationale: The patient's breathing takes priority over other problems. Suctioning when signs of dyspnea appear is the priority action.

12. Nursing goals are derived from the
    a. problem statement of the nursing diagnosis*
    b. etiology statement of the nursing diagnosis
    c. manifestation of the nursing diagnosis
    d. independent of the nursing diagnosis

Reference: p. 273

Descriptors:

1. 17	2. 05	3. Knowledge
4. I-1	5. Nursing Process	6. Easy

Rationale: Goals are derived from the problem statement of the nursing diagnosis.

13. The patient will have complete healing of the decubitus ulcer on his coccyx within 1 month. This is considered a/an
    a. short-term goal
    b. long-term goal*
    c. achieved etiology
    d. nursing evaluation

Reference: p. 273

Descriptors:

1. 17	2. 06	3. Comprehensive
4. IV-3	5. Nursing Process	6. Easy

Rationale: The long-term goal reflects the desired result for the patient.

14. The patient and nurse are developing the nursing care plan related to the education of the patient on colostomy care. This is an example of
    a. physiologic goals
    b. psychomotor goals
    c. cognitive goals*
    d. affective goals

Reference: p. 273

Descriptors:

1. 17	2. 06	3. Application
4. IV-1	5. Teach/Learn	6. Moderate

Rationale: Cognitive goals describe increases in patient knowledge or intellectual behaviors.

15. The patient will value health promotion activities implemented in her life by 12/06/2002. This goal represents the domain termed
    a. physiologic
    b. psychomotor
    c. cognitive
    d. affective*

Reference: p. 273

Descriptors:

1. 17	2. 06	3. Application
4. II-2	5. Self Care	6. Moderate

Rationale: Affective goals describe changes in patient's values, beliefs, and attitudes.

16. The *most* important consideration in goal development is
    a. physician involvement
    b. nursing involvement
    c. patient involvement*
    d. family involvement

Reference: p. 274

Descriptors:

1. 17	2. 08	3. Knowledge
4. I-1	5. Nursing Process	6. Easy

Rationale: The most important person to be involved in goal development with the nurse is the patient, followed by the family.

17. In the development of the patient goal, the nurse must be certain it is
    a. identifiable
    b. medical
    c. measurable*
    d. obtainable

Reference: p. 274

Descriptors:

1. 17	2. 08	3. Knowledge
4. I-1	5. Nursing Process	6. Easy

Rationale: The nurse must be certain that the goal is measurable to be properly written.

18. Which of the following is an example of a patient goal for the nursing diagnosis "Alteration in Comfort related to abdominal surgery pain and immobility"? Within the next 4 hours, the patient will
    a. be able to perform relaxation exercises*
    b. have his prescribed pain medication administered
    c. do passive range-of-motion exercises in the bed
    d. have a visit from his wife and adult children

Reference: p. 274

Descriptors:

1. 17	2. 05, 06	3. Application
4. I-1	5. Nursing Process	6. Moderate

Rationale: The patient goal should be measurable. The best goal is that the patient will be able to perform relaxation exercises, which should help the patient better tolerate the pain.

19. Nurse-initiated interventions are directed at the
    a. problem statement of the nursing diagnosis
    b. etiology statement of the nursing diagnosis*
    c. manifestation statement of the nursing diagnosis
    d. independent of the nursing diagnosis

Reference: p. 275

Descriptors:

1. 17	2. 07	3. Knowledge
4. IV-1	5. Nursing Process	6. Moderate

Rationale: The etiology statement of the nursing diagnosis suggests the appropriate nurse-initiated interventions.

20. Nursing interventions assist the
    a. physician in provision of orders
    b. physical therapist in goal development
    c. patient to meet specific goals/outcomes*
    d. development of a nursing diagnosis

Reference: p. 276

Descriptors:

1. 17	2. 07	3. Knowledge
4. IV-1	5. Nursing Process	6. Easy

Rationale: Nursing interventions assist the patient to meet specific goals/outcomes that are related directly to one goal/outcome.

21. The most effective plan of care for a patient with severe pain following chest surgery is for the nurse to
    a. assess the quality of the patient's pain
    b. administer the pain medication as ordered
    c. encourage the patient to ambulate before the medication is given
    d. give the patient a backrub 30 minutes before bedtime*

Reference: p. 276

Descriptors:

1. 17	2. 01, 04	3. Application
4. IV-1	5. Nursing Process	6. Moderate

Rationale: Although the pain medication is important, it may not be working for this patient for a number of reasons. A backrub prior to the patient's bedtime should help the patient relax.

22. When selecting appropriate nursing interventions to help achieve a patient goal, which of the following statements is true?
    a. Task oriented interventions are best for optimal care.
    b. Communication skills are helpful only for psychological concerns.
    c. Individualization is necessary for optimal care.*
    d. Only by involving significant others can the patient's goal be met.

Reference: p. 276

Descriptors:

1. 17	2. 07	3. Application
4. I-1	5. Nursing Process	6. Moderate

Rationale: Individualization is necessary and may require a number of nursing interventions to achieve the goal.

23. The nurse will instruct the patient with every dressing change to the right foot, the procedure to cleanse the wound with soap and water, and apply a dry sterile dressing. This is an example of a nursing
    a. evaluation
    b. procedure
    c. assessment
    d. intervention*

Reference: p. 277

Descriptors:

1. 17	2. 07	3. Application
4. IV-1	5. Nursing Process	6. Moderate

Rationale: A properly worded nursing intervention will provide for continuity of care and goal attainment.

24. Nursing intervention that involves medication administration is a/an
    a. collaboratively initiated intervention
    b. independently initiated intervention
    c. physician-initiated intervention*
    d. nurse-initiated intervention

Reference: p. 277

Descriptors:

1. 17	2. 07	3. Comprehensive
4. IV-2	5. Nursing Process	6. Moderate

Rationale: A physician-initiated intervention is an intervention initiated by a physician in response to a medical diagnosis but carried out by the nurse in response to a doctor's order.

25. In providing care to a 70-year-old woman who is overweight with severe arthritic pain and immobility, the nurse determines the need for nutrition education for the patient. The nurse should consult with the
    a. physician
    b. dietitian*
    c. physical therapist
    d. clinical nurse specialist

Reference: p. 277

Descriptors:

1. 17	2. 07	3. Application
4. IV-3	5. Teach/Learn	6. Moderate

Rationale: To provide thorough nursing care the nurse may consult with other healthcare professionals. In regard to nutrition the dietitian or nutritionist will provide the most knowledgeable expertise.

CHAPTER 18

Implementing

1. The nurse assists the patient in the achievement of healthcare goals during
   a. assessment
   b. evaluation
   c. planning
   d. implementation*

   Reference: p. 290

   Descriptors:

   1. 18   2. 01   3. Knowledge
   4. I-1   5. Nursing Process 6. Easy

   Rationale: The purpose of implementation is to assist the patient in achieving desired health goals: promote wellness, prevent disease and illness, restore health, and facilitate coping with altered functioning.

2. Who is legally accountable in nurse-initiated interventions?
   a. nurse*
   b. physician
   c. hospital
   d. administrator

   Reference: p. 290

   Descriptors:

   1. 18   2. 02   3. Knowledge
   4. I-1   5. Nursing Process 6. Easy

   Rationale: Nurses are legally responsible for assessments and nursing responses.

3. A physician orders morphine 10 mg intramuscular injection for a postoperative patient. Following administration of the injection, which of the following interventions is most appropriate? The nurse should
   a. call the physician and report its response
   b. assess the patient's reaction to the medication*
   c. place the bedpan near the patient's side
   d. keep the side rails down so the patient can ambulate

   Reference: p. 290

   Descriptors:

   1. 18   2. 02   3. Application
   4. IV-2   5. Nursing Process 6. Moderate

   Rationale: The nurse is legally responsible to assess the patient's reactions to all physician-initiated interventions, for example, medications.

4. A rehabilitation division participates in rounds on their patients every day. Those who are present include the patient, family, physical therapist, occupational therapist, and physiatrist. During rounds they determine that the patient should ambulate 50 feet with the assistance of one person beginning tomorrow. This constitutes a/an
   a. patient-initiated intervention
   b. collaboratively initiated intervention*
   c. physician-initiated intervention
   d. nurse-initiated intervention

   Reference: p. 290

   Descriptors:

   1. 18   2. 02   3. Application
   4. IV-3   5. Nursing Process 6. Moderate

   Rationale: Collaborative interventions are interdependent nursing interventions performed jointly by nurses and other members of the healthcare team.

5. When the nurse administers a prescribed intravenous solution to a patient, this type of intervention is termed
   a. independent
   b. physician initiated*
   c. nurse initiated
   d. collaborative

   Reference: p. 290

   Descriptors:

   1. 18   2. 01, 02   3. Application
   4. IV-2   5. Nursing Process 6. Easy

   Rationale: Administration of a prescribed intravenous solution to a patient is termed a physician-initiated nursing intervention.

6. The withholding of a medication of a patient due to a severe allergic reaction to the previous dose is a type of intervention termed
   a. dependent
   b. physician initiated
   c. collaborative
   d. nurse initiated*

   Reference: p. 290

   Descriptors:

1. 18	2. 01, 02	3. Application
4. IV-2	5. Nursing Process	6. Moderate

   Rationale: The withholding of a medication of a patient due to a severe allergic reaction to the previous dose is a type of intervention termed nurse initiated. The nurse should notify the physician of the intervention and seek additional orders.

7. Creating an environment in which the patient can commit energies toward rehabilitation and health promotion are implemented in the
   a. nurse–patient relationship*
   b. nurse–patient–family relationship
   c. nurse–nurse relationship
   d. nurse–healthcare team relationship

   Reference: p. 291

   Descriptors:

1. 18	2. 03	3. Comprehensive
4. IV-3	5. Nursing Process	6. Easy

   Rationale: Nurse–patient interventions provide a repertoire of therapeutic interpersonal behaviors to establish a trusting relationship with the patient.

8. In regard to insurance guidelines, the Nursing Interventions Taxonomy Structure, ensures
   a. continuity of care
   b. nursing reimbursement*
   c. evaluation of care
   d. nursing knowledge

   Reference: p. 291

   Descriptors:

1. 18	2. 03	3. Knowledge
4. I-1	5. Nursing Process	6. Moderate

   Rationale: The Nursing Interventions Taxonomy Structure ensures appropriate reimbursement for nursing services.

9. The liver function laboratory results for a 60-year-old male patient have been received on the floor. The results are noted to be abnormal. It is important for the nurse to
   a. place the results in the chart
   b. inform the patient of results
   c. call results to the physician*
   d. repeat the liver function test

   Reference: p. 292

   Descriptors:

1. 18	2. 04	3. Application
4. IV-3	5. Nursing Process	6. Moderate

   Rationale: It is the responsibility of the nurse to notify the physician of all pertinent medical information.

10. Standing orders include all of the following *except*
    a. surgical explanation*
    b. overdose agents
    c. bowel preparations
    d. dietary guidelines

    Reference: p. 292

    Descriptors:

1. 18	2. 01	3. Comprehensive
4. I-1	5. Nursing Process	6. Difficult

    Rationale: It is the responsibility of the physician to explain a surgical procedure with its risks and benefits. The nurse may witness the patient's signature on the consent form.

11. Two physicians caring for a 70-year-old patient with nephrotic syndrome write conflicting orders. The nurse notifies the physicians and the orders are changed. In this role, the nurse is the
    a. evaluator
    b. coordinator*
    c. assessor
    d. planner

    Reference: p. 292

    Descriptors:

1. 18	2. 05	3. Application
4. I-1	5. Nursing Process	6. Moderate

    Rationale: The nurse becomes the coordinator of the patient's care, and must stay abreast of the services and orders from all members of the healthcare team.

12. A home health nurse is visiting an 85-year-old woman who has had a cerebrovascular accident (stroke) with left-side paralysis. To assist with home maintenance the nurse must
   a. make daily visits to administer the patient's medication
   b. assess the patient's vital signs and neurologic function
   c. suggest ways to make the home structurally accessible*
   d. make arrangements for daily meals on wheels

   Reference: p. 293

   Descriptors:

1. 18	2. 04	3. Application
4. IV-3	5. Self-Care	6. Moderate

   Rationale: The Nursing Intervention Classification can be used to implement care for a patient and family who require assistance to maintain the home as a clean, safe, structurally accessible, and pleasant place.

13. What is the most appropriate intervention to implement when a child diagnosed with leukemia is preparing for discharge? The nurse should
   a. assess the home for accessibility
   b. educate the parents in all aspects of care*
   c. contact the Make-A-Wish Foundation
   d. assess the caregivers financial status

   Reference: p. 293

   Descriptors:

1. 18	2. 06	3. Application
4. I-1	5. Teach/Learn	6. Moderate

   Rationale: Nurses must be sensitive to the importance of the parent's learning to direct and manage all aspects of their child's care.

14. While instructing a patient about his care, the patient says to you, "I don't understand how the Jobst sleeve will help the swelling in my arm." It is important for the nurse to
   a. proceed with teaching, then answer any questions
   b. give the patient a brochure and let him read it
   c. stop teaching, and answer the question asked*
   d. provide the patient with the pathophysiology

   Reference: p. 293

   Descriptors:

1. 18	2. 07	3. Application
4. IV-3	5. Teach/Learn	6. Difficult

   Rationale: Timing is very important in patient education. The nurse should revise the plan of care to meet patient needs and stop teaching and answer the questions before continuing further.

15. Critical thinking skills that assist the nurse in appropriately setting care priorities are a type of nursing skill termed
   a. technical
   b. interpersonal
   c. cognitive*
   d. behavioral

   Reference: p. 293

   Descriptors:

1. 18	2. 05	3. Knowledge
4. None	5. None	6. Moderate

   Rationale: Critical thinking skills that assist the nurse in appropriately setting care priorities are a type of nursing skill termed cognitive.

16. During the patient's dressing change the patient's daughter asks for an explanation of the dressing change. What intervention should the nurse implement?
   a. Answer the daughter's question and assess the information needed.*
   b. Ask the daughter if she intends to care for the patient at home.
   c. Ignore the daughter's request and continue with the dressing change.
   d. Assess if the daughter has any experience with dressing changes.

   Reference: p. 293

   Descriptors:

1. 18	2. 07	3. Application
4. IV-3	5. Teach/Learn	6. Moderate

   Rationale: Provide all the information regarding patient care that the patient and family are requesting.

17. During a home visit, a 66-year-old male cancer patient seems very quiet and his eyes are downcast. When asked by the nurse if anything was bothering him, he stated, "I now have cancer in the bone. I don't know what decisions to make." In this situation, what is the nurse's best response?
    a. "Has the doctor told you about any treatment?"
    b. "Are you going back into the hospital?"
    c. "Have you spoken with any family members?"*
    d. "How do you feel about your diagnosis?"

    Reference: p. 300

    Descriptors:

    1. 18   2. 07   3. Application
    4. III-1   5. Communication   6. Difficult

    Rationale: In this scenario it is important to ascertain the support on whom the patient can rely during this period. Through the use of the focused question the nurse can assess areas of patient support.

18. What nursing intervention can be implemented to enhance the well-being of the nurse? The nurse should
    a. have wine with dinner
    b. remain at home nightly
    c. not speak with colleagues
    d. implement stress-relief measures*

    Reference: p. 300

    Descriptors:

    1. 18   2. 07   3. Application
    4. I-1   5. Caring   6. Easy

    Rationale: To adequately prepare for professional practice nurses should practice psychological care interventions.

19. The staff member who is an unlicensed assistive personnel (UAP) has been assigned by the charge nurse to give an enema to a 72-year-old woman who has an impaction. The nurse assessed the patient's blood pressure and determined it was 92/60. The nurse should
    a. allow the UAP to administer the enema as ordered
    b. call the doctor to rescind the order for the enema
    c. administer the enema, with frequent assessments*
    d. wait an hour then have the UAP give the enema

    Reference: p. 299

    Descriptors:

    1. 18   2. 04   3. Application
    4. IV-3   5. Nursing Process   6. Moderate

    Rationale: Because the nurse is legally responsible for all the care given by UAP, it is important to delegate tasks the UAP is capable of performing. Because the patient's blood pressure is low, and an enema can cause further hypotension, the nurse should not delegate this task.

20. The primary purpose of ongoing data collection in nursing care planning is to
    a. determine if a previous intervention solved the problem
    b. revise and update the nursing care plan as necessary*
    c. develop a comprehensive, researchable database
    d. ensure data collection from all relevant sources

    Reference: p. 300

    Descriptors:

    1. 18   2. 07   3. Application
    4. I-1   5. Nursing Process   6. Moderate

    Rationale: The primary purpose of ongoing data collection in nursing care planning is to revise and update the nursing care plan as necessary.

CHAPTER 19

Evaluating

1. Determination by the patient and the nurse on how well the patient goals were achieved is termed
   a. assessment
   b. planning
   c. implementation
   d. evaluation*

   Reference: p. 304

   Descriptors:

   1. 19   2. 01   3. Knowledge
   4. I-1   5. Nursing Process   6. Easy

   Rationale: The evaluation stage of the nursing process constitutes the determination of how well the patient goals were achieved.

2. A patient being cared for at home has a wound on her coccyx. The goal established stated that the wound would be healed in 1 month. After 1 month, the wound is half its previous size. Based on this information the
   a. goal is met
   b. goal is unmet*
   c. goal is unattainable
   d. intervention is met

   Reference: p. 304

   Descriptors:

   1. 19   2. 02   3. Application
   4. IV-4   5. Nursing Process   6. Moderate

   Rationale: If the goals of the nursing care plan are unmet, then the plan should be reevaluated and modified.

3. When the goal is unmet the nurse may need to modify the
   a. assessments
   b. diagnoses
   c. interventions*
   d. evaluations

   Reference: p. 304

   Descriptors:

   1. 19   2. 02   3. Application
   4. I-1   5. Nursing Process   6. Moderate

   Rationale: For the goal to be achieved, alternative nursing interventions may need to be implemented.

4. In the evaluation phase of the nursing process, the nurse should decide whether the
   a. medical interventions have been carried out
   b. goals have been prioritized with the patient
   c. assessments have been completed accurately
   d. patient goals have been achieved or unmet*

   Reference: p. 304

   Descriptors:

   1. 19   2. 01, 02   3. Application
   4. I-1   5. Nursing Process   6. Moderate

   Rationale: In the evaluation phase of the nursing process, the nurse should decide whether the patient goals have been achieved or unmet.

5. A 55-year-old woman is in her first postoperative day following a hysterectomy. The nurse would like her to sit up in the chair for 30 minutes then return to bed. After the patient was up for 10 minutes she became nauseated and dizzy and returned to bed. In this scenario the expected outcome was for the patient to
   a. sit up for 10 minutes
   b. experience dizziness
   c. abstain from vomiting
   d. sit up for 30 minutes*

   Reference: p. 304

   Descriptors:

   1. 19   2. 02   3. Application
   4. IV-3   5. Nursing Process   6. Moderate

   Rationale: The nurse must provide ongoing assessment and evaluation to determine if the expected outcome is met.

6. The measurable qualities for which nursing care is evaluated are defined as
   a. standard
   b. outcome
   c. criteria*
   d. intervention
   Reference: p. 305
   Descriptors:

1. 19	2. 01	3. Knowledge
4. None	5. None	6. Easy

   Rationale: Criteria are measurable qualities, attributes, or characteristics that specify skills, knowledge, or health states.

7. The level of performance accepted and expected by the nursing staff or other health team members is defined as
   a. standard*
   b. outcome
   c. criteria
   d. intervention
   Reference: p. 305
   Descriptors:

1. 19	2. 01	3. Knowledge
4. None	5. None	6. Easy

   Rationale: Standards are the levels of performance accepted and expected by the nursing staff or other health team members.

8. The nurse and patient have established a goal, which states, "The patient will properly draw up and administer his insulin within 3 days." This is an example of a goal termed
   a. cognitive
   b. psychomotor*
   c. affective
   d. task oriented
   Reference: p. 305
   Descriptors:

1. 19	2. 03	3. Application
4. IV-2	5. Teach/Learn	6. Moderate

   Rationale: Psychomotor goals describe the patient's achievement of new skills.

9. Psychomotor skills are best evaluated by
   a. asking the patient to describe the skill
   b. asking the patient to assess the outcome
   c. allowing the patient to verbalize the need
   d. assessing the patient's skill demonstration*
   Reference: p. 305
   Descriptors:

1. 19	2. 03	3. Comprehensive
4. I-1	5. Teach/Learn	6. Moderate

   Rationale: Evaluation of psychomotor skills occurs through assessment of the patient's demonstration of the skill.

10. A common mistake made in the acute care setting regarding the evaluation of outcome criteria is
    a. determining care provided during the patient discharge
    b. determining outcome achievement during discharge*
    c. developing unattainable patient goals at admission
    d. having the patient goals fail to resolve the nursing diagnosis
    Reference: p. 306
    Descriptors:

1. 19	2. 04	3. Knowledge
4. I-1	5. Nursing Process	6. Moderate

    Rationale: The most common mistake nurses make in evaluation in acute care settings is waiting until the day the patient is to be discharged before evaluating goal/outcome achievement.

11. A patient with diabetes is unable to draw up the insulin properly by the expected date. Revision of the nursing care plan should include
    a. observing the patient during mealtimes
    b. assessing the patient's visual acuity*
    c. ordering an in-depth learning assessment
    d. asking the physician to change the patient's medication
    Reference: p. 306
    Descriptors:

1. 19	2. 05	3. Application
4. IV-2	5. Nursing Process	6. Difficult

    Rationale: Revision of the nursing care plan should include assessing the patient's visual acuity because this may be the reason for the patient's inability to draw up the medication.

12. A 36-year-old patient has begun a low-fat diet to reduce his cholesterol. The patient currently consumes 150 grams of fat per day. The patient's goal was to eat no more than 60 grams of fat per day. At the end of the week he consumed 70 grams of fat per day. At the evaluative stage it was determined that the goal was
   a. met
   b. unmet
   c. unattainable
   d. partially met*

Reference: p. 306

Descriptors:

1. 19   2. 03   3. Application
4. II-2   5. Self Care   6. Moderate

Rationale: The nurse has three decision options for how goals have been met: met, partially met, and not met. In this case, the goal was partially met.

13. When evaluation reveals that the patient has made little or no progress toward goal/outcome achievement then the nurse should
   a. proceed with the care plan as written
   b. think critically about the nursing plan
   c. reevaluate each nursing process step*
   d. develop a new care plan with the patient

Reference: p. 306

Descriptors:

1. 19   2. 05   3. Application
4. I-1   5. Nursing Process   6. Moderate

Rationale: When reevaluation reveals that the patient has made little or no progress toward goal/outcome achievement, the nurse should attempt to identify the contributing factors pointing to the problems with the plan of care. Then the nurse needs to reevaluate each preceding step of the nursing process.

14. The nurse and patient have developed a nursing care plan with Impaired Physical Mobility related to left hemiparesis as the nursing diagnosis. The patient goal of properly transferring from bed to chair has been attained. The next goal should read
   a. The patient will ambulate 10 feet with a walker in 3 days.*
   b. The nurse will instruct the patient on safe ambulation.
   c. The nurse will observe the patient's ability to ambulate safely.
   d. The patient will exercise with passive and active range of motion.

Reference: p. 306

Descriptors:

1. 19   2. 05   3. Application
4. IV-3   5. Nursing Process   6. Difficult

Rationale: When the plan of care has been attained, it is important to increase the complexity of the goal.

15. Nurses' personal satisfaction of knowing that they are actually making a difference versus merely wishing things were different is termed
   a. adequate staffing
   b. evaluative programs
   c. quality assurance
   d. performance improvement*

Reference: p. 311

Descriptors:

1. 19   2. 06   3. Knowledge
4. I-1   5. Nursing Process   6. Easy

Rationale: Performance improvement includes discovering a problem, planning a strategy, implementing a change, and assessing that change.

16. Quality assurance programs in nursing assist nurses to provide effective care in that they
   a. enable the profession to be accountable to society*
   b. identify values and standards inherent to healthcare
   c. provide equal access to healthcare for all individuals
   d. help contain excessive costs of illness care

Reference: p. 312

Descriptors:

1. 19   2. 06   3. Application
4. I-1   5. Nursing Process   6. Difficult

Rationale: Quality assurance programs in nursing assist nurses to provide effective care in that they enable the nursing profession to be accountable to society through continuous improvements.

17. Maintaining statistics on the number of falls by patients in an institution constitutes
   a. adequate staffing
   b. evaluative programs
   c. quality assurance*
   d. performance improvement

Reference: p. 312

Descriptors:

| 1. 19 | 2. 06 | 3. Comprehensive |
| 4. I-1 | 5. Nursing Process | 6. Moderate |

Rationale: Quality assurance programs enable nursing to be accountable to society for the quality of nursing care. The least number of patient falls in an institution records the adequacy of the nursing care.

18. The seven-step quality assurance program was developed by the
    a. National League for Nursing
    b. American Nurses Association*
    c. World Health Organization
    d. Centers for Disease Control and Prevention

Reference: p. 312

Descriptors:

| 1. 19 | 2. 07 | 3. Knowledge |
| 4. None | 5. None | 6. Easy |

Rationale: The ANA model is used to develop and implement quality assurance nursing programs within institutions.

19. The commitment and approach used to continuously improve every process in every part of the organization defines
    a. quality assurance
    b. quality improvement*
    c. self-evaluation
    d. healthcare reform

Reference: p. 314

Descriptors:

| 1. 19 | 2. 07 | 3. Knowledge |
| 4. I-1 | 5. Nursing Process | 6. Easy |

Rationale: The commitment and approach used to continuously improve every process in every part of an organization, with the intent of meeting and exceeding customer expectations and outcomes, is termed quality improvement.

20. A method of evaluating nursing care that involves reviewing patient records to assess the outcomes of nursing care is termed a nursing
    a. retrospection
    b. documentation
    c. audit*
    d. standard

Reference: p. 315

Descriptors:

| 1. 19 | 2. 07 | 3. Application |
| 4. I-1 | 5. Nursing Process | 6. Moderate |

Rationale: A method of evaluating nursing care that involves reviewing patient records to assess the outcomes of nursing care is termed a nursing audit. Successful audits depend on accurate documentation in the patient's record.

21. A nurse involved in a hospital's quality assurance committee is assigned to telephone recently hospitalized patients at their home and use a postdischarge questionnaire. This nurse is conducting a review termed
    a. concurrent review
    b. mandate summary
    c. focused review
    d. retrospective evaluation*

Reference: p. 312

Descriptors:

| 1. 19 | 2. 06 | 3. Application |
| 4. I-1 | 5. Nursing Process | 6. Moderate |

Rationale: When a nurse is involved in a hospital's quality assurance committee and is assigned to telephone recently hospitalized patients at their home and use a postdischarge questionnaire, this nurse is conducting a review termed retrospective evaluation.

CHAPTER 20

Documenting, Reporting, and Conferring

1. Management information systems are being designed to assist nurses with
   a. documentation*
   b. information
   c. responsibility
   d. assessments
   Reference: p. 318
   Descriptors:

1. 20	2. 01	3. Knowledge
4. I-1	5. Documentation	6. Easy

   Rationale: Management information systems are being designed to assist nurses with documentation. Documentation is the legal record of all patient interactions.

2. The written, legal record of all pertinent interactions with the patient is termed
   a. evaluation
   b. assessment
   c. implementation
   d. documentation*
   Reference: p. 318
   Descriptors:

1. 20	2. 01	3. Knowledge
4. I-1	5. Documentation	6. Easy

   Rationale: Documentation data are used to facilitate patient care, serve as a financial and legal record, help in clinical research, and support decision analysis.

3. The nurse's best defense against negligence is the patient
   a. assessment
   b. care
   c. record*
   d. goals
   Reference: p. 318
   Descriptors:

1. 20	2. 04	3. Comprehensive
4. I-1	5. Documentation	6. Moderate

   Rationale: The patient record is the only permanent legal document that details the nurse's interactions with the patient and is the nurse's best defense if a patient or patient's surrogate alleges nursing negligence.

4. When viewing a patient record, the student nurse must maintain
   a. responsibility
   b. accountability
   c. confidentiality*
   d. punctuality
   Reference: p. 319
   Descriptors:

1. 20	2. 07	3. Knowledge
4. I-1	5. Documentation	6. Easy

   Rationale: All patient information is confidential. The student nurse maintains the same standards of practice as an RN.

5. A nursing student submits a clinical assignment with the patient's name on it. The nursing instructor should remind the student of
   a. patient confidentiality*
   b. patient care
   c. nursing intervention
   d. nursing assessment
   Reference: p. 319
   Descriptors:

1. 20	2. 07	3. Comprehensive
4. I-1	5. Documentation	6. Moderate

   Rationale: The student must assume the responsibility to hold patient information in confidence.

6. A nursing audit is conducted to determine whether the
   a. patient's insurance has been billed
   b. unlicensed personnel have charted
   c. patient's family is represented
   d. quality of care meets standards*

   Reference: p. 319

   Descriptors:

   | 1. 20 | 2. 04 | 3. Comprehensive |
   | 4. I-1 | 5. Documentation | 6. Moderate |

   Rationale: Charts are randomly selected for an audit to ascertain whether the standards of care have been met.

7. Healthcare agencies communicate information from the patient record to insurance companies for the purpose of
   a. reimbursement*
   b. research
   c. education
   d. quality assurance

   Reference: p. 319

   Descriptors:

   | 1. 20 | 2. 04 | 3. Knowledge |
   | 4. None | 5. None | 6. Easy |

   Rationale: Patient records are used to demonstrate to payers that patients received the care for which reimbursement is sought.

8. Based on incident reports filed, it has been determined that the skilled nursing facility has had a number of employee back injuries in the last 6 months. Based on this information, the facility should
   a. discourage patient lifting
   b. instruct on back safety*
   c. research the type of injury
   d. increase employee numbers

   Reference: p. 319

   Descriptors:

   | 1. 20 | 2. 04 | 3. Comprehensive |
   | 4. I-2 | 5. Teach/Learn | 6. Difficult |

   Rationale: Based on the data from the incident reports, the facility should instruct the staff members about back injuries and safety.

9. A method of documentation that groups data according to the personnel who are documenting is termed
   a. source oriented*
   b. problem oriented
   c. charting by exception
   d. focus charting

   Reference: p. 322

   Descriptors:

   | 1. 20 | 2. 05 | 3. Knowledge |
   | 4. I-1 | 5. Documentation | 6. Moderate |

   Rationale: In source-oriented charting the entries are made chronologically with each discipline charting in a separate section.

10. Of the following documented findings, which is *not* an appropriate description of the patient's status?
    a. Lung sounds are clear in all lobes of the lungs.
    b. Bowel sounds are audible in all four quadrants.
    c. The lub, dub sound of the heart is normal.*
    d. Peripheral pulses are palpable at a rate of 70 beats/min.

    Reference: p. 320

    Descriptors:

    | 1. 20 | 2. 06 | 3. Application |
    | 4. I-1 | 5. Documentation | 6. Moderate |

    Rationale: The use of the word normal is not descriptive of the assessment information.

11. The nurse caring for a 76-year-old patient has not charted since the shift began 5 hours ago. The patient begins to complain of chest pain and shortness of breath, and is diaphoretic. Following the administration of emergency medications the patient is to be transferred to the intensive care unit. The nurse is now responsible for charting all the relevant patient information. What might occur regarding documentation?
    a. The nurse will document all information with regard to time and care provided.
    b. The nurse is at risk of missing information based on the changes in his condition.*
    c. The information the nurse has compiled will be easily documented prior to transfer.
    d. During the patient's transfer the nurse will need a coworker to help with charting.

Reference: p. 320
Descriptors:
1. 20   2. 06   3. Application
4. IV-3   5. Documentation 6. Moderate
Rationale: Charting should be completed in a timely manner to prevent the loss of pertinent information.

12. Which of the following nursing documentation entries reflects a potential legal risk?
    a. "Skin pink, warm, dry over bilateral extremities."
    b. "Patient smelled like urine and is really dirty."*
    c. "Patient indicated he is happy to be going home."
    d. "Ambulated in hallway 3X with one assist."

Reference: p. 320
Descriptors:
1. 20   2. 07   3. Application
4. IV-1   5. Documentation 6. Moderate
Rationale: When the nurse documents "Patient smelled like urine and is really dirty" the nurse is writing about a subjective judgment and could be liable in a court of law.

13. Physician's records and notes, nurse's notes, graphic sheets, and laboratory results describe which type of documentation? Medical records termed
    a. source oriented*
    b. case management
    c. problem oriented
    d. focus oriented

Reference: p. 322
Descriptors:
1. 20   2. 05   3. Application
4. I-1   5. Documentation 6. Moderate
Rationale: These types of medical records are termed source oriented because each discipline has a place for documentation.

14. The documentation of the nurse's assessment of a patient's skin condition during the admission process is typically found in which documentation form?
    a. nursing care plan
    b. Kardex
    c. initial nursing assessment*
    d. progress notes

Reference: p. 326
Descriptors:
1. 20   2. 06   3. Application
4. I-1   5. Documentation 6. Moderate
Rationale: The nursing assessment performed during a patient's admission is typically documented in the initial nursing assessment form.

15. In an institution that uses the SOAP method of documentation, the nurse should document the patient's discharge status on the
    a. problem list
    b. final evaluation form
    c. home care referral form
    d. discharge notes*

Reference: p. 326
Descriptors:
1. 20   2. 06   3. Application
4. IV-1   5. Documentation 6. Moderate
Rationale: When using the SOAP format, the discharge summary is written in the discharge notes.

16. In PIE charting
    a. only the significant findings are documented
    b. all healthcare members chart on the same forms
    c. the plan of care is documented on the problem list*
    d. the focus of care is on the patient's concerns

Reference: p. 327
Descriptors:
1. 20   2. 05   3. Knowledge
4. I-1   5. Documentation 6. Easy
Rationale: In PIE charting the care plan is incorporated into the problem list in which problems are identified with numbers.

17. When a patient fails to meet an expected outcome or a planned intervention is not implemented in the case management model, what documentation should be made?
    a. evaluative charting
    b. variance charting*
    c. problematic charting
    d. interpretive charting

Reference: p. 327

Descriptors:

1. 20   2. 05   3. Comprehensive

4. I-1   5. Documentation   6. Moderate

Rationale: The usual format for variance charting is the unexpected event, the cause of the event, actions taken in response to the event, and discharge planning when appropriate.

18. To communicate the patient's plan of care to be implemented, healthcare facilities use
    a. flow sheets
    b. progress notes
    c. narrative notes
    d. Kardex care plans*

Reference: p. 333

Descriptors:

1. 20   2. 01   3. Knowledge

4. I-1   5. Documentation   6. Easy

Rationale: The Kardex care plan provides healthcare providers with information pertinent to patient care.

19. A disadvantage of charting by exception is it
    a. is less helpful for patients with multiple variances
    b. is time consuming and difficult to ascertain problems
    c. does not address preventive/wellness nursing functions*
    d. has no formal care plan to determine care provided

Reference: p. 334

Descriptors:

1. 20   2. 05   3. Comprehensive

4. I-1   5. Documentation   6. Moderate

Rationale: Preventive and wellness-promoting functions of nursing are not documented on this format because they do not address problems.

20. In an intensive care unit, an appropriate method of charting for critically ill patients with multiple problems requiring highly individualized plans of care is the
    a. SOAP format*
    b. case management model
    c. charting by exception
    d. PIE format

Reference: p. 334

Descriptors:

1. 20   2. 05   3. Application

4. I-1   5. Documentation   6. Moderate

Rationale: Patients with multiple problems requiring highly individualized plans of care are best documented using the SOAP format.

21. The nurse for the evening shift notes that a patient's blood pressure medication was not charted as being administered. The nurse should
    a. give the medication
    b. call the day nurse*
    c. notify the physician
    d. take the blood pressure

Reference: p. 337

Descriptors:

1. 20   2. 08   3. Application

4. IV-2   5. Documentation   6. Moderate

Rationale: The nurse should contact the day nurse to determine if the medication was administered.

22. Medicare requires that home health documentation certify that the patient is
    a. ill for 60 days
    b. terminally ill
    c. homebound*
    d. living alone

Reference: p. 337

Descriptors:

1. 20   2. 06   3. Knowledge

4. IV-1   5. Documentation   6. Moderate

Rationale: Medicare requires that the patient is homebound and still needs skilled nursing care.

23. A postoperative patient has saturated his surgical dressing with blood and fluid. The nurse should
    a. change the dressing
    b. call the physician*
    c. increase IV fluids
    d. recheck it in 1 hour

Reference: p. 338

Descriptors:

1. 20   2. 08   3. Comprehensive

4. IV-3   5. Communication   6. Difficult

Rationale: This may be a sign of hemorrhage and warrants calling the physician. When calling the physician the nurse should have all information well documented.

24. Telephone orders must be
   a. lengthy and understandable
   b. cosigned in a set amount of time by the physician*
   c. transcribed in the progress notes by medical records
   d. repeated to the nurse's supervisor

Reference: p. 338

Descriptors:

1. 20   2. 01   3. Knowledge
4. I-1   5. Documentation   6. Moderate

Rationale: Telephone orders must be cosigned by a physician in a set amount of time, usually within 24 hours.

25. To discuss and coordinate patient care with other health team members, the nurse must schedule a
   a. request
   b. referral
   c. nursing rounds
   d. nursing care conference*

Reference: p. 340

Descriptors:

1. 20   2. 01   3. Knowledge
4. I-1   5. Communication   6. Easy

Rationale: Nurses and other healthcare entities confer in groups to plan and coordinate patient care in a nursing care conference.

26. The form used to chart vital signs is termed the
   a. graphic sheet*
   b. progress notes
   c. critical pathway
   d. medical record

Reference: p. 333

Descriptors:

1. 20   2. 01   3. Knowledge
4. I-1   5. Documentation   6. Easy

Rationale: The graphic sheet is to record specific patient variables such as temperature, pulse, respirations, and blood pressure.

27. Which type of report will be given when a nurse arrives on the unit to begin work?
   a. laboratory
   b. change of shift report*
   c. medication history
   d. census of the unit

Reference: p. 338

Descriptors:

1. 20   2. 01   3. Comprehensive
4. I-1   5. Communication   6. Moderate

Rationale: Change of shift report is given by the primary nurse to the replacing nurse for continuing care of the patient.

28. The nurse is employed by a healthcare setting that uses the problem-oriented medical record. The patient states, "I have a sore throat, feel awful, and I think I have a temperature of 102°F." The above data would be classified as
   a. objective
   b. subjective*
   c. factual
   d. assessment

Reference: p. 326

Descriptors:

1. 20   2. 03   3. Comprehensive
4. IV-1   5. Nursing Process   6. Moderate

Rationale: Subjective data are what the patient says and cannot be directly observed by the nurse.

29. Using the case management model for documentation promotes all of the following *except*
   a. collaboration
   b. communication
   c. teamwork among caregivers
   d. time management*

Reference: pp. 322, 334

Descriptors:

1. 20   2. 05   3. Comprehensive
4. I-1   5. Communication   6. Moderate

Rationale: A case management model focuses care on carefully developed outcomes and requires teamwork, communication, and collaboration.

UNIT V

Roles Basic to Nursing Care

CHAPTER 21

Communicator

1. A student nurse is conducting an admission interview with a patient. To maintain the patient's personal space and maximize communication, the nurse should be at a distance from the patient that is approximately
   a. 10–12 inches
   b. 1.5–4 feet*
   c. 5–6 feet
   d. 7–8 feet

   Reference: p. 334

   Descriptors:

1. 21	2. 01	3. Knowledge
4. IV-1	5. Communication	6. Easy

   Rationale: The optimal space for communication with patients is 18 inches to 4 feet.

2. In effective communication, the source sends a message to the receiver. Which of the following describes the process by which reception and comprehension are verified?
   a. noise
   b. feedback*
   c. channel
   d. validation

   Reference: p. 348

   Descriptors:

1. 21	2. 01, 02	3. Knowledge
4. IV-1	5. Communication	6. Moderate

   Rationale: The process by which reception and comprehension are verified is termed feedback.

3. The building block of professional relationships is
   a. therapeutic touch
   b. patient assessment
   c. holistic health
   d. communication skills*

   Reference: p. 348

   Descriptors:

1. 21	2. 02	3. Comprehensive
4. I-1	5. Communication	6. Easy

   Rationale: Communication skills are the building blocks of professional relationships between nurse and patient, nurse and nurse, and nurse and other health team members.

4. The process of sharing information and the process of generating and transmitting meaning is
   a. communication*
   b. answering
   c. conveying
   d. transcribing

   Reference: p. 348

   Descriptors:

1. 21	2. 01	3. Knowledge
4. I-1	5. Communication	6. Easy

   Rationale: Communication is the process of sharing information and the process of generating and transmitting meaning.

5. The nurse caring for the patient is asking how she feels. The nurse is the
   a. encoder*
   b. decoder
   c. receiver
   d. analyzer

   Reference: p. 348

   Descriptors:

1. 21	2. 01	3. Comprehensive
4. I-1	5. Communication	6. Moderate

   Rationale: The source (encoder) prepares and sends to the receiver a message that can be accurately decoded.

6. Feedback in interpersonal communication occurs when the receiver does which of the following? The receiver
   a. evaluates the behavior of the sender
   b. shares one's interpretation of the message with the sender*
   c. listens attentively to the sender's remarks
   d. summarizes the sender's remarks following the interaction

   Reference: p. 348

   Descriptors:

1. 21	2. 02	3. Comprehensive
4. I-1	5. Communication	6. Moderate

   Rationale: Sharing one's interpretation of the message is termed feedback.

7. While communicating with the patient the nurse observes the patient's eyes as downcast. The lack of eye contact is a communication
   a. skill
   b. channel*
   c. expression
   d. outcome

   Reference: p. 348

   Descriptors:

1. 21	2. 02	3. Application
4. I-1	5. Communication	6. Moderate

   Rationale: The channel is the medium, which conveys the message. The nurse needs to interpret the patient's lack of eye contact.

8. The nursing student is preparing for her first day of clinical practice. During her preparation she is telling herself things she will need to accomplish. This is an example of communication termed
   a. interpersonal
   b. extrapersonal
   c. intrapersonal*
   d. organizational

   Reference: p. 349

   Descriptors:

1. 21	2. 01	3. Application
4. I-1	5. Communication	6. Moderate

   Rationale: Intrapersonal communication, or self-talk, is the communication that happens within an individual.

9. The nurse, other healthcare providers, the patient, and the patient's family are involved in a discharge planning meeting. This meeting is an example of communication termed
   a. intrapersonal
   b. interpersonal
   c. organization
   d. small-group*

   Reference: p. 350

   Descriptors:

1. 21	2. 01	3. Application
4. I-1	5. Communication	6. Moderate

   Rationale: Small-group communication occurs when nurses interact with two or more individuals face to face or use a medium like a conference call. To be effective the members must communicate to achieve a goal.

10. Members of groups who focus on changing the admission forms of a healthcare agency are involved in roles termed
    a. evaluative
    b. maintenance
    c. task-oriented*
    d. self-serving

    Reference: p. 350

    Descriptors:

1. 21	2. 01	3. Application
4. I-1	5. Communication	6. Difficult

    Rationale: Task-oriented roles focus on the work to be completed.

11. Within a group, one member states, "I am not going to do the work I need to do for this group. I think the whole job is irrelevant." This member of the group is the
    a. withdrawer
    b. blocker*
    c. tension reliever
    d. coordinator

    Reference: p. 350

    Descriptors:

1. 21	2. 02	3. Application
4. I-1	5. Communication	6. Difficult

    Rationale: The blocker is a self-serving role, which advances the needs of an individual member at the group's expense.

12. A patient states to the nurse that he feels better. However, his facial expression is noted with a grimace. What does this tell you about the patient? The patient's
    a. verbal communication is congruent with his nonverbal communication
    b. nonverbal communication is incongruent with verbal communication*
    c. denial means that he feels uncomfortable with his surroundings
    d. uncomfortable with the doctor and his present course of treatment

    Reference: p. 351

    Descriptors:

    1. 21   2. 08   3. Application
    4. IV-1   5. Communication   6. Difficult

    Rationale: The nurse must assess that the patient's verbal and nonverbal communication are congruent.

13. When a barrier to facilitative communication occurs, the nurse's *first* goal or task is to
    a. identify the purpose of the barrier
    b. recognize that the barrier exists*
    c. change the subject using a facilitative technique
    d. identify the desired alternative response

    Reference: p. 351

    Descriptors:

    1. 21   2. 01   3. Comprehensive
    4. I-1   5. Communication   6. Moderate

    Rationale: The barrier must be identified so facilitative communication can ensue.

14. While talking with a patient, you observe her body posture, facial expressions, and gestures. These behaviors make up what kind of communication?
    a. verbal
    b. perceptual
    c. cultural
    d. nonverbal*

    Reference: p. 351

    Descriptors:

    1. 21   2.03   3. Knowledge
    4. IV-1   5. Communication   6. Easy

    Rationale: Nonverbal communication consists of body posture, movement, and gestures, all communication except what is spoken.

15. Which one of the following behaviors demonstrates that the nurse is receptive to the patient during a discussion?
    a. leaning forward*
    b. staying in the intimate zone
    c. having constant eye contact
    d. maintaining silence

    Reference: p. 352

    Descriptors:

    1. 21   2. 03   3. Comprehensive
    4. IV-1   5. Communication   6. Moderate

    Rationale: Receptive behaviors are leaning forward, at a distance of 1 to 3 feet, and frequent eye contact.

16. A form of nonverbal communication includes
    a. daydreaming about a boyfriend
    b. calling the patient's name
    c. posturing with elbows in front*
    d. validating the patient's comments

    Reference: p. 351

    Descriptors:

    1. 21   2. 03   3. Application
    4. IV-1   5. Communication   6. Easy

    Rationale: Posturing with elbows in front is a form of negative nonverbal communication.

17. Characteristics of an effective group process include all of the following *except*
    a. all group members possess mutual trust
    b. group commitment to decision making is low*
    c. group goals are more important than personal goals
    d. aims and goals are clearly understood by all members

    Reference: p. 351

    Descriptors:

    1. 21   2. 08   3. Application
    4. I-1   5. Communication   6. Easy

    Rationale: When group commitment to decision-making is low, the group will not be effective.

18. A 10-year-old boy is staring into space during his school class. The school nurse determines he is
    a. thinking
    b. bored
    c. inattentive*
    d. confused

Reference: p. 352

Descriptors:

| 1. 21 | 2. 08 | 3. Comprehensive |
| 4. II-1 | 5. Nursing Process | 6. Moderate |

Rationale: A blank stare by a child indicates inattentiveness.

19. A patient is walking with a rigid unsteady gait. This is indicative of
    a. fear*
    b. comfort
    c. encouragement
    d. strength

Reference: p. 352

Descriptors:

| 1. 21 | 2. 08 | 3. Application |
| 4. IV-4 | 5. Nursing Process | 6. Moderate |

Rationale: It is important for the nurse to assess the patient's gait because it is indicative of the patient's physical and emotional status.

20. The nurse enters the room and walks to the patient's bedside to speak with the patient. As the nurse approaches, the patient backs away from the nurse. This is indicative of the patient's
    a. lack of the nurse's trust
    b. fear of the unknown
    c. invasion of territoriality*
    d. inability to communicate

Reference: p. 354

Descriptors:

| 1. 21 | 2. 04 | 3. Comprehensive |
| 4. IV-1 | 5. Communication | 6. Difficult |

Rationale: People are generally more comfortable in areas they claim as their own. In this scenario the nurse had invaded the territory of the patient's room.

21. When interviewing a preschool child during the hospital admission phase, it is important to
    a. interview the child only
    b. obtain an open room
    c. let the parents assist*
    d. wait until the next day

Reference: p. 354

Descriptors:

| 1. 21 | 2. 04 | 3. Application |
| 4. II-1 | 5. Communication | 6. Easy |

Rationale: It is easier to interview children if a parent is nearby.

22. Verbal and nonverbal communication skills are essential for an accurate
    a. assessment*
    b. diagnosis
    c. implementation
    d. plan

Reference: p. 355

Descriptors:

| 1. 21 | 2. 04 | 3. Knowledge |
| 4. IV-1 | 5. Nursing Process | 6. Easy |

Rationale: The major focus of the assessment step is information gathering; verbal and nonverbal communication are essential nursing tools.

23. As a nurse walks by the patient's room she sees that the patient is crying. What is the most appropriate question or response for the nurse to make?
    a. "I see you are crying. Are you in pain?"
    b. "Has someone made you feel uncomfortable?"
    c. "What seems to be bothering you?"
    d. " You are crying. Can I help with something."*

Reference: p. 356

Descriptors:

| 1. 21 | 2. 04 | 3. Application |
| 4. III-1 | 5. Communication | 6. Difficult |

Rationale: It is important to acknowledge the patient's crying, then attempt to ascertain what is bothering the patient.

24. Silence is an effective communication technique because it
    a. gives both communicators time to relax
    b. allows time for reorganization of thoughts*
    c. allows the patient to have time for himself
    d. builds up emotional tension

Reference: p. 356

Descriptors:

| 1. 21 | 2. 03 | 3. Comprehensive |
| 4. IV-1 | 5. Communication | 6. Easy |

Rationale: Silence allows both the patient and the nurse time to reorganize and review their thoughts.

25. To ensure the continuity of care the nurse must
    a. inform the physician of the patient's status frequently
    b. document thoroughly for the health team*
    c. report patient findings to the next shift
    d. communicate patient status to the family

Reference: p. 356

Descriptors:

1. 21   2. 04   3. Comprehensive

4. I-1   5. Communication   6. Difficult

Rationale: The most appropriate nursing action to ensure continuity of care is to thoroughly document all aspects of patient care.

26. When a nurse enters a room and presents with a rough demeanor stating that she is in charge and the patient must follow her orders, she will
    a. make the patient compliant
    b. give the patient a sense of trust
    c. allow the patient to feel secure
    d. cause the patient to feel fear*

Reference: p. 357

Descriptors:

1. 21   2. 07   3. Comprehensive

4. IV-1   5. Communication   6. Moderate

Rationale: The use of ineffective communication techniques will leave the patient with feelings of fear and anxiety.

27. Which of the following behaviors by the nurse demonstrates an ability to be trusted and to keep information confidential?
    a. Gently refusing to discuss other patients*
    b. Initiating each conversation on a social level
    c. Answering all personal questions
    d. Testing patients' trust on a regular basis

Reference: p. 360

Descriptors:

1. 21   2. 05   3. Comprehensive

4. IV-1   5. Communication   6. Moderate

Rationale: Confidentiality must be maintained at all times.

28. A male patient states he is "dizzy" when he gets out of bed. The nurse's *best* response is to say
    a. "Tell me about your dizziness."*
    b. "The dizziness will go away."
    c. "I'll be sure to report it to your doctor."
    d. "You're really worried about that?"

Reference: p. 360

Descriptors:

1. 21   2. 01   3. Comprehensive

4. IV-1   5. Communication   6. Difficult

Rationale: The nurse needs to ask an open-ended question to allow the patient to explain further about the dizziness.

29. An appropriate goal for the orientation phase of the helping relationship between the nurse and the patient includes
    a. evaluating the relationship between the participants
    b. completing clarification of each others' roles*
    c. introducing the caregiver to the patient's family
    d. assisting the patient in receiving prompt medical treatment

Reference: p. 357

Descriptors:

1. 21   2. 05   3. Application

4. IV-1   5. Communication   6. Moderate

Rationale: During the orientation phase, the primary goal is to clarify the roles of both the patient and the nurse.

30. The nurse is in the working phase of the helping relationship with a patient who has had a cast applied for a fractured femur. An appropriate goal in this phase of the helping relationship includes
    a. turning, coughing, and deep-breathing exercises
    b. demonstration of appropriate cast care*
    c. identification of progress toward goals
    d. evaluation of the effectiveness of the relationship

Reference: p. 35

Descriptors:

1. 21   2. 05   3. Application

4. IV-3   5. Teach/Learn   6. Moderate

Rationale: During the working phase of the relationship, it is important to use nursing interventions to achieve a goal, such as demonstration and return demonstration of cast care.

31. During the termination stage of a helping relationship, the nurse and the patient should
    a. establish mutually agreed on goals
    b. cooperate with one another in goal-related activities
    c. explore the patient's prognosis and future healthcare needs
    d. identify progress toward mutually established goals*

Reference: p. 358

Descriptors:

1. 21	2. 05	3. Application
4. IV-1	5. Communication	6. Moderate

Rationale: During the termination stage of a helping relationship, the nurse and the patient should identify progress toward mutually established goals.

32. Nursing guidelines when caring for a patient from a different culture should include
    a. assuming the patient's background can relate to the nurse
    b. referring all patients to an interpreter before explaining care
    c. validating understanding to avoid misinterpretation*
    d. determining whether nonverbal communication is the same in both cultures

Reference: p. 360

Descriptors:

1. 21	2. 06	3. Application
4. IV-1	5. Culture	6. Moderate

Rationale: Nursing guidelines when caring for a patient from a different culture should include validating understanding to avoid misinterpretation. In many cultures, nonverbal communication is universal.

33. When the nurse is interviewing the patient, the nurse should
    a. remain focused on patient questions
    b. use little eye contact with the patient
    c. allow no time for pauses in questions
    d. let the patient set the pace of the interview*

Reference: p. 361

Descriptors:

1. 21	2. 09	3. Comprehensive
4. IV-1	5. Nursing Process	6. Moderate

Rationale: To obtain an adequate nursing history the patient should set the pace of the conversation.

34. The patient offers to tell the nurse a secret as long as the nurse promises not to tell anyone. Which of the following responses would be *most* appropriate for the nurse to make?
    a. "A secret? You can trust me. I'd never tell anyone about you."
    b. "I will listen, but I may need to share the information if it endangers life or health."*
    c. "I don't think you should tell just me, I'll definitely have to tell the staff."
    d. "I'll listen to what you have to say and keep it under my hat."

Reference: p. 362

Descriptors:

1. 21	2. 05	3. Comprehensive
4. IV-1	5. Communication	6. Moderate

Rationale: Confidentiality must be maintained in a nurse–patient relationship, unless the information pertains to life or health (eg, suicide contemplation).

35. The nurse finds an adolescent patient crying because of pain, but both realize that it is too early for his next pain medication. The nurse states, "I understand you're hurting; let me help you get into a more comfortable position." The nurse's response is an example of
    a. reflection
    b. empathy*
    c. warmth
    d. sympathy

Reference: pp. 359, 366

Descriptors:

1. 21	2. 05	3. Comprehensive
4. III-1	5. Caring	6. Moderate

Rationale: The nurse gives an empathic response by putting herself in the patient's position and tries alternative comfort measures.

36. During the patient interview the nurse notes that the patient's arms and legs are crossed. What can the nurse assess from the patient's stance? The patient is
    a. cold
    b. closed*
    c. relaxed
    d. comfortable

Reference: p. 362

Descriptors:

1. 21	2. 08	3. Comprehensive
4. IV-1	5. Communication	6. Easy

Rationale: The crossing of arms and legs is indicative of the patient being closed to the conversation.

37. A patient with whom the nurse has established a positive helping relationship appears agitated when the nurse enters the room. When the nurse asks the patient what is the matter, the patient says "Oh, nothing's wrong. Not really anything." The nurse should
   a. sit beside the patient's bedside and wait a few minutes in silence*
   b. leave the patient alone and return in about an hour
   c. tell the patient "okay" and discuss her next treatment
   d. ask the patient to tell you what is wrong and why she is upset

Reference: p. 363

Descriptors:

1. 21	2. 06	3. Comprehensive
4. III-1	5. Communication	6. Moderate

Rationale: An agitated patient may just need time to recompose herself or try to cope on her own. Sitting in silence may give the patient time to cope and then share the source of the agitation.

38. Before obtaining the patient's signature on the operative permit, the nurse asks, "I have been told that the doctor has explained the surgery to you. Did the surgeon explain everything to you?" This is an example of a
   a. directing question
   b. sequencing question
   c. reflective question
   d. validating question*

Reference: p. 365

Descriptors:

1. 21	2. 09	3. Comprehensive
4. IV-1	5. Communication	6. Difficult

Rationale: The use of validation allows the nurse to ascertain if the patient has been informed of the surgery. These types of questions should be used sparingly.

39. A male patient says to his wife in a matter-of-fact tone of voice, "I'm angry because you were late again." This demonstrates which type of communication behavior by the patient?
   a. passive
   b. passive aggressive
   c. assertive*
   d. aggressive

Reference: p. 366

Descriptors:

1. 21	2. 01	3. Comprehensive
4. III-2	5. Communication	6. Moderate

Rationale: The patient is being assertive.

40. A nurse asks a hospitalized patient "Did you have a good lunch?" Which one of the following types of responses to this question is the patient most likely to give?
   a. brief yes or no response*
   b. complaint about what was served
   c. description of the food that was served
   d. comparison with the patient's usual type of lunch

Reference: p. 367

Descriptors:

1. 21	2. 06	3. Comprehensive
4. IV-1	5. Communication	6. Moderate

Rationale: When a closed question is asked, a yes or no response is the usual answer.

41. Of the following questions, which question will block a conversation?

   a. "Have you taken your medication today?"*
   b. "Would you like your lunch now?"
   c. "Why didn't you call me before arising?"
   d. "Is your family coming in to see you today?"

Reference: p. 367

Descriptors:

1. 21	2. 08	3. Comprehensive
4. IV-1	5. Communication	6. Moderate

Rationale: Questions using why and how are intimidating to patients and can block the conversation.

42. A 68-year-old patient is in severe pain due to bone cancer. He states, "I am so uncomfortable. It makes me so depressed." The nurse responds, "You will be fine, your family will be here, and you don't need to feel depressed." This is an example of
    a. false assurance*
    b. changing the subject
    c. assertiveness
    d. directing comment

Reference: p. 368

Descriptors:

1. 21	2. 08	3. Comprehensive
4. III-1	5. Communication	6. Moderate

Rationale: False assurance may give patients the impression that the nurse is not interested in their pain or problems.

43. The most effective way for a nurse to communicate with a patient who has a hearing impairment is to
    a. raise the voice and pitch of the conversation
    b. sit directly in front of the patient when speaking*
    c. increase the lighting in the patient's room
    d. exaggerate mouth movements so the patient can lip-read

Reference: p. 370

Descriptors:

1. 21	2. 09	3. Application
4. IV-1	5. Communication	6. Moderate

Rationale: The most effective way for a nurse to communicate with a patient who has a hearing impairment is to sit directly in front of the patient when speaking to allow the patient to lip-read if he desires.

CHAPTER 22

Teacher and Counselor

1. The primary purpose of patient teaching is to provide the
   a. family with emotional support
   b. health team with less work
   c. patient with self-care development*
   d. nurse with continuity of care
   Reference: p. 374
   Descriptors:

1. 22	2. 01	3. Comprehensive
4. IV-1	5. Teach/Learn	6. Moderate

   Rationale: The basic purpose of teaching and counseling is to help patients and families develop self-care abilities.

2. Teaching the elderly exercises to reduce disability is an example of
   a. promotion of wellness*
   b. knowledge of illness
   c. restoration of health
   d. treatment of diseases
   Reference: p. 374
   Descriptors:

1. 22	2. 02	3. Application
4. II-2	5. Teach/Learn	6. Easy

   Rationale: Teaching a patient exercises promotes a high level of wellness.

3. Effective patient teaching will facilitate
   a. patient evaluation
   b. patient coping*
   c. nurse advocacy
   d. nurse autonomy
   Reference: p. 375
   Descriptors:

1. 22	2. 03	3. Comprehensive
4. III-1	5. Teach/Learn	6. Moderate

   Rationale: Health teaching facilitates patient coping, thus enhancing self-concept.

4. The process by which a person acquires or increases knowledge or changes behavior defines
   a. learning*
   b. teaching
   c. evaluation
   d. assessment
   Reference: p. 375
   Descriptors:

1. 22	2. 01	3. Knowledge
4. II-1	5. Teach/Learn	6. Easy

   Rationale: Learning is the process by which a person acquires or increases knowledge or changes behavior in a measurable way as a result of an experience.

5. A parent of a child with asthma can state the signs and symptoms of an acute asthma attack. This is an example of
   a. psychomotor learning
   b. pathophysiologic learning
   c. affective learning
   d. cognitive learning*
   Reference: p. 375
   Descriptors:

1. 22	2. 01	3. Application
4. II-1	5. Teach/Learn	6. Moderate

   Rationale: Cognitive learning involves acquisition of knowledge.

6. A patient's mother demonstrates the use of an epinephrine syringe to treat the patient's allergic reactions to bee stings. This type of learning is
   a. psychomotor*
   b. cognitive
   c. affective
   d. preventive

Reference: p. 375

Descriptors:

1. 22	2. 01	3. Application
4. IV-2	5. Teach/Learn	6. Moderate

Rationale: Learning a physical skill involving the integration of mental and muscular activity is called psychomotor learning.

7. An example of cognitive learning is a/an
   a. demonstration of correct lifting techniques
   b. successful completion of a test on diabetes*
   c. realizing that one is angry because of the diagnosis of diabetes
   d. expression of excitement over learning how to self-inject insulin

Reference: p. 375

Descriptors:

1. 22	2. 01	3. Application
4. II-1	5. Teach/Learn	6. Moderate

Rationale: Cognitive learning involves the storing and recalling of new knowledge and information in the brain.

8. A nurse is teaching an 8-year-old child about the administration of an inhaler for bronchodilation. The nurse should explain
   a. all aspects of asthma care
   b. inhaler administration*
   c. medication action
   d. effect on vital capacity

Reference: p. 376

Descriptors:

1. 22	2. 05	3. Application
4. IV-2	5. Teach/Learn	6. Difficult

Rationale: When educating young children about a disease process and its treatment, the nurse must simplify the material to facilitate understanding.

9. Which of the following patients has the developmental maturity and capability to self-catheterize? A
   a. 16-year-old patient with a fractured dominant arm
   b. 12-year-old patient with full range of motion in both hands*
   c. 10-year-old severely mentally retarded patient with good motor skills
   d. healthy 8-year-old patient with bilateral hemiplegia

Reference: p. 376

Descriptors:

1. 22	2. 02	3. Application
4. II-1	5. Teach/Learn	6. Moderate

Rationale: A 12-year-old child with full range of motion should be able to self-catheterize. The patient with a fracture, mental retardation, or hemiplegia will most likely not be able to self-catheterize.

10. Teaching a 9-year-old child about healthy nutrition is termed
    a. androgogy
    b. pedagogy*
    c. formal teaching
    d. developmental norms

Reference: p. 377

Descriptors:

1. 22	2. 01	3. Comprehensive
4. II-2	5. Teach/Learn	6. Easy

Rationale: Pedagogy refers to teaching children and adolescents.

11. A patient, who has been diagnosed with diabetes, does not see the importance of being compliant with the diabetic diet. The nurse should
    a. explain all aspects of the care of the diabetic patient
    b. motivate the patient in understanding the diabetic diet*
    c. instruct the family in the importance of the diet
    d. communicate to the patient the side effects of diabetes

Reference: p. 377

Descriptors:

1. 22	2. 05	3. Application
4. IV-3	5. Teach/Learn	6. Difficult

Rationale: The adult patient must understand the necessity of learning new information and may need to be motivated to be in compliance.

12. A prenatal patient has developed preterm labor and after 5 hours her contractions have stopped. She is being instructed on medication administration and home monitoring for stopping the contractions should they resume. The nurse must
    a. present the material in a nonthreatening manner*
    b. review the material only one time in the home
    c. explain the information to the patient only
    d. instruct the home monitoring in the first session

Reference: p. 377

Descriptors:

| 1. 22 | 2. 05 | 3. Application |
| 4. IV-3 | 5. Teach/Learn | 6. Moderate |

Rationale: Material taught to patients is often difficult and must be presented in a nonthreatening manner.

13. The teaching–learning process is more effective when the
    a. material is presented in lecture format
    b. family is present during the teaching
    c. patient is fearful related to past failure
    d. nurse and patient plan the objectives*

Reference: p. 377

Descriptors:

| 1. 22 | 2. 03 | 3. Knowledge |
| 4. IV-1 | 5. Teach/Learn | 6. Moderate |

Rationale: The teaching–learning process is more effective when the patient is included in planning learning objectives.

14. When learning objectives have not been met, the nurse should
    a. increase the difficulty of the material
    b. instruct the family instead of the patient
    c. reassess and change the teaching plan*
    d. introduce the patient to written material

Reference: p. 378

Descriptors:

| 1. 22 | 2. 05 | 3. Comprehensive |
| 4. IV-1 | 5. Teach/Learn | 6. Easy |

Rationale: When learning objectives have not been met, careful reassessment provides ideas for changing the teaching plan for subsequent implementation.

15. The primary consideration for the nurse who is planning to teach a patient how to care for his colostomy is the patient's
    a. ability to read
    b. supportive family members
    c. readiness to learn*
    d. need for independence

Reference: p. 378

Descriptors:

| 1. 22 | 2. 03 | 3. Application |
| 4. IV-3 | 5. Teach/Learn | 6. Moderate |

Rationale: The primary consideration is the patient's readiness to learn a new skill. If the patient is not ready, retention of knowledge will not occur.

16. A new mother is having difficulty diapering her newborn infant and repeatedly asks the nurses for assistance related to care of the circumcision site. The priority nursing diagnosis for this patient is
    a. Risk for Altered Parenting related to inexperience and anxiety*
    b. Ineffective Coping, Individual, related to childbirth experience
    c. Knowledge Deficit related to change in roles and need for care
    d. Risk for Hemorrhage: Infant Care related to circumcision site

Reference: p. 379

Descriptors:

| 1. 22 | 2. 04 | 3. Application |
| 4. II-1 | 5. Nursing Process | 6. Moderate |

Rationale: The priority nursing diagnosis is Risk for Altered Parenting related to inexperience and anxiety. The mother needs support and praise for her efforts.

17. The nurse is planning to teach a 10-year-old patient how to perform self-care related to diabetes. The nurse's plan of care should include
    a. teaching the patient how to weigh his own food and prepare it
    b. showing the patient a pamphlet about patients with diabetes
    c. assessing the patient's ability to hold and manipulate a syringe*
    d. determining if the patient's parents understand the significance of diabetes

Reference: p. 378

Descriptors:

| 1. 22 | 2. 05 | 3. Application |
| 4. II-1 | 5. Teach/Learn | 6. Difficult |

Rationale: The nursing care plan should include an assessment of the child's motor skill and developmental maturity level related to self-injection techniques.

18. A 55-year-old patient is diagnosed with cancer of the bowel. His surgery included removal of the diseased colon and a colostomy. With regard to patient education, an appropriate nursing diagnosis would be
    a. Knowledge Deficit related to disease process
    b. Knowledge Deficit related to colostomy care*
    c. Altered Bowel Elimination related to cancer
    d. Diarrhea related to postoperative period

    Reference: p. 379

    Descriptors:

1. 22	2. 09	3. Application
4. IV-1	5. Nursing Process	6. Moderate

    Rationale: This nursing diagnosis identifies knowledge deficit as the primary problem followed by the etiology of caring for the patient's colostomy.

19. When teaching an elderly woman who lives with her family about her diabetic diet, it is important for the nurse to
    a. teach the patient all aspects of diabetic care
    b. have the dietitian teach the patient's diet
    c. teach the diet to the patient and family*
    d. use team teaching with diet instruction

    Reference: p. 379

    Descriptors:

1. 22	2. 09	3. Application
4. IV-3	5. Teach/Learn	6. Moderate

    Rationale: Teaching plans must be developed according to the needs of the patient.

20. When the nurse decides what information the patient needs to complete a skill successfully, it should be noted in the
    a. content*
    b. learning objectives
    c. diagnosis
    d. patient's record

    Reference: p. 380

    Descriptors:

1. 22	2. 05	3. Comprehensive
4. IV-1	5. Teach/Learn	6. Easy

    Rationale: After the learner objectives are written, the nurse must decide what information the patient needs to complete them successfully. This information is the content of the teaching plan.

21. The nurse is teaching a preschool class about bicycle safety. What is the best teaching method for this age group?
    a. videotape of bicycle safety
    b. interactive bicycle presentation*
    c. lecture followed by testing
    d. computer-assisted interaction

    Reference: p. 381

    Descriptors:

1. 22	2. 02	3. Application
4. I-2	5. Teach/Learn	6. Difficult

    Rationale: The preschool-aged child will learn most effectively with a hands-on presentation.

22. The nurse who is most effective in teaching health promotion is a nurse who
    a. has a master's degree in community health
    b. has worked in intensive care units
    c. performs physical assessments on adults
    d. practices health promotion*

    Reference: p. 381

    Descriptors:

1. 22	2. 10	3. Comprehensive
4. I-1	5. Teach/Learn	6. Easy

    Rationale: Role-modeling is the most effective way to enhance a patient's positive health behavior.

23. The home health nurse visiting an 80-year-old woman needs to teach the family to administer her insulin injections. The most appropriate teaching strategy is
    a. programmed instruction
    b. printed material
    c. role-play
    d. demonstration*

    Reference: p. 382

    Descriptors:

1. 22	2. 05	3. Application
4. IV-2	5. Teach/Learn	6. Moderate

    Rationale: Demonstration is the most appropriate strategy to instruct a patient and family on the administration of medication.

24. When the nurse implements patient education, the nurse must consider
    a. that printed material must be understandable*
    b. that audiovisual material be used alone
    c. role-playing with most education sessions
    d. computer-assisted instruction for home health

Reference: p. 382

Descriptors:

1. 22	2. 02	3. Application
4. IV-1	5. Teach/Learn	6. Moderate

Rationale: Print materials should be carefully evaluated on the effectiveness of the explanation of healthcare information.

25. To increase the effectiveness of patient education, it is important to establish a/an
    a. method for testing
    b. contractual agreement*
    c. evaluative form
    d. return demonstration

Reference: p. 383

Descriptors:

1. 22	2. 05	3. Comprehensive
4. IV-1	5. Teach/Learn	6. Difficult

Rationale: The contractual agreement is a pact between two people made for the achievement of mutually set goals. The agreement can increase the effectiveness of patient education.

26. The most effective teaching sessions for adult patients should be
    a. 15–30 minutes*
    b. 30–45 minutes
    c. 45–60 minutes
    d. 1–2 hours

Reference: p. 385

Descriptors:

1. 22	2. 05	3. Knowledge
4. IV-1	5. Teach/Learn	6. Easy

Rationale: Sessions of 15 to 30 minutes are generally well tolerated.

27. A patient states to the nurse that his feet are swelling after eating barbecue pork. The nurse explains the effect of increased salt intake and edema. This is an example of
    a. formal teaching
    b. group teaching
    c. informal teaching*
    d. role playing

Reference: p. 386

Descriptors:

1. 22	2. 06	3. Application
4. IV-3	5. Teach/Learn	6. Moderate

Rationale: Informal teaching is unplanned teaching sessions that deal with the patient's immediate learning needs.

28. A 59-year-old patient is admitted for evaluation of hypertension. He was first diagnosed with hypertension last year. It is important for the nurse to
    a. assess his blood pressure before teaching
    b. assess his current knowledge of hypertension*
    c. instruct on all aspects of hypertension
    d. provide group teaching with other patients

Reference: p. 386

Descriptors:

1. 22	2. 06	3. Application
4. IV-3	5. Teach/Learn	6. Difficult

Rationale: It is important that the nurse assess the patient's previous learning to enhance the education of new material.

29. The nurse is planning to teach a group of elderly individuals with rheumatoid arthritis how to perform low-impact exercises in the senior citizen center. Which of the following would be a primary consideration for this group of patients?
    a. easy first floor accessibility*
    b. sophisticated treadmill equipment
    c. weight-lifting equipment to increase strength
    d. dim lighting in the area to decrease eye strain

Reference: p. 386

Descriptors:

1. 22	2. 05	3. Application
4. II-1	5. Teach/Learn	6. Moderate

Rationale: Elderly individuals with arthritis need easy first floor access to the area and bright lighting. Sophisticated equipment is not necessary.

30. The nurse has instructed a postoperative patient how to change his abdominal dressing. The best method for the nurse to use in evaluating the teaching is to have the patient
   a. tell the nurse the steps used in the dressing change
   b. write down the steps used in the dressing change
   c. change the dressing while the nurse observes the demonstration*
   d. take an oral test about the steps used in changing the dressing

   Reference: p. 387

   Descriptors:

1. 22	2. 06	3. Application
4. IV-1	5. Teach/Learn	6. Moderate

   Rationale: A return demonstration of the dressing change while the nurse observes the patient is the best method to evaluate psychomotor skills.

31. The nurse demonstrated crutch walking to a patient prior to foot surgery and the patient returned the demonstration successfully. Appropriate documentation of the nurse's teaching should include
   a. "crutch walking performed well while nurse observed"
   b. "patient provided with crutch-walking demonstration"
   c. "crutch-walking demonstration given with appropriate return demonstration by patient"*
   d. "thirty minutes spent teaching patient crutch-walking technique before foot surgery with return demonstration"

   Reference: p. 388

   Descriptors:

1. 22	2. 07	3. Application
4. IV-3	5. Documentation	6. Moderate

   Rationale: An appropriate way to document the teaching provided is "crutch-walking demonstration given with appropriate return demonstration by patient."

32. Counseling by the nurse includes
   a. formulating the patient's problem
   b. telling the patient how to solve the problem
   c. bringing in all family members to help with the problem
   d. assisting the patient in the problem-solving process*

   Reference: p.

   Descriptors:

1. 22	2. 08	3. Application
4. III-1	5. Communication	6. Moderate

   Rationale:

33. When educating a patient on the application of a colostomy bag, the most appropriate evaluative method is
   a. return demonstration*
   b. question and answer
   c. positive reinforcement
   d. written examination

   Reference: p. 387

   Descriptors:

1. 22	2. 06	3. Application
4. IV-1	5. Teach/Learn	6. Moderate

   Rationale: The psychomotor domain of teaching is best evaluated by return demonstration.

34. A cancer patient is sharing his fears about his diagnosis. The nurse must
   a. introduce the patient to the pathophysiology of disease
   b. provide the patient with the resources for treatment
   c. introduce the patient to a cancer survivor for help
   d. provide the patient with a warm, caring environment*

   Reference: p. 389

   Descriptors:

1. 22	2. 10	3. Application
4. III-2	5. Caring	6. Difficult

   Rationale: The interpersonal skills of warmth, friendliness, openness, and empathy are necessary for successful counseling.

35. The nurse is acting in a counseling role for a patient who is having marital difficulties. The nurse should
   a. identify the patient's problems
   b. document the patient's uncertain feelings
   c. assist the patient in the problem-solving process*
   d. contact the patient's minister to help her

Reference: p. 389

Descriptors:

1. 22   2. 08   3. Application

4. III-2   5. Caring   6. Moderate

Rationale: As a counselor, it is the nurse's role to teach the patient and to assist the patient in the problem-solving process.

36. The nurse is caring for a hospitalized postoperative patient when the patient learns that his 10-year-old son has fractured his right forearm and has had a cast applied. The type of counseling that the nurse should provide for this patient is termed
    a. long-term
    b. situational
    c. short-term*
    d. motivational

    Reference: p. 392

    Descriptors:

    1. 22   2. 08   3. Application

    4. III-2   5. Caring   6. Moderate

    Rationale: The nurse should provide short-term counseling for a patient experiencing a situational crisis.

37. The nurse is caring for a diabetic patient who has been in and out of the hospital because her diabetes is out of control. The patient does not seem willing to care for herself effectively. The type of counseling that the nurse should provide to the patient is
    a. short-term
    b. cultural
    c. referral
    d. motivational*

    Reference: pp. 392–393

    Descriptors:

    1. 22   2. 10   3. Application

    4. III-1   5. Caring   6. Moderate

    Rationale: The type of counseling that the nurse should provide to this patient is termed motivational because the patient does not seem to want to care for herself.

38. A teenage patient is admitted to the emergency room for abdominal pain. She is 6 weeks pregnant. The nurse has stated she will stay with the patient when she tells her parents. This is an example of a
    a. developmental crisis
    b. motivational crisis
    c. situational crisis*
    d. cultural crisis

    Reference: p. 392

    Descriptors:

    1. 22   2. 10   3. Application

    4. III-1   5. Caring   6. Moderate

    Rationale: A situational crisis is when a patient faces an event or situation that causes a disruption of life.

CHAPTER 23

Leader, Researcher, and Advocate

1. Leadership skills necessary for nurses include the ability to
   a. criticize another staff member
   b. aggressively seek additional help
   c. establish positive relationships*
   d. critique a peer's performance skills

   Reference: p. 398

   Descriptors:

1. 23	2. 02	3. Application
4. I-1	5. Communication	6. Moderate

   Rationale: Leadership skills necessary for nurses include the ability to establish positive relationships and think critically, to show assertiveness and flexibility, and to have a vision.

2. The unit director calls a mandatory nursing staff meeting to discuss the problem of the recent staffing shortage. The group devises a short-term and long-term strategy for solving the problem. In this situation, the unit director is using a style of leadership termed
   a. motivational
   b. laissez-faire
   c. autocratic
   d. democratic*

   Reference: p. 398

   Descriptors:

1. 23	2. 02	3. Application
4. I-1	5. Communication	6. Moderate

   Rationale: The unit director is using a democratic leadership style when the director allows the staff to formulate both short-term and long-term solutions to the problem.

3. An example of an ineffective nursing management style on a busy surgical unit of a hospital is for the nurse manager to
   a. maintain the current staffing ratio even though more nurses are needed*
   b. engage the staff members in decisions related to equipment purchases
   c. provide the staff with information about the latest research findings
   d. plan for greater numbers of staff members when the census increases

   Reference: p. 399

   Descriptors:

1. 23	2. 03	3. Application
4. I-1	5. Communication	6. Moderate

   Rationale: Laissez-faire leadership is rarely effective. An example of an ineffective nursing management style on a busy surgical unit of a hospital is for the nurse manager to maintain the current staffing ratio even though more nurses are needed.

4. A nurse is concerned about the healthcare needs of pregnant women in a low-income neighborhood. After receiving funding from various community agencies, a nursing center is established to meet the needs of these patients. This type of nursing leadership is termed
   a. transformational*
   b. visionary
   c. situational
   d. democratic

   Reference: p. 399

   Descriptors:

1. 23	2. 02	3. Application
4. I-1	5. Caring	6. Moderate

   Rationale: This type of leadership is termed transformational because these leaders are able to create revolutionary change.

5. A hospital unit comprised of staff nurses and ancillary personnel uses a decentralized method of management. In this type of system there is
   a. top-down decision making
   b. little input by the staff into decisions
   c. greater responsibility and accountability*
   d. greater expense involved in the decision-making process

Reference: p. 400

Descriptors:

1. 23	2. 01, 03	3. Application
4. I-1	5. Communication	6. Moderate

Rationale: A decentralized method of management involves greater responsibility and accountability by the staff members.

6. The unit director is planning a change in the way that nurses perform charting and documentation to make it more efficient. To overcome the possible resistance to the change by the staff, the unit director should
   a. introduce the change rapidly
   b. involve a few of the nurses at first
   c. identify the advantages of the change*
   d. obtain support from the physicians for the change

Reference: p. 402

Descriptors:

1. 23	2. 04	3. Application
4. I-1	5. Documentation	6. Moderate

Rationale: To overcome the possible resistance to the change by the staff, the unit director should introduce the change slowly, involve all of the affected nursing staff, and identify the advantages of the change.

7. The difference between a mentorship and a preceptorship arrangement is
   a. preceptors are paid employees of the hiring institution*
   b. selection of a mentor is done by the institution
   c. preceptors assist the orientee in networking
   d. mentors provide research assistance when needed

Reference: p. 404

Descriptors:

1. 23	2. 05	3. Application
4. I-1	5. Communication	6. Difficult

Rationale: Mentorship involves a relationship between an experienced individual and the protégé, and provides support and networking without a financial reward. Preceptors are paid employees of the hiring institution to facilitate an orientee's transition.

8. Revising an intravenous solution change procedure due to a recent research review is an example of which source of knowledge?
   a. authoritative
   b. scientific*
   c. traditional
   d. verified

Reference: p. 406

Descriptors:

1. 23	2. 06	3. Application
4. I-1	5. Communication	6. Moderate

Rationale: Revising an intravenous solution change procedure due to a recent research review is an example of a source of knowledge termed scientific.

9. Basic research skills that nurses in a caregiver role use include
   a. relating research findings to clinical practice*
   b. advising patients to participate in research projects
   c. determining the dates of clinical trials
   d. performing statistical processes for validation

Reference: p. 407

Descriptors:

1. 23	2. 07	3. Application
4. I-1	5. Communication	6. Difficult

Rationale: Basic research skills that nurses in a caregiver role use include relating research findings to clinical practice, identifying researchable problems, and protecting patient rights.

10. The nurse determines that a hospitalized patient understands living wills and advance directives when the patient
    a. makes his own decisions related to his care*
    b. asks his family to make decisions for him
    c. repeatedly asks the nurse if he should donate an organ
    d. states that his decisions are irreversible

Reference: p. 410

Descriptors:

1. 23	2. 10	3. Application
4. I-1	5. Self Care	6. Easy

Rationale: The nurse determines that a hospitalized patient understands living wills and advance directives when the patient makes his own decisions related to his care.

11. A hospitalized patient tells the nurse that he is not sure he should have the surgery that is scheduled for the next morning. The best action by the nurse is to
   a. assure the patient that the surgery is for the best
   b. further explore the patients feelings and fears about the surgery*
   c. ask the patient if the nurse should contact the physician
   d. call the surgeon and ask to cancel the patient's surgery

Reference: p. 410–411

Descriptors:

1. 23	2. 08	3. Application
4. IV-1	5. Communication	6. Moderate

Rationale: The best action by the nurse is to further explore the patient's feelings and fears about the surgery. If the patient is convinced that he does not want the surgery performed the nurse should contact the surgeon immediately and ask the surgeon for further orders.

UNIT VI

Actions Basic to Nursing Care

CHAPTER 24

Vital Signs

1. The body temperature is regulated by the
   a. medulla
   b. thalamus
   c. hypothalamus*
   d. cerebrum
   Reference: p. 418
   Descriptors:

1. 24	2. 04	3. Knowledge
4. None	5. None	6. Easy

   Rationale: The hypothalamus is responsible for thermoregulation.

2. A 76-year-old patient hospitalized following abdominal surgery has a temperature of 38°C (100.4°F). The nurse plans to assess the patient's vital signs every
   a. 30 minutes
   b. 60 minutes
   c. 2 hours
   d. 4 hours*
   Reference: p. 418
   Descriptors:

1. 24	2. 02	3. Application
4. IV-3	5. Nursing Process	6. Easy

   Rationale: In most institutions, the typical period for taking a patient's vital signs is every 4 hours, unless there is a need to take the vital signs more frequently.

3. A patient is admitted to the hospital from the emergency room with a temperature of 105.8°F. The nurse determines that the patient is experiencing
   a. hyperpyrexia*
   b. hypopyrexia
   c. hyperemia
   d. hypothermia
   Reference: p. 420
   Descriptors:

1. 24	2. 01	3. Knowledge
4. IV-3	5. Nursing Process	6. Easy

   Rationale: Hyperpyrexia is a fever of 105.8°F or higher.

4. The emergency room nurse examines an adult patient who has intense shivering, rigid muscles, dilated pupils, and bluish skin. The nurse determines that the patient is most likely experiencing
   a. hypothermia*
   b. hyperthermia
   c. circulatory collapse
   d. shock
   Reference: p. 421
   Descriptors:

1. 24	2. 02	3. Comprehensive
4. IV-3	5. Nursing Process	6. Moderate

   Rationale: The patient is most likely experiencing symptoms of hypothermia, which include shivering, rigid muscles, dilated pupils, and bluish skin.

5. A patient with a convulsive disorder is admitted from the emergency room. Which type of thermometer or route of temperature monitoring should the nurse select?
   a. oral glass thermometer to produce the least trauma
   b. disposable thermometer to maintain infection control
   c. electronic rectal probe to ensure a safe, accurate reading
   d. tympanic thermometer for rapid results*

Reference: p. 422

Descriptors:

1. 24	2. 02	3. Comprehensive
4. IV-3	5. Nursing Process	6. Moderate

Rationale: A patient with a convulsive disorder should not have his temperature taken with an oral thermometer. The tympanic thermometer will give the most rapid results.

6. The nurse is preparing to assess an adult patient's oral temperature using an electronic thermometer. The nurse explains the procedure to the patient and determines that she understands the instructions when she says electronic thermometers
   a. measure body temperature in 25 to 50 seconds*
   b. are less accurate when used with children
   c. reduce infection because all of the equipment is disposable
   d. are usually more accurate than rectal thermometers

Reference: p. 422

Descriptors:

1. 24	2. 03	3. Application
4. IV-1	5. Teach/Learn	6. Moderate

Rationale: The patient understands the instructions when she says that electronic thermometers measure body temperature in 25 to 50 seconds.

7. The nurse instructs the mother of a 2-week-old infant about checking her child's temperature. The nurse determines that the mother needs further instructions when she says
   a. "I should check the temperature using the axillary site."
   b. "A glass thermometer should be left in place for at least 3 minutes."
   c. "A digital thermometer can determine the temperature quickly."
   d. "I can use a tympanic membrane device to check the temperature."*

Reference: p. 422

Descriptors:

1. 24	2. 06	3. Application
4. II-1	5. Teach/Learn	6. Moderate

Rationale: The mother needs further instructions when she says she can use the tympanic membrane device to check the 2-week-old infant's temperature. These are not appropriate for infants.

8. Before obtaining an axillary temperature of an adult patient with a glass thermometer, the nurse explains to the patient that the
   a. thermometer will remain in place for 5 minutes
   b. axillary temperature is 1° higher than the rectal site
   c. method is not used with children under 6 years of age
   d. deepest area of the axilla provides the most accuracy*

Reference: p. 427

Descriptors:

1. 24	2. 05	3. Application
4. IV-1	5. Teach/Learn	6. Moderate

Rationale: For an axillary temperature, the deepest area of the axilla provides the most accuracy and the thermometer should remain in place up to 10 minutes.

9. After assessing an adult patient's rectal temperature, the nurse documents both the temperature and the site in the patient's record because
   a. different readings will be obtained from each site*
   b. constipation is common following a rectal temperature
   c. infections can influence the temperature at each site
   d. the oral route is the most commonly used site

Reference: p. 429

Descriptors:

1. 24	2. 03	3. Application
4. IV-1	5. Documentation	6. Moderate

Rationale: It is important for the nurse to document both the temperature and the site used because different readings will be obtained from each site.

10. The nurse is caring for several patients on a surgical unit of a hospital. The nurse should assess a patient's temperature using the rectal site if the patient is
    a. receiving oxygen by mask*
    b. receiving oxygen by nasal cannula
    c. recovering from thoracic surgery
    d. cannot speak clearly

Reference: p. 430

Descriptors:

1. 24	2. 02	3. Application
4. IV-1	5. Nursing Process	6. Moderate

Rationale: A patient who is receiving oxygen by face mask should not have the oxygen mask removed for temperature assessment.

11. The nurse is planning to instruct a family member about taking her mother's temperature at home. Which of the following would be important to include in the teaching plan?
    a. Wash a glass thermometer after use with hot, soapy water.
    b. Place a glass thermometer under the tongue for 5 minutes.
    c. Shake the thermometer before use to 98.6°F.
    d. Wait 30 minutes after she eats before taking the temperature.*

References: p. 430

Descriptors:

1. 24	2. 06	3. Application
4. IV-1	5. Teach/Learn	6. Moderate

Rationale: The nurse should instruct the family member to wait at least 30 minutes after the patient eats before taking the temperature, because eating can affect the temperature.

12. A patient has a rate of breathing that is abnormally slow but regular in rhythm. The term that *best* describes this is
    a. tachypnea
    b. eupnea
    c. dyspnea
    d. bradypnea*

Reference: p. 431

Descriptors:

1. 24	2. 04	3. Knowledge
4. IV-1	5. Nursing Process	6. Moderate

Rationale: The term for abnormally slow breathing that is regular in rhythm is bradypnea.

13. The nurse notes that a hospitalized adult patient has orthopnea. The nurse plans to assess the patient's respirations while the patient
    a. lies in a side-lying position in bed
    b. sits upright in a chair*
    c. lies in a prone position
    d. lies supine in bed

Reference: p. 431

Descriptors:

1. 24	2. 02	3. Application
4. IV-1	5. Nursing Process	6. Easy

Rationale: A patient with orthopnea has difficulty breathing in a supine or prone position, so the nurse should assess the patient while he is sitting in a chair.

14. The nurse assesses an elderly patient with terminal cancer and determines that the patient's respirations gradually increase, then decrease, and then there is a period of apnea. The nurse determines that the patient is experiencing respirations termed
    a. Cheyne-Stokes*
    b. Biot's
    c. bradypnea
    d. eupnea

Reference: p. 431

Descriptors:

1. 24	2. 02	3. Knowledge
4. IV-1	5. Nursing Process	6. Easy

Rationale: Respirations that increase, decrease, and have apnea are termed Cheyne-Stokes.

15. Of the following sets of vital signs, which one represents normal vital signs for an average adult at rest?
    a. BP 190/70, P 120, R 36, T 99.6
    b. BP 120/80, P 72, R 18, T 98.2*
    c. BP 130/74, P 150, R 16, T 101.6
    d. BP 116/68, P 42, R 24, T 97.6

Reference: pp. 435, 437

Descriptors:

1. 24	2. 04	3. Comprehensive
4. IV-1	5. Nursing Process	6. Moderate

Rationale: Baseline values are established for vital signs to monitor each patient individually. Normal blood pressure should be in the range of 120/80, pulse 60 to 80, temperature 97° to 99°, and respirations of 16-20 breaths per minute.

16. The nurse notifies the physician when it is determined that an adult male patient's pulse is 56 beats/min because the patient is experiencing
    a. cardiovascular collapse
    b. bradycardia*
    c. hypocardia
    d. dysrhythmia

Reference: p. 435

Descriptors:

1. 24	2. 03	3. Comprehensive
4. IV-1	5. Nursing Process	6. Easy

Rationale: A patient with a pulse of 56 beats/min is experiencing bradycardia.

17. Four hours after knee surgery, an 88-year-old patient has a pulse rate of 110 beats/min and is squirming in the bed. The nurse should assess the patient for
    a. decubitus formation
    b. hypothermia
    c. pain*
    d. dysrhythmia

Reference: p. 435

Descriptors:

1. 24	2. 02	3. Application
4. II-1	5. Nursing Process	6. Easy

Rationale: Four hours after knee surgery, this patient is most likely experiencing pain.

18. The apical pulse rate is the number of pulsations felt in what period of time?
    a. 15 seconds
    b. 30 seconds
    c. 60 seconds*
    d. 90 seconds

Reference:

p. 436

Descriptors:

1. 24	2. 06	3. Knowledge
4. IV-1	5. Nursing Process	6. Easy

Rationale: The apical pulse is auscultated with a stethoscope for a full minute to detect any abnormalities.

19. When assessing the pedal pulse, the nurse should
    a. count the pulse for 2 minutes
    b. ask another nurse to verify the pulse
    c. monitor the pulse on both extremities of the patient*
    d. check the pulse at 15-minute intervals

Reference: p. 436

Descriptors:

1. 24	2. 06	3. Knowledge
4. IV-1	5. Nursing Process	6. Moderate

Rationale: Comparing pulses in both extremities is important to detect abnormalities.

20. A patient's temperature is 100°F, pulse is 80 beats/min, respirations are 22 breaths per minute, and blood pressure is 120/80. Which is the systolic pressure?
    a. 22
    b. 120*
    c. 80
    d. 40

Reference: p. 437

Descriptors:

1. 24	2. 01	3. Knowledge
4. IV-1	5. Nursing Process	6. Easy

Rationale: Systolic pressure is the pressure of the blood through the artery as the blood pressure cuff is released. It is recorded as the top/first number.

21. Which of the following nursing actions when taking vital signs will be *most* helpful in encouraging patient cooperation and reduction of patient apprehension?
    a. Wash your hands before and after the procedure.
    b. Gather all equipment before beginning.
    c. Wear disposable gloves for all procedures.
    d. Explain the procedure to the patient.*

Reference: p. 438

Descriptors:

1. 24	2. 02	3. Comprehensive
4. IV-1	5. Communication	6. Moderate

Rationale: Explaining the procedure to the patient will help to relieve the patient's anxiety.

22. To assess pulse deficit of an adult patient, the nurse taking the apical pulse plans to
    a. place the stethoscope at the patient's third intercostal space
    b. place the patient in a side-lying position
    c. ask the patient to sit in a chair*
    d. ask the patient to take a deep breath

Reference: p. 439

Descriptors:

1. 24	2. 05	3. Application
4. IV-1	5. Nursing Process	6. Easy

Rationale: The nurse should ask the patient to sit in a chair so the nurse can place the stethoscope between the fifth and sixth ribs.

23. Any constriction (narrowing) of the blood vessels will have what effect on the patient's blood pressure?
    a. decreased blood pressure
    b. increased blood pressure*
    c. have no effect on the blood pressure
    d. initially increase followed by a dramatic decrease

    Reference: p. 440

    Descriptors:

    | 1. 24 | 2. 04 | 3. Comprehensive |
    | 4. IV-1 | 5. Nursing Process | 6. Moderate |

    Rationale: When the blood vessel is constricted, more force is required for the blood to flow, causing the blood pressure to rise.

24. The nurse has instructed a group of adults at a local senior citizens center about blood pressure and hypertension. The nurse determines that one of the members of the group understands the instructions when she says
    a. "Blood pressure increases as one ages due to decreased elasticity of the arteries."*
    b. "Women usually have a higher blood pressure than men."
    c. "Blood pressure is the highest during the late morning."
    d. "After eating, blood pressure usually falls, then rises before sleep."

    Reference: p. 441

    Descriptors:

    | 1. 24 | 2. 06 | 3. Application |
    | 4. II-2 | 5. Teach/Learn | 6. Moderate |

    Rationale: The instructions have been understood when one of the members says that blood pressure increases as one ages because of decreased elasticity of the arteries.

25. The nurse is preparing to assist a patient to ambulate for the first time after a period of bedrest following gallbladder surgery. Before ambulation, the nurse should assess the patient for
    a. decreased respiratory rate
    b. increased pulse pressure
    c. orthostatic hypotension*
    d. secondary hypertension

    Reference: p. 442

    Descriptors:

    | 1. 24 | 2. 03 | 3. Application |
    | 4. IV-4 | 5. Nursing Process | 6. Easy |

    Rationale: Orthostatic hypotension may occur if the patient stands up suddenly after being in bed for a while.

26. An adult patient received a dose of meperidine hydrochloride (Demerol) 30 minutes ago. Before ambulation, the nurse should assess the patient for
    a. tachycardia
    b. hypertension
    c. hypotension*
    d. tachypnea

    Reference: p. 442

    Descriptors:

    | 1. 24 | 2. 01 | 3. Application |
    | 4. IV-2 | 5. Nursing Process | 6. Moderate |

    Rationale: Meperidine hydrochloride can cause hypotension.

27. The nurse is preparing to assess a patient's blood pressure. To identify the first Korotkoff sound accurately, the nurse should
    a. place the cuff about 3 inches above the patient's elbow
    b. reinflate the cuff once air is released to recheck rate
    c. repeat any suspicious reading within 10 seconds
    d. inflate the cuff while palpating the artery and note the reading where the pulse disappears*

    Reference: p. 446

    Descriptors:

    | 1. 24 | 2. 02 | 3. Application |
    | 4. IV-1 | 5. Nursing Process | 6. Moderate |

    Rationale: To note the first Korotkoff sound accurately, the nurse should inflate the cuff while palpating the artery and note the reading where the pulse disappears.

28. A patient diagnosed with hypertension asks the nurse about blood pressure monitoring equipment for home use. The nurse should instruct the patient that
    a. digital blood pressure monitoring equipment is not very accurate
    b. if there is difficulty hearing the blood pressure sounds, lower the arm for 15 seconds'
    c. home monitoring of a patient's blood pressure is not recommended

d. cuff sizes vary and a poorly fitting cuff can produce an inaccurate measurement*

Reference: p. 448

Descriptors:

1. 24   2. 06   3. Application
4. IV-1   5. Teach/Learn   6. Moderate

Rationale: Cuff sizes vary and a poorly fitting cuff can produce an inaccurate measurement.

29. The nurse has instructed an adult patient how to monitor her blood pressure while at home. The nurse determines that the patient has understood the instructions when she says
    a. "A cuff that is too small will result in falsely high readings."*
    b. "I can record the systolic and diastolic measurement by the sensory detection method."
    c. "Misplacing the bell beyond the direct area of the artery can result in falsely high readings."

d. "Monitoring my blood pressure at home means that I don't need to have it checked periodically by a nurse."

Reference: pp. 448, 434

Descriptors:

1. 24   2. 06   3. Application
4. IV-1   5. Teach/Learn   6. Moderate

Rationale: A cuff that is too small will cause falsely high readings.

30. When taking a blood pressure, estimation of systolic pressure is *most* accurately made by
    a. checking previous blood pressure readings
    b. estimating according to body build and age
    c. palpating for obliteration of the radial pulse*
    d. using 20 mm Hg as the usual systolic pressure

Reference: p. 450

Descriptors:

1. 24   2. 06   3. Knowledge
4. IV-1   5. Nursing Process   6. Easy

Rationale: Estimation of systolic pressure is *most* accurate when the nurse palpates for obliteration of the radial pulse.

CHAPTER 25

Health Assessment

1. The major purpose of a health assessment of an adult patient by the nurse is to
   a. identify patient weaknesses
   b. focus on a specific body system
   c. evaluate the effects of the aging process
   d. establish a nurse–patient relationship*

Reference: p. 458

Descriptors:

| 1. 25 | 2. 02 | 3. Knowledge |
| 4. IV-1 | 5. Nursing Process | 6. Easy |

Rationale: Purposes of the health assessment include establishing a nurse–patient relationship, identifying patient strengths, and collecting data about the patient.

2. The nurse is planning to perform an examination of an adult patient's internal eye structures. The nurse should explain to the patient that the purpose of the numbers on the rotating dial of the ophthalmoscope is to
   a. determine if the lens is illuminated
   b. adjust magnification power of the lens*
   c. determine visual acuity
   d. test intraocular movements

Reference: p. 459

Descriptors:

| 1. 25 | 2. 04 | 3. Application |
| 4. IV-1 | 5. Nursing Process | 6. Moderate |

Rationale: The numbers on the rotating dial adjust the magnification power of the lens. Red numbers are used for myopic patients, and black numbers are used for hyperopic patients.

3. To examine an adult patient's external ear canal and tympanic membrane, the nurse should obtain a/an
   a. tuning fork
   b. cotton swab
   c. inspection probe
   d. otoscope*

Reference: p. 459

Descriptors:

| 1. 25 | 2. 05 | 3. Application |
| 4. IV-1 | 5. Nursing Process | 6. Easy |

Rationale: An otoscope is used to examine a patient's external ear canal and tympanic membrane.

4. To assess full lung expansion of an adult patient, the nurse plans to place the patient in which position?
   a. dorsal recumbent
   b. side-lying
   c. knee–chest
   d. sitting*

Reference: p. 461

Descriptors:

| 1. 25 | 2. 06 | 3. Application |
| 4. IV-1 | 5. Nursing Process | 6. Moderate |

Rationale: To assess full lung expansion of an adult patient, the nurse should ask the patient to assume a sitting position.

5. To assess an adult patient's abdomen and peripheral pulses, the nurse begins by placing the patient in a
   a. supine position*
   b. side-lying position
   c. Sims' position
   d. sitting position

Reference: p. 461

Descriptors:

| 1. 25 | 2. 06 | 3. Application |
| 4. IV-1 | 5. Nursing Process | 6. Moderate |

Rationale: To assess an adult patient's abdomen and peripheral pulses, the nurse begins by placing the patient in a supine position so that the abdomen and pulses are easily accessible.

6. When performing a pelvic examination, the position for the patient to assume is
   a. prone
   b. Sims
   c. lithotomy*
   d. supine

   Reference: p. 461

   Descriptors:

1. 25	2. 06	3. Knowledge
4. IV-1	5. Nursing Process	6. Easy

   Rationale: Lithotomy position allows the healthcare provider to have the patient's legs in stirrups, with the hips at the end of the examination table; the examiner is then able to examine pelvic organs.

7. The nurse is planning to perform a physical assessment on an adult patient. Before the examination, the nurse should ask the patient to
   a. remove her jewelry
   b. empty the bladder*
   c. practice relaxation exercises
   d. take several deep breaths

   Reference: p. 463

   Descriptors:

1. 25	2. 04	3. Application
4. IV-1	5. Nursing Process	6. Moderate

   Rationale: Emptying the bladder is necessary to allow for greater comfort for the patient during the examination.

8. During a physical examination, the patient complains to the nurse that she has pain in her left calf. The nurse should
   a. examine both legs for tenderness*
   b. palpate the left calf deeply at the area
   c. ask the patient if she has varicosities
   d. have the patient move the leg in a swinging motion

   Reference: p. 463

   Descriptors:

1. 25	2. 03	3. Application
4. IV-3	5. Nursing Process	6. Easy

   Rationale: Even though the patient is only complaining of pain in the left calf, the nurse should examine both extremities to compare the two legs.

9. During a health assessment, the patient indicates to the nurse that she has a small mass on her forearm. To assess whether or not the mass is fluid filled, the nurse palpates with the
   a. palm of the hand
   b. index finger of dominant hand
   c. fingers and finger pads*
   d. dorsal surface of the hand

   Reference: p. 463

   Descriptors:

1. 25	2. 03	3. Application
4. IV-1	5. Nursing Process	6. Easy

   Rationale: To determine if a mass is fluid filled, the nurse should palpate with the fingers and finger pads.

10. While performing a health assessment of an adult patient, the nurse should exercise utmost caution when using
    a. deep palpation*
    b. intermittent palpation
    c. light palpation
    d. focused palpation

    Reference: p. 463

    Descriptors:

1. 25	2. 03	3. Application
4. IV-1	5. Nursing Process	6. Moderate

    Rationale: The nurse should use utmost caution when performing deep palpation because of the risk of possible internal injury.

11. The nurse is planning to percuss a patient's stomach to assess for tympany. The nurse should
    a. place the dominant hand over the area and strike with the other hand
    b. use the middle finger of the dominant hand as the striking force*
    c. use both hands to determine vibration in the stomach area
    d. place the patient's nondominant hand over the stomach area

    Reference: pp. 463–464, 490

    Descriptors:

1. 25	2. 03	3. Application
4. IV-1	5. Nursing Process	6. Moderate

    Rationale: To perform percussion of the patient's abdomen, the nurse should use the middle finger of the dominant hand as the striking force to assess vibrations.

12. The assessment technique that uses a stethoscope is termed
    a. inspection
    b. palpation
    c. percussion
    d. auscultation*
    Reference: p. 464
    Descriptors:
    1. 25   2. 03   3. Knowledge
    4. IV-1   5. Nursing Process   6. Easy
    Rationale: A stethoscope is used to amplify sounds for auscultation.

13. When performing a general survey of a patient, all of the following characteristics are assessed *except*
    a. hygiene
    b. age*
    c. affect
    d. orientation
    Reference: p. 464
    Descriptors:
    1. 25   2. 03   3. Comprehensive
    4. IV-1   5. Nursing Process   6. Moderate
    Rationale: A general survey is an assessment used to evaluate the appearance, behavior, and orientation, not necessarily a patient's age.

14. The integumentary structures include all of the following *except*
    a. skin
    b. nails
    c. hair
    d. heart*
    Reference: pp. 466–468
    Descriptors:
    1. 25   2. 03   3. Knowledge
    4. IV-1   5. Nursing Process   6. Easy
    Rationale: The heart is not part of the integumentary system.

15. Pallor in dark-skinned patients is seen as
    a. ashen gray*
    b. pink tinged
    c. pasty white
    d. cream colored
    Reference: p. 467
    Descriptors:
    1. 25   2. 01   3. Knowledge
    4. IV-1   5. Nursing Process   6. Easy
    Rationale: Pallor appears as an ashen gray on dark-skinned patients on lips and mucous membranes.

16. The nurse performed a health assessment on a 79-year-old patient. The nurse documents which of the following findings as abnormal for a patient of this age?
    a. decreased skin turgor
    b. thinning hair on scalp
    c. tympany over the abdomen
    d. jaundiced skin*
    Reference: p. 467
    Descriptors:
    1. 25   2. 08   3. Application
    4. IV-1   5. Documentation   6. Moderate
    Rationale: Jaundiced skin is an abnormal finding in an adult of any age and could indicate liver problems.

17. The nurse assesses a dark-skinned patient for cyanosis by observing the color of the patient's
    a. mucous membrane of the mouth*
    b. abdominal tissue
    c. skin around the head and neck
    d. ankles and feet
    Reference: p. 467
    Descriptors:
    1. 25   2. 03   3. Application
    4. IV-1   5. Nursing Process   6. Moderate
    Rationale: In dark-skinned patients, cyanosis is observed by looking at the mucous membrane of the patient's mouth.

18. The nurse is performing a health assessment on a 10-year-old child. The nurse observes a bluish purple discoloration on the child's left elbow. The nurse should document this as
    a. bruit
    b. keloid
    c. desquamation
    d. ecchymosis*

Reference: p. 467

Descriptors:

1. 25   2. 08   3. Application

4. IV-1   5. Nursing Process 6. Easy

Rationale: Ecchymosis is the term used to describe bruising that is bluish purple.

19. Edema is characterized by all of the following *except*
    a. swelling
    b. shiny
    c. taut
    d. elasticity*

    Reference: p. 467

    Descriptors:

    1. 25   2. 01   3. Knowledge

    4. IV-1   5. Nursing Process 6. Easy

    Rationale: Edema in tissues causes the skin to swell, become shiny and taut, and be pulled tightly from expansion. Elasticity applies to skin turgor.

20. The nurse is assessing a patient's skin during an office visit. What technique should the nurse use to best assess the temperature of his skin? The nurse should use the
    a. fingertips because they are more sensitive to small changes in temperature
    b. palmar surface of the hand because an increased nerve supply is present
    c. dorsal surface of the hand because the skin is thinner there than the palms*
    d. ulnar portion of the hand for enhanced temperature sensitivity

    Reference: p. 467

    Descriptors:

    1. 25   2. 07   3. Knowledge

    4. IV-1   5. Nursing Process 6. Moderate

    Rationale: The dorsal surface is more sensitive to temperature because the skin is thinner.

21. The nurse is examining a patient's lower leg and notes a draining ulceration. Which of the following actions is most appropriate in this situation?
    a. Continue to examine the ulceration, then wash your hands.
    b. Wash your hands, put on gloves, and continue with the examination of the ulceration.*
    c. Wash your hands and put a dressing on the wound.

d. Wash your hands, proceed with the examination, then go back to the ulceration.

Reference: p. 467

Descriptors:

1. 25   2. 07   3. Application

4. I-2   5. Nursing Process 6. Moderate

Rationale: Wash your hands before putting on gloves, then proceed with the examination.

22. An adult patient tells the nurse during a health assessment that he has had vitiligo for several years. The nurse anticipates that the patient will have
    a. pale mucous membranes
    b. white patchy areas on the skin*
    c. red marks on the face
    d. pallor in the ankle area

    Reference: p. 468

    Descriptors:

    1. 25   2. 08   3. Application

    4. IV-1   5. Nursing Process 6. Moderate

    Rationale: Vitiligo is a condition that results in white patchy areas on the skin.

23. The nurse conducts a health assessment on a 22-year-old man and observes fissures in both feet. The nurse should ask the patient if he has ever been treated for
    a. athlete's foot*
    b. impetigo
    c. arthritis
    d. wheals

    Reference: p. 469

    Descriptors:

    1. 25   2. 08   3. Application

    4. IV-1   5. Nursing Process 6. Moderate

    Rationale: When the nurse observes fissures on the patient's feet, the patient is most likely experiencing athlete's foot.

24. While performing a physical assessment of an 84-year-old patient, the nurse notes that the angle between the skin and the nailbed is flat and at 180 degrees, with the skin tissue feeling springy and floating. The nurse documents this as
    a. spoon nails
    b. onycholysis
    c. early clubbing*
    d. late clubbing

Reference: pp. 468, 470

Descriptors:

1. 25	2. 08	3. Application
4. IV-1	5. Nursing Process	6. Moderate

Rationale: When the nailbed is flat and at 180 degrees with the skin tissue feeling springy and floating, the nurse should document this as early clubbing.

25. While inspecting the eyes of a hospitalized patient, the nurse observes that the patient has unequal pupils. The nurse determines that this is symptomatic of
    a. mydriasis
    b. cataracts
    c. coma
    d. central nervous system injury*

Reference: p. 470

Descriptors:

1. 25	2. 08	3. Application
4. IV-1	5. Nursing Process	6. Easy

Rationale: Unequal pupils are indicative of central nervous system injuries.

26. To assess an adult patient's consensual reflex, the nurse should
    a. shine a penlight on one pupil and then the other*
    b. hold a cotton swab about 4 inches from the patient's nose
    c. move one finger away from the patient's nose
    d. use an ophthalmoscope to find the red reflex

Reference: p. 470

Descriptors:

1. 25	2. 05	3. Application
4. IV-1	5. Nursing Process	6. Moderate

Rationale: To assess the adult patient's consensual reflex of the eyes, the nurse should shine a penlight on one pupil and then the other pupil.

27. The nurse is planning to assess a 30-month-old patient who has had frequent ear infections. The nurse plans to
    a. use the smallest cotton swab that will fit into the patient's ear
    b. instruct the mother to hold the patient's head downward
    c. straighten the ear canal by gently pulling the pinna up and back
    d. straighten the ear canal by gently pulling the pinna down and back*

Reference: p. 474

Descriptors:

1. 25	2. 07	3. Application
4. II-2	5. Nursing Process	6. Moderate

Rationale: For a 30-month-old child, the nurse should assess the child's ears by straightening the ear canal by gently pulling the pinna down and back.

28. The nurse explains the purpose of Weber's test to an adult patient. The nurse determines that the patient has understood the instructions when the patient says
    a. "This test is used to test bone conduction."*
    b. "This test is used to test air conduction."
    c. "You will place the tuning fork close to my ear."
    d. "You will place the tuning fork near my forehead."

Reference: p. 475

Descriptors:

1. 25	2. 04	3. Application
4. IV-1	5. Teach/Learn	6. Moderate

Rationale: Weber's test is used to test bone conduction during an examination of the patient's hearing. The tuning fork is placed on the top of the patient's head.

29. The nurse has completed a physical examination of an adult patient's head and neck. Which of the following would be considered an abnormal finding?
    a. small pink symmetric tonsils
    b. nonpalpable thyroid gland
    c. neck vein distention*
    d. nonpalpable lymph nodes

Reference: p. 478

Descriptors:

1. 25	2. 08	3. Knowledge
4. IV-1	5. Nursing Process	6. Easy

Rationale: Neck vein distention is indicative of cardiac disease.

30. When auscultating the lung sounds in an adult, the nurse should
    a. use the bell of the stethoscope held lightly against the chest
    b. instruct the patient to breathe in and out through the nose
    c. use the diaphragm of the stethoscope held firmly against the chest*
    d. instruct the patient to take deep, rapid breaths with mouth wide open

    Reference: pp. 480–481

    Descriptors:

    1. 25   2. 07   3. Comprehensive
    4. IV-1   5. Nursing Process   6. Moderate

    Rationale: The diaphragm of the stethoscope amplifies lung sounds, and for an adult, the diaphragm is pressed firmly against the chest.

31. The most important technique when progressing from one auscultatory site on the thorax to another is to compare
    a. top to bottom
    b. side to side*
    c. posterior to anterior
    d. interspace to interspace

    Reference: pp. 479–482

    Descriptors:

    1. 25   2. 03   3. Knowledge
    4. IV-1   5. Nursing Process   6. Moderate

    Rationale: Side-to-side comparison is used to determine on which side of the chest there may be adventitious sounds.

32. The nurse determines that an adult patient has a very loud, low-pitched sound with a booming quality over the left lung. The nurse documents this as
    a. tympany
    b. resonance
    c. hyperresonance*
    d. hollowness

    Reference: p. 484

    Descriptors:

    1. 25   2. 08   3. Application
    4. IV-1   5. Nursing Process   6. Moderate

    Rationale: A very loud, low-pitched sound with a booming quality is termed hyperresonance.

33. While auscultating lung sounds, the nurse hears a grating sound. The nurse documents this finding as
    a. pleural friction rub*
    b. stridor
    c. wheezes
    d. bronchiole rales

    Reference: p. 481

    Descriptors:

    1. 25   2. 08   3. Knowledge
    4. IV-1   5. Nursing Process   6. Moderate

    Rationale: A pleural friction rub is a grating sound caused by an inflamed pleura rubbing against the chest wall.

34. The nurse is caring for a 12-month-old infant who has been hospitalized with croup. While assessing the infant's lung sounds, the nurse notes a harsh, high-pitched sound on inspiration. The nurse should document this finding as
    a. wheezes
    b. crackles
    c. stridor*
    d. stertorous

    Reference: p. 481

    Descriptors:

    1. 25   2. 08   3. Application
    4. II-1   5. Nursing Process   6. Difficult

    Rationale: High-pitched, harsh sounds on inspiration, particularly with children diagnosed with croup, are termed stridor.

35. To auscultate cardiac sounds and hear the S_1 sound most clearly in an adult patient, the nurse plans to place the stethoscope at the area known as
    a. tricuspid
    b. pulmonic
    c. ventricular
    d. apical*

    Reference: p. 483

    Descriptors:

    1. 25   2. 03   3. Application
    4. IV-1   5. Nursing Process   6. Easy

    Rationale: To hear the S_1 heart sound clearly, the nurse should plan to place the stethoscope at the apical area of the chest.

36. An S$_1$ heart sound is made by the closing of the
_____ valves.
a. aortic and tricuspid
b. pulmonary and aortic
c. mitral and tricuspid*
d. mitral and pulmonary
Reference: pp. 482–485
Descriptors:

1. 25   2. 07   3. Knowledge
4. None   5. None   6. Moderate

Rationale: The S$_1$ heart sound is made by the closing of the mitral and tricuspid valves.

37. The base of the heart is located at the
a. top of the heart*
b. bottom of the heart
c. end of the left ventricle
d. left of the sternal border
Reference: pp. 482–485
Descriptors:

1. 25   2. 07   3. Knowledge
4. None   5. None   6. Moderate

Rationale: The base of the heart is located at the top, the apex of the heart is located at the bottom.

38. The heart is assessed in all of the following areas
except
a. mitral
b. tricuspid
c. carotid*
d. Erb's point
Reference: pp. 482–485
Descriptors:

1. 25   2. 03   3. Knowledge
4. IV-1   5. Nursing Process   6. Easy

Rationale: The carotid is not part of the actual heart assessment. In a systematic head to toe assessment, the carotids are assessed before the heart.

39. The main reason auscultation precedes palpation of the abdomen is to
a. allow the patient more time to relax and be more comfortable
b. prevent distortion of vascular sounds that might be heard
c. prevent distortion of bowel sounds that might occur after palpation*
d. determine specific areas of tenderness before palpation

Reference: pp. 488–498
Descriptors:

1. 25   2. 07   3. Comprehensive
4. IV-1   5. Nursing Process   6. Difficult

Rationale: Auscultation must precede palpation because palpation may distort bowel sounds.

40. The nurse is preparing to perform a vaginal examination and obtain specimens of an adult patient. After explaining the procedure to the patient, and putting on clean gloves, the nurse should then
a. apply a water-soluble lubricant
b. warm the speculum with warm water*
c. wash the perineal area
d. observe for lesions on the labia
Reference: p. 491
Descriptors:

1. 25   2. 07   3. Application
4. IV-1   5. Nursing Process   6. Moderate

Rationale: After explaining the procedure, and putting on gloves, the nurse should then warm the speculum.

41. The nurse plans to assess a female patient's vagus nerve by asking the patient to
a. shrug her shoulders against the nurse's resistance
b. protrude her arms forward
c. raise her eyelids
d. swallow and speak*
Reference: p. 498
Descriptors:

1. 25   2. 07   3. Application
4. IV-1   5. Nursing Process   6. Moderate

Rationale: The vagus nerve is intact if the patient can swallow and speak.

42. During a health assessment, the nurse asks the patient to open and clench her jaws to assess the
a. hypoglossal nerve
b. facial nerve
c. trigeminal nerve*
d. accessory nerve
Reference: p. 497
Descriptors:

1. 25   2. 07   3. Application
4. IV-1   5. Nursing Process   6. Moderate

Rationale: When the patient can open and clench her jaws, the nurse is assessing the trigeminal nerve.

43. The nurse has instructed an adult patient about nuclear scanning for a possible brain tumor. The nurse determines that the patient understands the instructions when the patient says
    a. "I will be without food or fluids for 4 hours after the test."
    b. "This test is similar to having an MRI."
    c. "Electrical impulses will be recorded on a graph."
    d. "I will receive a radionuclide for this test."*

Reference: p. 503

Descriptors:

1. 25	2. 09	3. Application
4. II-2	5. Teach/Learn	6. Moderate

Rationale: The patient has understood the instructions when the patient says he will receive a radionuclide for this test.

CHAPTER 26

Safety

1. A nurse working in an operating room has just learned that she is pregnant. The nurse should
   a. consider a temporary transfer to another area of the healthcare facility*
   b. use caution when administering intravenous fluids to patients
   c. discontinue seat belt use until after delivery
   d. take frequent rest breaks after lengthy operations

   Reference: p. 507

   Descriptors:

1. 26	2. 02	3. Application
4. I-2	5. Self Care	6. Moderate

   Rationale: Because there are many hazards to pregnant women in the operating room setting, the nurse should request a temporary transfer until after the delivery.

2. The nurse recognizes that the developmental task of old age is to
   a. foster dependence
   b. maintain independence*
   c. lose self-esteem
   d. gain courage

   Reference: pp. 508–509

   Descriptors:

1. 26	2. 04	3. Knowledge
4. II-2	5. Nursing Process	6. Moderate

   Rationale: Integrity versus despair is Erickson's developmental task of old age. Maintenance of independence would foster integrity.

3. The first priority when a fire occurs it to
   a. rescue anyone in immediate danger*
   b. notify the appropriate persons
   c. close doors and windows
   d. get the fire extinguisher ready

   Reference: p. 510

   Descriptors:

1. 26	2. 09	3. Application
4. I-2	5. Caring	6. Easy

   Rationale: The first priority is to rescue anyone in danger.

4. A nurse is liable if a hospitalized patient falls if the nurse's behavior is
   a. reasonable
   b. prudent
   c. similar to behavior found in other nurses
   d. irresponsible and unreasonable*

   Reference: pp. 509–510

   Descriptors:

1. 26	2. 03	3. Knowledge
4. I-1	5. Caring	6. Easy

   Rationale: The nurse is liable if he is not responsible and is unreasonable in behavior.

5. Most drowning victims are children under the age of 5 due to
   a. inadequate supervision in the bathtub or small pool*
   b. boating accidents involving speed boats
   c. improper flotation devices near pools
   d. lack of lifeguards on duty during pool hours

   Reference: p. 511

   Descriptors:

1. 26	2. 04	3. Knowledge
4. I-2	5. Caring	6. Easy

   Rationale: Inadequate supervision in any type of water is the main cause of drowning in children under age 5 years.

6. The most important health promotion tactic for accident prevention is
   a. assessment
   b. planning
   c. helping
   d. teaching*

Reference: p 17

Descriptors:

1. 26	2. 07	3. Knowledge
4. I-2	5. Teach/Learn	6. Easy

Rationale: Teaching is the most important tool for accident prevention.

7. The number one cause of death for school-aged children, adolescents, and young adults is
   a. drowning
   b. alcohol intoxication
   c. motor vehicle accidents*
   d. huffing

Reference: p. 513

Descriptors:

1. 26	2. 04	3. Knowledge
4. I-2	5. None	6. Easy

Rationale: Motor vehicle accidents are the number one cause of death for school-aged children, adolescents, and young adults.

8. The nurse is caring for a pregnant patient in the clinic when the patient tells the nurse that she is trying to stop smoking. The nurse instructs the patient that smoking while pregnant can lead to
   a. severe congenital anomalies
   b. congenital blindness
   c. decreased weight loss after pregnancy
   d. low birthweight in the newborn*

Reference: p. 513

Descriptors:

1. 26	2. 02	3. Application
4. II-1	5. Teach/Learn	6. Moderate

Rationale: Smoking during pregnancy is associated with low-birthweight infants.

9. The nurse is planning to instruct a group of high school students on the topic of safety. Which of the following would be important to include in the teaching plan?
   a. Many motor vehicle accident fatalities are alcohol related.*
   b. Domestic violence is common in this age group.
   c. Falls and sports injuries are the primary cause of fatalities.
   d. Poisonings contribute to the majority of suicides for this age group.

Reference: p. 513

Descriptors:

1. 26	2. 02	3. Application
4. I-2	5. Teach/Learn	6. Moderate

Rationale: The important teaching aspect for adolescents is that motor vehicle accidents that result in fatalities are frequently alcohol related.

10. An 80-year-old patient is participating in a stroke rehabilitation program. A primary concern for the patient is
    a. love and belonging
    b. self-actualization
    c. safety*
    d. self-esteem

Reference: pp. 512–519

Descriptors:

1. 26	2. 04	3. Comprehensive
4. I-2	5. Self Care	6. Moderate

Rationale: According to Maslow, safety needs must be met first. After a stroke, there is a potential for falls, accidents, injuries due to altered mobility.

11. The nurse is planning a class related to safety issues for children for a group of new mothers. Which of the following would be important to include in the teaching plan?
    a. Small pillows may be used for newborns in their cribs.
    b. Toddlers should be put to sleep on their stomachs after eating.
    c. Carbon monoxide poisoning is common among young children.
    d. Drowning is a common cause of mortality among young children.*

Reference: p. 514

Descriptors:

1. 26	2. 02	3. Application
4. I-2	5. Teach/Learn	6. Moderate

Rationale: Drowning is a common cause of mortality among young children, primarily due to accidents.

12. The nurse has instructed a new mother about the use of infant car seats. The nurse determines that the patient understood the instructions when she says
    a. "I should use a rear-facing car seat placed in the back seat of the car."*
    b. "A rear-facing car seat can be used in the front seat if I have a car with airbags."
    c. "There are some states in the United States that do not require infant car seats be used."
    d. "If my child is over 25 pounds, the child can use a seat belt."

Reference: p. 513

Descriptors:

1. 26	2. 03	3. Application
4. I-2	5. Teach/Learn	6. Moderate

Rationale: The mother has understood the instructions when she says that the rear-facing car seat should be placed in the back seat of the car. All states have child car seat safety laws.

13. The nurse is assessing a 4½-year-old child while the mother is nearby. The nurse should explain to the mother that a major safety threat for preschoolers is
    a. fires
    b. dog bites
    c. ingestion of poisons*
    d. flammable toys

Reference: p. 513

Descriptors:

1. 26	2. 02	3. Application
4. II-1	5. Teach/Learn	6. Moderate

Rationale: A major safety threat to preschoolers is ingestion of poisons. All parents should have syrup of ipecac on hand and the emergency poison control number near the telephone.

14. An 84-year-old patient lives alone in a one-room apartment. The safety assessment reveals many scatter rugs and no hand rails in the bathroom. A priority nursing diagnosis is
    a. Risk for Injury related to use of scatter rugs and no hand rails in bathroom*
    b. Potential for Falls related to living alone in an apartment
    c. Self-Care Deficit related to age and immobility
    d. Impaired Mobility related to advanced age and being alone

Reference: p. 516

Descriptors:

1. 26	2. 02	3. Comprehensive
4. I-2	5. Nursing Process	6. Moderate

Rationale: A priority nursing diagnosis is stated as Risk for Injury related to use of scatter rugs and no hand rails in the bathroom.

15. The leading cause of accidental death in persons aged 79 years or older is
    a. motor vehicle accidents
    b. fires
    c. poisoning
    d. falls*

Reference: p. 516

Descriptors:

1. 26	2. 03	3. Knowledge
4. I-2	5. None	6. Easy

Rationale: Falls are the leading cause of accidental death in persons aged 79 years and older.

16. All of the following interventions are necessary with the use of restraints except
    a. skin assessment
    b. use of least restrictive device
    c. monitor behavior of patient
    d. call family member to sit with patient*

Reference: p. 517–520

Descriptors:

1. 26	2. 09	3. Comprehensive
4. I-2	5. Nursing Process	6. Moderate

Rationale: Family members are usually not able to come and sit with the patient at all times.

17. The nurse has instructed a group of certified nursing assistants about the use of restraints within the healthcare facility. The nurse determines that one of the assistants needs further instructions when she says
    a. "Using restraints on confused patients usually leads to fewer fractures."*
    b. "In some situations, temporary restraints may be the only solution."
    c. "There is danger of suffocation when restraints are used."
    d. "Pressure ulcers and fractures have been associated with use of restraints."

Reference: p. 518

Descriptors:

1. 26	2. 03	3. Application
4. I-2	5. Teach/Learn	6. Moderate

Rationale: The nursing assistant needs further instructions when the assistant says that using restraints on confused patients leads to fewer fractures. Fracture rates increase when restraints are used.

18. The nurse discovers a fire with smoke in the bathroom of a patient's hospital room. After evacuating the patients and visitors from the room, the nurse should
    a. get the fire extinguisher ready
    b. activate the hospital's fire code system*
    c. call the fire department
    d. place wet sheets under the closed door

Reference: p. 520

Descriptors:

1. 26	2. 08	3. Application
4. I-2	5. Communication	6. Moderate

Rationale: The nurse should remove the patients and visitors and then immediately activate the hospital's fire code system.

19. The nurse removes the vest restraint of an 81-year-old patient. While the patient is free of the restraint, the nurse plans to
    a. keep the restraint tied to the bed rails
    b. feed the patient a snack or fruit juice
    c. leave the patient alone in bed for a while
    d. encourage the patient to exercise*

Reference: p. 524

Descriptors:

1. 26	2. 05	3. Application
4. IV-3	5. Nursing Process	6. Easy

Rationale: The nurse should not leave the patient alone, but should encourage the patient to stretch and get some exercise.

20. The nurse is completing an incident report after a hospitalized patient fell in the hallway while walking. No injuries are apparent. The nurse plans to
    a. document who was responsible for walking the patient
    b. provide details about the patient's response after the incident*
    c. send the incident report to the medical records department after it is completed
    d. ask the physician to document the patient's condition in the medical record after the incident

Reference: p. 525

Descriptors:

1. 26	2. 03	3. Application
4. IV-3	5. Communication	6. Moderate

Rationale: The nurse completing the incident report should document the patient's response after the fall. This does not become part of the medical record.

21. The nurse is caring for an 82-year-old apparently healthy patient who has recently moved into a two-story house with his 55-year-old son. The nurse plans to discuss safety issues with the son. Which of the following should be included in the nurse's teaching plan?
    a. Throw rugs should have nonskid backing.
    b. All medications should be locked up.
    c. A cane would be useful to prevent falls.
    d. The area around the stairs should be kept clear.*

Reference: p. 526

Descriptors:

1. 26	2. 05	3. Application
4. I-2	5. Teach/Learn	6. Moderate

Rationale: To prevent falls, the area around the stairs should be kept clear at all times.

22. The nurse makes a home visit to an 86-year-old patient with limited financial resources. While discussing fire safety with the patient, the nurse should first assess
    a. how the patient plans to escape a fire
    b. how the patient heats the house*
    c. the frequency of checking whether the oven is off
    d. if the patient knows the telephone number for emergencies

Reference: p. 526

Descriptors:

1. 26	2. 02	3. Application
4. I-2	5. Teach/Learn	6. Moderate

Rationale: Patients with limited resources may overload electrical sockets from space heaters, or perhaps use kerosene heaters to conserve resources.

23. The nurse is caring for an 80-year-old patient who is taking numerous daily medications for arthritis, hypertension, and a urinary tract infection. The nurse should suggest to the patient that he
    a. take the medicine for arthritis first to relieve pain
    b. take all of the daily medications at the same time
    c. ask the doctor if he can stop taking some of the medications
    d. use a medication calendar or diary to keep track of the medications*

Reference: p. 527

Descriptors:

1. 26	2. 03	3. Application
4. IV-2	5. Teach/Learn	6. Moderate

Rationale: The appropriate suggestion by the nurse is to suggest to the patient that he use a medication calendar or diary to keep track of the medications.

CHAPTER 27

Asepsis

1. A patient is seen in the emergency room following an outdoor picnic and is diagnosed with Lyme disease from a deer tick. The nurse should explain to the patient that this type of infection is transmitted by
   a. vehicle
   b. vector*
   c. airborne
   d. indirect contact

   Reference: p. 536
   Descriptors:

1. 27	2. 02	3. Knowledge
4. IV-3	5. Teach/Learn	6. Moderate

   Rationale: Lyme disease from a deer tick is considered a vector.

2. The nurse has instructed a group of healthcare workers about prevention of the virus that transmits hepatitis B. The nurse determines that one of the workers needs further instructions when she says that the virus is transmitted by
   a. blood
   b. feces
   c. bodily fluids
   d. sweat*

   Reference: p. 536
   Descriptors:

1. 27	2. 02	3. Application
4. I-2	5. Teach/Learn	6. Moderate

   Rationale: The worker needs further instructions when she says that the hepatitis B virus is transmitted by sweat. It is transmitted by blood, feces, and other bodily fluids, but not in sweat.

3. The interval between the invasion of the body by the pathogen and appearance of symptoms of infection is called a
   a. prodromal stage
   b. full-stage illness
   c. convalescent period
   d. incubation period*

   Reference: p. 537
   Descriptors:

1. 27	2. 08	3. Knowledge
4. None	5. None	6. Moderate

   Rationale: During the incubation stage the organisms are growing and multiplying.

4. An adult male patient has a sore throat, fever, and chills. These symptoms indicate
   a. full-stage illness*
   b. prodromal stage
   c. convalescent period
   d. incubation period

   Reference: p. 537
   Descriptors:

1. 27	2. 04	3. Knowledge
4. IV-3	5. Nursing Process	6. Moderate

   Rationale: Full-stage illness is the presence of specific signs and symptoms.

5. An adult female patient complains of feeling achy all over and being tired. This stage of infection is called
   a. convalescent period
   b. full-stage illness
   c. prodromal stage*
   d. incubation period

   Reference: p. 537
   Descriptors:

1. 27	2. 04	3. Knowledge
4. IV-3	5. Nursing Process	6.. Moderate

   Rationale: In the prodromal stage, early signs and symptoms are present but they are vague and nonspecific. A person is most infectious at this time.

6. Return of the patient to a healthy state occurs in the
   a. prodromal stage
   b. full-stage illness
   c. convalescent period*
   d. incubation period

Reference: p. 537

Descriptors:

1. 27   2. 04   3. Knowledge

4. None   5. None   6. Easy

Rationale: Recovery occurs in the convalescent period. Signs and symptoms disappear.

7. An 80-year-old female patient is diagnosed with chronic urinary tract infections. The nurse plans to instruct the patient that one of the reasons for increased urinary tract infections in older adults is that
   a. there is less intact skin
   b. the bladder is not completely emptied*
   c. changes occur in the skin's pH
   d. there is an increase in estrogen production

Reference: p. 538

Descriptors:

1. 27   2. 05   3. Application

4. IV-3   5. Teach/Learn   6. Moderate

Rationale: Urinary tract infections are more common in older adults because of decreased estrogen production, relaxation of the pelvic floor, and the bladder not emptying completely.

8. An 85-year-old patient is hospitalized with pneumonia and a urinary tract infection. The patient has an indwelling urinary catheter and appears malnourished. The nurse caring for the patient determines that the patient's priority nursing diagnosis is
   a. Risk for Chronic Infections and Anxiety due to advanced age
   b. Risk for Further Infection related to malnutrition and urinary catheter*
   c. Immobility related to urinary catheter and infection
   d. Social Isolation related to presence of disease

Reference: p. 538

Descriptors:

1. 27   2. 08   3. Comprehensive

4. IV-3   5. Nursing Process   6. Moderate

Rationale: The priority nursing diagnosis is Risk for infection related to malnutrition and urinary catheter.

9. Nosocomial infections are usually
   a. genetic
   b. contagious
   c. vector attained
   d. hospital acquired*

Reference:

p. 540

Descriptors:

1. 27   2. 01   3. Knowledge

4. I-2   5. Nursing Process   6. Easy

Rationale: Nosocomial infections are hospital acquired from personnel or equipment.

10. When treating patients with pneumonia, the handwashing product for healthcare workers to use should contain which ingredient?
    a. antimicrobial*
    b. emollient
    c. antiseptic
    d. detergent

Reference: p. 541

Descriptors:

1. 27   2. 06   3. Knowledge

4. I-2   5. Nursing Process   6. Easy

Rationale: Antimicrobial or antibacterial soap kills the bacteria or suppresses their growth.

11. A 70-year-old patient has had an indwelling urinary catheter for 8 hours following surgery. Before removing the catheter, the nurse sends a urine sample for analysis, culture, and sensitivity to determine if the patient has developed an infection termed
    a. exogenous
    b. viral
    c. microbial
    d. iatrogenic*

Reference: p. 540

Descriptors:

1. 27   2. 01   3. Knowledge

4. IV-1   5. Nursing Process   6. Moderate

Rationale: Iatrogenic infections are acquired through a treatment or a diagnostic procedure such as a urinary catheter.

12. The nurse has conducted a class for healthcare workers on the topic of infection control. The nurse determines that one of the workers needs further instructions when he says that
    a. "Most hospital-acquired infections are due to bacteria."
    b. "Indwelling catheters have been implicated in a large percentage of infections."
    c. "Hospital-acquired infections are relatively easy to treat with antibiotics."*
    d. "Frequent handwashing is the best method of preventing hospital-acquired infections."

Reference: p. 540

Descriptors:

1. 27	2. 03	3. Application
4. I-1	5. Teach/Learn	6. Moderate

Rationale: The worker needs further instructions when he says that hospital-acquired infections are relatively easy to treat with antibiotics. Many disease-causing organisms are becoming resistant to antibiotic therapy.

13. A hospitalized patient has developed a severe enterococci infection following abdominal surgery. The nurse plans to administer
    a. methicillin
    b. cleocin
    c. streptomycin
    d. vancomycin*

Reference: pp. 540–541

Descriptors:

1. 27	2. 06	3. Application
4. IV-2	5. Nursing Process	6. Moderate

Rationale: At the present time, vancomycin is the drug of choice; however, some strains of *Escherichia coli* are becoming resistant to the drug. Newer drugs are coming on the market to treat these resistant organisms.

14. The nurse has instructed a group of newly employed nursing assistants about medical asepsis. The nurse assesses the workers during morning care and determines that medical asepsis techniques have been broken by the employee who
    a. keeps soiled linens away from his clothing
    b. places soiled linens on the floor near the patient*
    c. uses a dampened cloth to dust the overhead table
    d. cleans the least soiled area near the patient first

Reference: p. 540

Descriptors:

1. 27	2. 03	3. Application
4. I-2	5. Nursing Process	6. Moderate

Rationale: Medical asepsis techniques have been broken by the employee who places soiled linens on the floor near the patient.

15. Before changing a clean dressing of a home care patient, the nurse should *first*
    a. wash the hands with an antibacterial soap*
    b. remove any nail polish on the fingernails
    c. put on a pair of sterile gloves
    d. remove any wedding rings or other jewelry

Reference: p. 541

Descriptors:

1. 27	2. 07	3. Application
4. I-2	5. Nursing Process	6. Easy

Rationale: Before changing a clean dressing of a home care patient, the nurse should *first* wash the hands with an antibacterial soap before donning gloves.

16. While caring for a patient who has intermittent diarrhea, the nurse plans to take precautions to prevent contamination from
    a. *Escherichia coli**
    b. *Clostridium difficile*
    c. *Staphylococcus aureus*
    d. *Neisseria meningitis*

Reference: p. 541

Descriptors:

1. 27	2. 09	3. Knowledge
4. I-2	5. Nursing Process	6. Moderate

Rationale: *Escherichia coli* are found in human feces.

17. The nurse is working in a gynecologic clinic. Before sending contaminated speculums to the central supply area for sterilization, the nurse plans to be certain that the items are
    a. washed first in hot soapy water
    b. sent in a basin of warm soapy water
    c. placed in a container designated for bodily fluids
    d. rinsed first in cold running water*

Reference: p. 545

Descriptors:

1. 27	2. 03	3. Application
4. I-2	5. Nursing Process	6. Moderate

Rationale: Equipment should be rinsed in cold running water before sending the contaminated equipment to the central supply area.

18. The nurse makes a home visit to care for a patient diagnosed with HIV. The nurse should instruct the patient that an effective disinfectant for home use is
    a. alcohol
    b. chlorine bleach*
    c. boiling water
    d. iodine

Reference: p. 545

Descriptors:

1. 27	2. 03	3. Application
4. I-2	5. Teach/Learn	6. Moderate

Rationale: An effective disinfectant is chlorine bleach.

19. The nurse is caring for a 68-year-old patient at home with a postoperative abdominal skin dressing and drain. The nurse assesses the patient and determines that the technique used for this dressing change should be
   a. clean
   b. antiseptic
   c. sterile*
   d. medically aseptic

Reference: p. 546

Descriptors:

1. 27	2. 10	3. Application
4. IV-3	5. Nursing Process	6. Easy

Rationale: Patients with wound dressings should have the dressing changed using sterile technique to prevent infection.

20. An adult patient has been instructed on the use of sterile technique to change his dressing. During a return demonstration, the nurse determines that the patient has understood the instructions when he
   a. puts on sterile gloves before beginning the procedure
   b. places the solution container at the back of the sterile field
   c. opens the sterile dressing package and drops it from a height of 16 inches
   d. opens the sterile dressing packages before donning the sterile gloves*

Reference: p. 547

Descriptors:

1. 27	2. 10	3. Application
4. I-2	5. Teach/Learn	6. Moderate

Rationale: The nurse determines that the patient has understood the instructions when the patient opens the sterile dressing packages before donning the sterile gloves. Putting on sterile gloves before beginning the procedure, placing the solution container at the back of the sterile field, and opening the sterile dressing package and dropping it from a height of 16 inches are all incorrect.

21. The nurse assesses a sterile field and determines that it has been contaminated when the nurse observes
   a. the outer 1 inch of the sterile towel over the side of the table
   b. sterile objects held above the waist of the practitioner
   c. sterile packages opened so that the first edge is away from the practitioner
   d. moisture on the sterile cloth on top of a nonsterile table*

Reference: p. 548

Descriptors:

1. 27	2. 10	3. Application
4. I-2	5. Nursing Process	6. Moderate

Rationale: Sterile technique has been broken when there is moisture or wetness on the sterile cloth on top of a nonsterile table.

22. The nurse is preparing to perform a normal saline wet-to-dry dressing change on a home care patient. The nurse notes that the capped, partially used bottle of saline at the patient's bedside was opened 4 hours ago today. The nurse should
   a. discard a small amount of the solution into the sink before using the solution*
   b. ask the patient if the bottle was really opened only 4 hours ago
   c. throw away the old bottle and open a new one before the dressing change
   d. clean the inside of the cap with alcohol before putting the contents on a sterile area

Reference: p. 548

Descriptors:

1. 27	2. 10	3. Application
4. IV-3	5. Nursing Process	6. Moderate

Rationale: Discarding a small amount of solution into the sink before using the solution will maintain sterility of the contents.

23. Surgical asepsis differs from medical asepsis in that surgical asepsis
   a. confines a specific microorganism to a specific area
   b. keeps an area or object free from all microorganisms*
   c. keeps an area or object free from pathogens
   d. limits the number of microorganisms in an area

Reference: p. 546–549

Descriptors:

| 1. 27 | 2. 01 | 3. Knowledge |
| 4. None | 5. None | 6. Easy |

Rationale: Surgical asepsis keeps an area free from all microorganisms.

24. Which of the following situations has the highest potential for contaminating a sterile field? The nurse
   a. diverts her head from the sterile field when talking
   b. holds her sterile gloved hands above the waist
   c. reaches around a sterile field
   d. turns her back on the sterile field*

Reference: pp. 546–549

Descriptors:

| 1. 27 | 2. 01 | 3. Application |
| 4. I-2 | 5. Nursing Process | 6. Moderate |

Rationale: The nurse should not turn her back on the sterile field because it causes the area to become contaminated.

25. Which of the following situations is an example of microorganism transmission via droplet contact?
   a. An infected wound drainage contacts the nurse's hand.
   b. A virus is transmitted through sexual intercourse.
   c. Infectious microorganisms contact a person's nasal mucosa when someone coughs nearby.*
   d. A contaminated stethoscope touches the skin of a patient.

Reference: pp. 546–549

Descriptors:

| 1. 27 | 2. 01 | 3. Comprehensive |
| 4. I-2 | 5. Nursing Process | 6. Moderate |

Rationale: Droplet transmission is by coughing, sneezing, or talking.

26. The nurse is planning to remove sterile gloves following a wet-to-dry dressing change. The nurse plans to
   a. use the dominant hand to grasp the other glove on the outside of the cuff*
   b. use the nondominant hand to grasp the other glove at the fingertips
   c. grasp the glove on the nondominant hand on the inside of the glove's cuff
   d. wash both hands with an antimicrobial solution before removal

Reference: p. 552

Descriptors:

| 1. 27 | 2. 10 | 3. Application |
| 4. I-2 | 5. Nursing Process | 6. Moderate |

Rationale: To remove sterile gloves correctly, the nurse should use the dominant hand to grasp the other glove on the outside of the cuff.

27. The nurse has instructed a group of new employees about universal precautions. The nurse determines that one of the employees needs further instructions when he says that universal precautions are necessary when handling items that are soiled with
   a. sweat*
   b. amniotic fluid
   c. cerebrospinal fluid
   d. urine

Reference: p. 552

Descriptors:

| 1. 27 | 2. 09 | 3. Application |
| 4. I-2 | 5. Teach/Learn | 6. Moderate |

Rationale: Universal body precautions apply to amniotic fluid, cerebrospinal fluid, urine, and feces, not sweat.

28. The nurse is notified that a patient with tuberculosis and a fractured leg will soon be admitted to the hospital unit. The nurse determines that this patient will require
   a. contact isolation
   b. droplet precautions*
   c. immunity precautions
   d. strict isolation

Reference: p. 556

Descriptors:

| 1. 27 | 2. 09 | 3. Application |
| 4. I-2 | 5. Nursing Process | 6. Moderate |

Rationale: A patient with tuberculosis requires droplet precautions because the disease is spread by contamination with sputum.

29. Healthcare providers can prevent needlestick injuries by
   a. not recapping needles*
   b. placing used needles in the trash
   c. donning sterile gloves before using the syringe
   d. carefully removing the needle from the syringe

Reference: p. 556

Descriptors:

1. 27	2. 09	3. Application
4. I-2	5. Nursing Process	6. Moderate

Rationale: Do not recap needles after injections to prevent injury. Dispose in sharps containers as soon as the nurse is finished with the syringe.

30. An elderly patient has been admitted to the hospital and is diagnosed with vancomycin-resistant enterococci (VRE). The nurse plans to instruct the patient that
    a. visitors are contraindicated
    b. all healthcare workers will wear masks before entering the room
    c. sterile gloves will be used when providing care
    d. frequently used equipment will be kept in the room*

Reference: p. 556

Descriptors:

1. 27	2. 10	3. Application
4. I-2	5. Nursing Process	6. Moderate

Rationale: The nurse should instruct the patient that frequently used equipment, such as a sphygmomanometer, will be kept in the room.

31. The nurse has demonstrated how to don sterile gloves to a group of nursing students. The nurse should instruct the students that
    a. vinyl glove punctures reseal automatically
    b. latex gloves are used primarily with major procedures
    c. vinyl gloves are less costly and easier to don
    d. latex gloves can result in allergic reactions*

Reference: p. 560

Descriptors:

1. 27	2. 10	3. Application
4. I-2	5. Teach/Learn	6. Moderate

Rationale: Latex gloves are less expensive than vinyl, but can result in allergic reactions.

32. The nurse is supervising a nursing student who is preparing to provide care for a patient with active tuberculosis. Before assisting the student in providing care to this patient, the nurse assesses the student's awareness of the necessity for wearing
    a. masks*
    b. sterile gloves
    c. sterile gowns
    d. clean gloves

Reference: p. 556

Descriptors:

1. 27	2. 09	3. Application
4. I-2	5. Teach/Learn	6. Moderate

Rationale: Masks are necessary when caring for patients with tuberculosis because it is spread by droplet transmission.

33. The nurse is planning to assist another nurse to perform tracheostomy suctioning on an adult patient. Before beginning the procedure, the nurse plans to
    a. double-bag all used equipment
    b. obtain a particulate respirator mask
    c. wear protective eyewear with sideshields*
    d. put on a sterile gown while in the room

Reference: p. 558

Descriptors:

1. 27	2. 10	3. Application
4. I-2	5. Nursing Process	6. Moderate

Rationale: Before performing tracheostomy suctioning, the nurse should protect the eyes from any splashing by donning protective eyewear with sideshields.

34. The infection control nurse becomes concerned when she inspects a unit in a hospital and observes
    a. double-bagging of soiled linens
    b. securely tied plastic trash bags
    c. a leaking urine specimen placed in a basket*
    d. clean gloves being worn by laundry personnel

Reference: p. 561

Descriptors:

1. 27	2. 09	3. Application
4. I-2	5. Nursing Process	6. Moderate

Rationale: Urine is a bodily fluid and should be placed in a sealed plastic bag or container before sending it to the laboratory.

35. A patient has been placed in isolation because he is diagnosed with a contagious illness. The nurse should instruct the patient that
    a. linens from the patient's bed will be double-bagged
    b. meals will be served on washable dishes*
    c. extensive isolation rarely causes psychological problems
    d. paper trays and plastic utensils prevent disease transmission

Reference: p. 561

Descriptors:

1. 27   2. 10   3. Application
4. I-2   5. Nursing Process   6. Moderate

Rationale: Washable dishes are recommended rather than disposable products.

36. If the nurse receives a needlestick following administration of an injection to a patient, the nurse should *first*
    a. wash the exposed area with soap and warm water*
    b. report the incident to the appropriate supervisor
    c. receive a blood test to determine HIV status
    d. ask the patient to consent to an HIV blood test

Reference: p. 562

Descriptors:

1. 27   2. 09   3. Application
4. I-2   5. Nursing Process   6. Moderate

Rationale: The nurse with a needlestick injury should first wash the exposed area with soap and warm water. After this, the incident should be reported to the supervisor or follow the institutional policies.

CHAPTER 28

Medications

1. The law enacted in 1970 to regulate the distribution of narcotics and other drugs of abuse is known as the
   a. Food and Drug Administration act
   b. Federal Narcotics act
   c. Pure Food and Drug act
   d. Controlled Substances act*

   Reference: p. 568

   Descriptors:

   1. 28   2. 02   3. Knowledge
   4. None   5. None   6. Easy

   Rationale: The Controlled Substances act was passed in 1970 to regulate the distribution of narcotics and other drugs of abuse.

2. When different manufacturers produce the same drug, the drug is usually sold by its
   a. generic name
   b. formulary name
   c. brand name*
   d. official name

   Reference: p. 569

   Descriptors:

   1. 28   2. 01   3. Knowledge
   4. None   5. None   6. Easy

   Rationale: When different manufacturers produce and sell the same drug, it is known by its brand name.

3. The name for the drug Tylenol is termed
   a. trade*
   b. generic
   c. chemical
   d. formulary

   Reference: p. 569

   Descriptors:

   1. 28   2. 03   3. Knowledge
   4. None   5. None   6. Easy

   Rationale: Tylenol is a trade, brand, or proprietary name selected by the drug company and is copyrighted.

4. The study of the movement of drug molecules in the body in relation to the drug's absorption, distribution, metabolism, and excretion is termed
   a. pharmacokinetics*
   b. pharmacology
   c. pharmacodynamics
   d. phramacoanthropology

   Reference: p. 569

   Descriptors:

   1. 28   2. 04   3. Knowledge
   4. None   5. None   6. Easy

   Rationale: The study of how drugs interact in the body is termed pharmacokinetics.

5. Patients with liver failure would most likely have problems with drug
   a. excretion
   b. absorption
   c. metabolism*
   d. distribution

   Reference: pp. 569–570

   Descriptors:

   1. 28   2. 04   3. Knowledge
   4. None   5. None   6. Moderate

   Rationale: Metabolism of drugs occurs in the liver.

6. The nurse is caring for a patient who is 12 weeks pregnant. The nurse should explain to the patient that drugs taken during pregnancy
   a. have the potential for harmful effects on the fetus*
   b. can have a synergistic effect on both the mother and fetus
   c. will typically cause fetal anomalies prior to delivery
   d. should only be taken in a water-soluble form

Reference: p. 571

Descriptors:

1. 28	2. 0	3. Knowledge
4. II-1	5. Teach/Learn	6. Easy

Rationale: Certain drugs can be teratogenic; therefore, there is potential harm for the fetus. The patient shouldn't take any drugs without first contacting the healthcare provider.

7. The majority of medications are metabolized in the
   a. gallbladder
   b. pancreas
   c. liver*
   d. small intestine

Reference: p. 571

Descriptors:

1. 28	2. 04	3. Knowledge
4. None	5. None	6. Easy

Rationale: Because the majority of medications are metabolized in the liver, the nurse should look for signs of liver malfunction, such as weight loss, jaundice, or lack of appetite.

8. A 10-year-old child weighing 115 pounds has an order for Demerol 50 mg IM q 3–4 hours following extensive abdominal surgery. The nurse caring for this patient determines that
   a. this dosage is appropriate for the child's weight*
   b. this dosage is not recommended for a 10-year-old child
   c. higher pain tolerances in children should not require Demerol
   d. the absorption rate of Demerol requires an increased dosage

Reference: p. 571

Descriptors:

1. 28	2. 05	3. Application
4. IV-2	5. Nursing Process	6. Difficult

Rationale: This dosage is appropriate for the child's age and weight.

9. A 75-year-old patient has been taking antihypertensive medications for 2 days. The nurse should assess the patient for symptoms of
   a. increased weight gain
   b. stomach irritation
   c. dizziness or light-headedness*
   d. diarrhea or runny stools

Reference: p. 572

Descriptors:

1. 28	2. 05	3. Application
4. IV-2	5. Nursing Process	6. Moderate

Rationale: Antihypertensives, when taken by elderly patients, may cause dizziness or light-headedness. If these symptoms persist, the patient may discontinue the medications.

10. The nurse is caring for an Asian American patient weighing 106 pounds who has been given a prescription for antihypertensive medication. The nurse should instruct the patient that
    a. Asian American patients may not be able to tolerate this medication
    b. the medication can be discontinued once the blood pressure stabilizes
    c. herbal remedies and teas may interfere with the drug's action*
    d. enzyme deficiencies in Asian American patients may interfere with the drug's effects

Reference: p. 572

Descriptors:

1. 28	2. 05	3. Application
4. IV-2	5. Culture	6. Moderate

Rationale: Herbal remedies and teas may interfere with the drug's action.

11. About an hour after administration of penicillin 500 mg PO, the patient complains of an itchy rash over his arms and abdomen. The nurse determines that the patient is most likely experiencing a reaction to the drug termed
    a. allergic*
    b. anaphylactic
    c. idiosyncratic
    d. antagonistic

Reference: p. 574

Descriptors:

1. 28	2. 05	3. Comprehensive
4. IV-2	5. Nursing Process	6. Moderate

Rationale: A rash or urticaria is typically present when the patient experiences a drug allergy.

12. The ability to breathe easier secondary to the administration of Theo-Dur is called a/an _____ effect.
    a. therapeutic*
    b. side
    c. secondary
    d. idiosyncratic

Reference: p. 574

Descriptors:

1. 28	2. 05	3. Comprehensive
4. IV-2	5. None	6. Moderate

Rationale: The desired effect of the drug is the therapeutic effect.

13. Within minutes after receiving an injection of penicillin, the patient complains of dyspnea and chest pain. The nurse notifies the patient's physician because this patient is most likely experiencing a drug reaction termed
    a. idiosyncratic
    b. overdose
    c. allergic
    d. anaphylactic*

Reference: p. 574

Descriptors:

1. 28	2. 05	3. Comprehensive
4. IV-2	5. Nursing Process	6. Moderate

Rationale: Chest pain and dyspnea following a medication administration are indicative of an anaphylactic reaction.

14. A 55-year-old patient has been taking Valium 2 mg PO twice daily for several months. In the last few days, the patient has become very agitated and restless. The nurse determines that the patient is most likely experiencing a drug reaction termed
    a. cumulative
    b. tolerant
    c. synergistic
    d. idiosyncratic*

Reference: p. 574

Descriptors:

1. 28	2. 05	3. Comprehensive
4. IV-2	5. None	6. Moderate

Rationale: When a drug has had a therapeutic effect for several months, and then the patient begins to have an opposite effect from the drug, this is termed idiosyncratic.

15. When combining Darvon and acetaminophen for pain relief, the effect would be
    a. combination
    b. doubled
    c. individualized
    d. synergistic*

Reference: p. 574

Descriptors:

1. 28	2. 01	3. Knowledge
4. IV-2	5. None	6. Easy

Rationale: The combination of both drugs produces a synergistic (positive) effect and more so than each drug alone.

16. The nurse is caring for a newly hospitalized patient who has been taking the drug Dilantin daily for several years to control his epilepsy. After admission, the nurse discovers that the physician has not written any medication orders for daily Dilantin. The nurse should
    a. document in the chart that the patient has been taking Dilantin at home
    b. contact the patient's physician for orders for the drug Dilantin*
    c. tell the patient's mother to give him the Dilantin brought from home
    d. contact the patient's physician for an order for Dilantin if the patient has a seizure

Reference: p. 576

Descriptors:

1. 28	2. 08	3. Application
4. IV-2	5. Communication	6. Easy

Rationale: The nurse should contact the patient's physician and request an order for Dilantin to prevent the patient from having a seizure while hospitalized.

17. The nurse is caring for a postoperative patient following chest surgery 4 hours ago. While reviewing the medication orders for the patient's pain medication, the nurse should review the orders termed
    a. single
    b. stat
    c. standing
    d. PRN*

Reference: p. 576

Descriptors:

1. 28	2. 08	3. Application
4. IV-2	5. Nursing Process	6. Easy

Rationale: Postoperative pain medications are typically written PRN or as needed.

18. The nurse is preparing to administer a narcotic to a postoperative patient. In reviewing the physician's order, the nurse should be certain that the order
    a. indicates what to do if the patient refuses the medication
    b. offers several choices for pain medication
    c. identifies the possible allergic reactions to the medication
    d. has a valid date, time, and signature by the order*

    Reference: p. 576

    Descriptors:

1. 28	2. 08	3. Application
4. IV-2	5. Nursing Process	6. Moderate

    Rationale: Narcotic medications must have the physician's date, time, and signature by the order for the medication.

19. The physician orders morphine sulfate, 10 mg IM stat. The nurse interprets this order to mean
    a. as needed
    b. when requested
    c. immediately*
    d. standing orders

    Reference: p. 576

    Descriptors:

1. 28	2. 03	3. Comprehensive
4. IV-2	5. Documentation	6. Easy

    Rationale: Stat means immediately.

20. A nurse prepared a patient's insulin injection of 10 units of Humulin. The nurse is then called to a "code blue" scene and asks another nurse to administer the patient's insulin. The second nurse should
    a. give the medication as soon as possible
    b. refuse to administer the medication*
    c. ask the patient to wait until his nurse returns
    d. call the unit director for advice on the administration

    Reference: p. 578

    Descriptors:

1. 28	2. 08	3. Comprehensive
4. IV-2	5. Nursing Process	6. Moderate

    Rationale: To prevent medication errors, the nurse should only administer medications that she has prepared herself.

21. A nurse is to give a patient a medication for pain. The order reads: "Demerol 500 mg IM" and the PDR states the normal dose is 100 mg. The nurse should
    a. administer the ordered amount
    b. administer the normal amount
    c. contact the physician concerning the written order*
    d. check with the head nurse about the safety of giving the ordered amount

    Reference: p. 578

    Descriptors:

1. 28	2. 09	3. Comprehensive
4. IV-2	5. Communication	6. Moderate

    Rationale: Any drug order suspected to be in error should be questioned.

22. An adult patient is scheduled for surgery in the morning. The physician has ordered a preoperative medication to be administered. The nurse learns that the patient has had an allergic reaction to this medication in the past. The nurse plans to
    a. administer the medication while observing the patient closely for a reaction
    b. contact the patient's physician and indicate that the patient has had a previous allergic reaction*
    c. withhold the medication and notify the nurse in the operating room
    d. ask the patient to describe the reaction he has had to the drug in the past

    Reference: p. 578

    Descriptors:

1. 28	2. 08	3. Application
4. IV-2	5. Communication	6. Moderate

    Rationale: When the patient tells the nurse he has had an allergic reaction to a particular medication, it is the nurse's responsibility to notify the physician. Most likely, the physician will order a different medication.

23. While reviewing a newly admitted patient's medication orders, the nurse has difficulty reading the exact dosage of the drug prescribed because of illegible handwriting. In this situation, the nurse should
    a. ask the other nurses on the unit about the dosage
    b. check the correct dosage in the hospital's Formulary
    c. contact the patient's physician for the correct dosage*
    d. tell the patient that the medication will not be given

Reference: p. 578

Descriptors:

1. 28	2. 08	3. Application
4. IV-2	5. Communication	6. Moderate

Rationale: The nurse's responsibility is to contact the physician for the correct dosage.

24. A physician orders 1000 mL lactated Ringer's solution with 10 mEq KCl to be administered over 8 hours. The tubing drop factor is 60 gtts/mL. How many mL/hr should the nurse administer?
    a. 12.5
    b. 60
    c. 125*
    d. 250

    Reference: p. 579

    Descriptors:

1. 28	2. 07	3. Application
4. IV-2	5. Nursing Process	6. Easy

    Rationale: To answer this, divide 1000 mL by 8 hours (60 gtts/min or 1 mL) and the number of mL/hr = 125.

25. The doctor has ordered: digoxin 0.125 mg/tabs. The nurse has on hand: digoxin 0.25 mg/tabs. The nurse should give
    a. ¼ tab
    b. ½ tab*
    c. 1 tab
    d. 2 tabs

    Reference: p. 580

    Descriptors:

1. 28	2. 07	3. Application
4. IV-2	5. Nursing Process	6. Easy

    Rationale: Divide 0.125 by 0.250 mg and the answer is ½ tab.

26. The physician orders phenobarbital 1 grain. The medication is available in 30-mg tablets. The nurse plans to administer
    a. ½ tablet
    b. 1 tablet
    c. 2 tablets*
    d. 3 tablets

    Reference: p. 580

    Descriptors:

1. 28	2. 07	3. Application
4. IV-2	5. Nursing Process	6. Easy

    Rationale: Two 30-mg tablets are equivalent to 1 grain or 60 mg.

27. The nurse is caring for a 9-year-old child on a pediatric unit. To calculate the appropriate medication dosage, the nurse uses the child's body surface area (BSA). The nurse should calculate the patient's dosage by calculating the
    a. child's BSA times the adult BSA divided by the adult dose equals the child's dose
    b. child's BSA divided by an adult's BSA times adult dose equals child's dose*
    c. adult's BSA divided by the child's BSA times the adult dose equals child's dose
    d. usual adult dose times the weight of the child divided by 150 equals the child's dose

    Reference: p. 580

    Descriptors:

1. 28	2. 05	3. Application
4. IV-2	5. Nursing Process	6. Moderate

    Rationale: To obtain the child's dose, the nurse should determine the child's BSA and divide by the adult's BSA times the adult dose, which equals the child's dose.

28. While preparing an oral medication for an adult patient, the nurse should check the label of the medication container
    a. one time
    b. two times
    c. three times*
    d. four times

    Reference: p. 581

    Descriptors:

1. 28	2. 08	3. Application
4. IV-2	5. Nursing Process	6. Easy

    Rationale: The nurse should check the medication container three times to prevent medication errors.

29. The five rights of medication administration are correct
    a. route, patient, time, signature, dose
    b. patient, time, signature, route, medication
    c. medication, route, patient, time, dosage*
    d. dosage, time, route, medication, doctor order

    Reference: p. 581

    Descriptors:

1. 28	2. 08	3. Knowledge
4. IV-2	5. Documentation	6. Easy

    Rationale: The five rights include correct medication, route, patient, time, and dosage.

30. The nurse is caring for a 78-year-old hospitalized patient. Before administering the ordered intravenous medication, the nurse plans to
    a. ask the patient to state his name
    b. check the patient's bedside tag for his name
    c. ask the patient if he has any allergies to this medication
    d. check the patient's name on his identification bracelet

    Reference: p. 582

    Descriptors:

1. 28	2. 08	3. Application
4. IV-2	5. Nursing Process	6. Moderate

    Rationale: The nurse should always validate the patient's name by checking the patient's identification bracelet.

31. The nurse is caring for a hospitalized adult patient who has several medications to be administered at the same time. The nurse should plan to
    a. determine if the patient can swallow the pills all at once
    b. leave the medications at the patient's bedside if he is out of the room
    c. ask the physician if the patient can be on a different medication schedule
    d. offer the patient one medication at a time while remaining with the patient*

    Reference: p. 582

    Descriptors:

1. 28	2. 08	3. Application
4. IV-2	5. Nursing Process	6. Easy

    Rationale: The nurse should remain with the patient at all times to be certain that the patient has taken the medications.

32. The nurse has instructed an adult patient about the enteric-coated aspirin tablets ordered by the physician. The nurse determines that the patient has understood the instructions when the patient says "Enteric-coated medications
    a. should be cut in half before I take them."
    b. can irritate the bowels."
    c. prevent stomach irritation."*
    d. can be dissolved in a liquid before I take them."

Reference: p. 582

Descriptors:

1. 28	2. 09	3. Application
4. IV-2	5. Teach/Learn	6. Moderate

Rationale: Enteric-coated medications can help to prevent stomach irritation. They do not need to be cut in half and should not be dissolved in a liquid.

33. An adult patient with a nasogastric tube is scheduled to be given a medication via the nasogastric tube. Before administering the medication, the nurse should
    a. flush the tubing with 5 mL of normal saline
    b. determine if the tube is connected to suctioning
    c. dissolve the medication in 15 mL of very cold water
    d. determine patency of the nasogastric tube*

    Reference: p. 587

    Descriptors:

1. 28	2. 08	3. Application
4. IV-2	5. Nursing Process	6. Moderate

    Rationale: The nurse should first ensure patency of the tube by flushing the tubing with 15 to 30 mL of water at room temperature. Cold fluids can cause discomfort.

34. Injecting medications into the body with a needle and syringe is known as the _____ route.
    a. intravenous
    b. parenteral*
    c. topical
    d. inhalation

    Reference: p. 587

    Descriptors:

1. 28	2. 10	3. Knowledge
4. IV-2	5. None	6. Easy

    Rationale: Injecting medications with a needle and syringe is the parenteral route.

35. An adult patient has been prescribed nitroglycerin tablets for chest pain. The nurse should instruct the patient to take the medication by the route termed
    a. sublingual*
    b. oral
    c. nasal
    d. topical

Reference: p. 587

Descriptors:

1. 28 2. 09 3. Application

4. IV-2 5. Teach/Learn 6. Moderate

Rationale: Nitroglycerin tablets should be placed under the tongue, that is, taken sublingually.

36. The nurse is planning to inject 2 mL of a viscous medication to an adult patient who is 6 feet tall and weighs 190 pounds. The nurse plans to use a 3-mL syringe with a needle that is
  a. 5/8 inch 25 gauge
  b. ½ inch 23 gauge
  c. 1½ inch 21 gauge*
  d. 2 inch 14 gauge

Reference: p. 588

Descriptors:

1. 28 2. 08 3. Application

4. IV-2 5. Nursing Process 6. Difficult

Rationale: For a patient of this weight and height and for a viscous 2 mL of medication to be injected, the nurse should select a 1½-inch needle at 21 gauge. The 5/8 and ½ inch needle are too small to reach the muscle; 14-gauge needles are to big for a routine injection.

37. A physician orders Demerol 50 mg IM for a postoperative patient. The medication is in a 10-ml vial. Before drawing the medication into a syringe, the nurse should *first*
  a. break the small neck of the container
  b. discard 1 mL of the medication to ensure sterility
  c. remove the rubber stopper on top of the vial
  d. inject an amount of air equal to the medication dose*

Reference: p. 589

Descriptors:

1. 28 2. 08 3. Application

4. IV-2 5. Nursing Process 6. Moderate

Rationale: Before drawing a medication from the vial, the nurse should wipe the top of the vial with an alcohol prep sponge and inject an amount of air equal to the medication dose.

38. When drawing up a medication from a glass ampule, the nurse should
  a. break the ampule toward the body
  b. consider the rim of the ampule as contaminated*
  c. wrap a paper towel around the ampule before breaking it
  d. inject 0.5 mL into the ampule before drawing up the medication

Reference: p. 590

Descriptors:

1. 28 2. 08 3. Application

4. IV-2 5. Nursing Process 6. Moderate

Rationale: The nurse should use a small alcohol prep sponge to wrap around the ampule before breaking the ampule away from the body. The rim of the ampule is considered contaminated. No air needs to be injected into an ampule.

39. The nurse is caring for a patient who will need to be given a medication before a lengthy diagnostic procedure. The nurse should explain to the patient that the medication route that has the longest absorption time is the route termed
  a. intravenous
  b. intramuscular
  c. intradermal*
  d. transdermal

Reference: p. 594

Descriptors:

1. 28 2. 08 3. Application

4. IV-2 5. Teach/Learn 6. Moderate

Rationale: The medication route that has the longest absorption time is the intradermal route.

40. The physician orders Lente insulin 10 units and Humulin (regular) 5 units SQ at 0700. To mix these two insulins, the nurse should
  a. draw up 10 units of Lente first and place it in the Humulin vial
  b. inject air in the Lente vial after the Humulin vial
  c. draw up the regular insulin last and recap the syringe
  d. put 10 units of air into the Lente prior to putting 5 units of air into the regular vial*

Reference: p. 594–595

Descriptors:

1. 28	2. 01	3. Application
4. IV-2	5. Nursing Process	6. Difficult

Rationale: The nurse should first put air into the cloudy (Lente) vial, then air into the clear vial. Draw the clear solution out first, then the cloudy solution to prevent contamination.

41. The nurse is preparing to inject 1.5 mL of a viscous medication intramuscularly to an adult patient. The nurse determines that the best site for the injection is the
    a. ventrogluteal site*
    b. deltoid site
    c. rectus femoris site
    d. dorsogluteal site

Reference: p. 599

Descriptors:

1. 28	2. 08	3. Application
4. IV-2	5. Nursing Process	6. Moderate

Rationale: The best site for this type of medication is the ventrogluteal site. Giving the medication in the other sites can cause severe patient discomfort.

42. The nurse is planning to give a variety of medication injections to several patients hospitalized on the surgical unit. For which of the following medications should aspiration be avoided after the needle has been inserted into the patient's administration site?
    a. penicillin
    b. streptomycin
    c. heparin*
    d. Depo-Provera

Reference: p. 601

Descriptors:

1. 28	2. 08	3. Application
4. IV-2	5. Nursing Process	6. Moderate

Rationale: Heparin, a blood thinner, has been known to cause bruising at the site if the site is aspirated before injection of the medication.

43. Before giving an intramuscular injection, the nurse should
    a. massage the site
    b. apply pressure to the site
    c. aspirate for blood return*
    d. squeeze the skin together

Reference: p. 601

Descriptors:

1. 28	2. 08	3. Application
4. IV-2	5. Nursing Process	6. Moderate

Rationale: Before injecting the IM medication, the nurse should aspirate for blood to be certain that the medication is going into the muscle and not a blood vessel.

44. The nurse is preparing to give a vitamin K injection to a 6½ pound infant. The nurse determines that the best site for the injection for this patient is the
    a. ventrogluteal site
    b. deltoid site
    c. dorsogluteal site
    d. vastus lateralis site*

Reference: p. 602

Descriptors:

1. 28	2. 08	3. Application
4. IV-2	5. Nursing Process	6. Difficult

Rationale: The best site to use for an infant injection is the vastus lateralis because the muscles of the other sites are not well developed and can result in injury.

45. When the nurse administers Vistaril 50 mg IM per Z-tract, the nurse should
    a. pull the skin to the side and hold the skin while injecting*
    b. push the skin closely together before injecting
    c. spread the skin and area tautly
    d. displace the tissues during the injection

Reference: p. 604

Descriptors:

1. 28	2. 01	3. Knowledge
4. IV-2	5. Nursing Process	6. Moderate

Rationale: Pulling the skin to one side and holding allows the injection of the medication to the deep muscle tissues.

46. The nurse is preparing to administer an injection using the Z-tract method. The nurse plans to
    a. put a small air bubble at the top of the syringe
    b. change the needle after withdrawing the medication*
    c. massage the site vigorously after the injection is given
    d. quickly withdraw the needle following the injection

Reference: p. 604

Descriptors:

1. 28	2. 08	3. Application
4. IV-2	5. Nursing Process	6. Difficult

Rationale: The nurse should plan to change the needle after withdrawing the medication to prevent tissue damage. There is no need for an air bubble, the site should not be massaged, and the needle should be withdrawn slowly.

47. The nurse is going to use the Z-tract method to inject medication. The *best rationale* for doing this is
   a. the patient has sufficient muscle for this type of injection
   b. it is the only method to use when giving an injection in the gluteus medius muscle
   c. the medication is highly irritating to subcutaneous and skin tissue*
   d. it is the safest and least painful way to give an injection

Reference: p. 604

Descriptors:

1. 28	2. 10	3. Comprehensive
4. IV-2	5. Nursing Process	6. Moderate

Rationale: The 2-tract method prevents irritation to the subcutaneous and skin tissue.

48. The physician has ordered an intravenous antibiotic for an adult patient to be administered via a heparin lock. The nurse plans to
   a. connect the patient to the regular intravenous fluids after the administration of the antibiotic
   b. administer the medication as a bolus infusion to avoid a reaction
   c. flush the heparin lock with normal saline after the administration of the antibiotic*
   d. administer intermittent infusions of heparin to maintain patency of the heparin lock

Reference: p. 618

Descriptors:

1. 28	2. 08	3. Application
4. IV-2	5. Nursing Process	6. Moderate

Rationale: Following the administration of the antibiotic, the nurse should plan to flush the heparin lock with normal saline solution to maintain patency of the lock. Reconnecting the patient to the intravenous fluids is not necessary, nor is intermittent heparin.

49. A patient has an order for Benadryl ointment for an itchy rash on his arms. To promote absorption of the drug, the nurse should
   a. apply an ice pack to the arms after application
   b. wash the area with mild soap and water before applying the ointment*
   c. wear sterile gloves before applying the ointment
   d. ask the patient to walk around the room after the application

Reference: p. 619

Descriptors:

1. 28	2. 08	3. Application
4. IV-2	5. Nursing Process	6. Moderate

Rationale: Washing the area with a mild soap and water will enhance absorption of the ointment.

50. An adult patient has an order for eyedrops t.i.d. in both eyes. The nurse should plan to
   a. wear sterile gloves prior to opening the eyedrop container
   b. ask the patient to look downward during the instillation
   c. cleanse the patient's eyelids from the outer canthus to the inner canthus
   d. administer the number of drops ordered into the conjunctival sacs*

Reference: p. 622

Descriptors:

1. 28	2. 08	3. Application
4. IV-2	5. Nursing Process	6. Difficult

Rationale: The nurse should plan to administer the number of drops ordered into the conjunctival sacs. Sterile gloves are not necessary. The patient should look upward. Eyes should always be cleansed from the inner to the outer canthus.

51. While making a home visit to an adult patient, the nurse observes the patient's wife administer the patient's required eardrops into his ears. The nurse determines that the patient's wife needs additional instructions when the nurse observes the wife
   a. instill the drops into the patient's second ear immediately after the first instillation*
   b. turn the patient to the unaffected side before instillation of the eardrops
   c. clean the external ear with cotton balls moistened with saline
   d. hold the ear dropper with its ear tip up above the auditory canal

Reference: p. 624

Descriptors:

1. 28	2. 09	3. Application
4. IV-2	5. Teach/Learn	6. Difficult

Rationale: The patient's wife needs further instructions when the nurse observes her instill the drops into the patient's second ear immediately after the first instillation. The wife should be instructed to wait 5 minutes before instilling the drops in the second ear.

52. The nurse is planning to administer eardrops to a 6-year-old child. The nurse should pull the ear
    a. out and back
    b. in and forward
    c. straight back*
    d. down and back

    Reference: p. 624

    Descriptors:

1. 28	2. 01	3. Application
4. II-1	5. Nursing Process	6. Moderate

Rationale: Pulling the child's ear straight back straightens the ear canal and allows the solution to reach all areas of the ear canal easily.

53. Prior to insertion of a vaginal suppository, it is important for the nurse to instruct the patient to
    a. breathe normally
    b. empty the bladder*
    c. have a bowel movement
    d. bear down gently

    Reference: p. 624

    Descriptors:

1. 28	2. 01	3. Application
4. IV-2	5. Nursing Process	6. Moderate

Rationale: The nurse should instruct the patient to empty her bladder prior to insertion of the suppository because the pressure of the suppository may cause the patient to feel the urge to urinate, and this can expel the suppository.

54. The nurse has instructed an adult patient how to instill prescribed nosedrops. The nurse determines that the patient has understood the instructions when he says
    a. "I should place the dropper as far back into the nose as I can."
    b. "I should blow my nose before instilling the nosedrops."*
    c. "I should be certain that the dropper is touching both nostrils."
    d. "I should sit forward immediately after I have administered the drops."

    Reference: p. 626

    Descriptors:

1. 28	2. 09	3. Application
4. IV-2	5. Nursing Process	6. Moderate

Rationale: The patient has understood the instructions when he says "I should blow my nose before instilling the nosedrops." The head should be tilted back and stay that way for a few minutes after instillation. The dropper should be held just at the tip of the nose. The patient should avoid touching the nostrils with the dropper because this may cause sneezing.

55. The nurse is preparing to administer prescribed antibiotics to an adult hospitalized patient suffering from a wound infection. When the nurse offers the oral medication to the patient, he says "I'm not taking those. Those pills make me nauseated and gaggy." The nurse should
    a. try to convince the patient of the need for the medications
    b. stay with the patient until he takes the medications
    c. document the patient's refusal in the medication record
    d. contact the patient's physician about the patient's refusal*

    Reference: p. 629

    Descriptors:

1. 28	2. 08	3. Application
4. IV-2	5. Communication	6. Moderate

Rationale: It is the responsibility of the nurse to contact the patient's physician when the patient refuses a medication that has been ordered.

56. During a home visit to an 80-year-old patient, the nurse has instructed the patient about his prescribed medications. The nurse determines that the patient has understood the instructions when he says
    a. "I can keep these medications in the freezer to ensure potency."
    b. "I shouldn't alter the dosage without contacting my doctor."*
    c. "I can continue to take these pills even if they become discolored."
    d. "If I miss a few of my hypertension pills, I should take an extra one to be safe."

Reference: p. 631

Descriptors:

1. 28	2. 09	3. Application
4. IV-2	5. Teach/Learn	6. Moderate

Rationale: The patient has understood the instructions when he says "I shouldn't alter the dosage without contacting my doctor." Keeping medications in the freezer is not recommended. Discolored pills should be discarded. Taking an extra antihypertensive medication is not recommended.

57. The nurse makes a home visit to a patient on Medicare who has limited financial resources, but is on several prescription medications. The nurse should instruct the patient to
    a. avoid borrowing from or loaning medications to other people*
    b. ask the physician to prescribe brand name drugs even if they are more costly
    c. avoid the use of over-the-counter medications sold in drug stores
    d. explore the use of herbal remedies that may cost less

Reference: p. 631

Descriptors:

1. 28	2. 09	3. Application
4. IV-2	5. Teach/Learn	6. Moderate

Rationale: The nurse should instruct the patient to avoid borrowing from or loaning medications to other people. Generic brands may be just as effective and are cheaper. Herbal remedies may be more costly and can interfere with some medications.

58. For which of the following activities would the nurse be responsible during the evaluation phase of drug administration?
    a. preparation and administration of medications safely and as ordered
    b. establishing goals and outcome criteria related to drug therapy
    c. monitoring the patient for therapeutic effects as well as adverse effects*
    d. gathering data on drug and diet history, particularly allergies

Reference: pp. 631–632

Descriptors:

1. 28	2. 09	3. Comprehensive
4. IV-2	5. Nursing Process	6. Moderate

Rationale: Monitoring the patient for therapeutic and adverse effects is part of the evaluation phase.

CHAPTER 29

Perioperative Nursing

1. The nurse is caring for a perioperative patient. The term "perioperative phase" refers to care given to a patient
   a. immediately before an operative procedure
   b. during the operative procedure and immediate recovery
   c. immediately after an operative procedure
   d. before, during, and after an operative procedure*

   Reference: p. 640

   Descriptors:

1. 29	2. 01	3. Knowledge
4. None	5. None	6. Easy

   Rationale: The perioperative phase refers to care given to a patient before, during, and after an operative procedure.

2. The nurse is caring for a patient who is scheduled for a radical mastectomy. The nurse should explain to the patient and family that this type of surgery is classified as
   a. minor
   b. major*
   c. ablative
   d. constructive

   Reference: p. 641

   Descriptors:

1. 29	2. 01	3. Knowledge
4. IV-1	5. Teach/Learn	6. Easy

   Rationale: A radical mastectomy is considered major surgery.

3. The nurse is caring for a patient scheduled for an appendectomy. The nurse should explain to the patient that this type of procedure is termed
   a. ablative*
   b. diagnostic
   c. therapeutic
   d. reconstructive

   Reference: p. 641

   Descriptors:

1. 29	2. 01	3. Application
4. IV-1	5. Teach/Learn	6. Easy

   Rationale: An appendectomy is considered an ablative surgery because it involves the removal of a diseased organ.

4. A patient is scheduled for a tubal ligation procedure following the delivery of her third child. The nurse should explain to the patient that this type of surgery is termed
   a. emergency
   b. cosmetic
   c. ablative
   d. elective*

   Reference: p. 641

   Descriptors:

1. 29	2. 01	3. Application
4. IV-1	5. Teach/Learn	6. Easy

   Rationale: A tubal ligation (sterilization) is considered an elective procedure.

5. The nurse is caring for a patient who will receive general anesthesia. The nurse should explain to the patient that general anesthesia
   a. is administered through the intravenous route
   b. allows the patient to remain awake and aware of the procedure
   c. is often used for brief surgical procedures
   d. can produce central nervous system depression*

   Reference: p.642

   Descriptors:

1. 29	2. 02	3. Application
4. IV-1	5. Teach/Learn	6. Moderate

   Rationale: General anesthesia can produce central nervous system depression.

6. A patient is scheduled for a cesarean section delivery under spinal anesthesia. The nurse determines that the patient understands the instructions given by the anesthesiologist when the patient says
   a. "This type of anesthesia injects a local anesthetic around a nerve trunk."
   b. "Central nervous system depression is a common side effect."
   c. "Following the surgery, I may develop a headache."*
   d. "My blood pressure may be elevated after the anesthesia is given."

   Reference: p. 642
   Descriptors:

1. 29	2. 02	3. Application
4. IV-1	5. Teach/Learn	6. Moderate

   Rationale: One of the complications of spinal anesthesia is a postspinal headache. Blood pressure tends to be lower, not elevated, with this type of anesthesia.

7. A patient is scheduled for a hernia repair under regional anesthesia. All of the following reactions occur with this type of anesthesia *except*
   a. loss of consciousness*
   b. analgesia
   c. relaxation
   d. reflex loss

   Reference: p. 642
   Descriptors:

1. 29	2. 01	3. Application
4. IV-2	5. Teach/Learn	6. Easy

   Rationale: Regional anesthesia produces the same effects as general anesthesia except the patient remains awake with no loss of consciousness.

8. All of the following are disadvantages of general anesthetics *except*
   a. circulatory depression
   b. postoperative nausea and vomiting
   c. alteration in thermoregulation
   d. lack of awareness of physical trauma*

   Reference: p. 642
   Descriptors:

1. 29	2. 01	3. Knowledge
4. IV-2	5. None	6. Moderate

   Rationale: Some advantages of general anesthesia are that it can be used for all ages and the patient is not aware of the physical trauma of surgery.

9. Which type of anesthesia has the advantage of rapid excretion and reversal of effects?
   a. controlled
   b. inhaled*
   c. intravenous
   d. regional

   Reference: p. 642
   Descriptors:

1. 29	2. 01	3. Knowledge
4. IV-2	5. None	6. Moderate

   Rationale: Inhaled anesthesia is rapidly excreted and is immediately reversed.

10. When a dentist performs a root canal on a patient's tooth, the type of anesthetic that is typically used is termed
    a. nerve block*
    b. spinal
    c. caudal
    d. epidural

    Reference: p. 642
    Descriptors:

1. 29	2. 01	3. Knowledge
4. IV-2	5. None	6. Easy

    Rationale: For a root canal on a tooth, the type of anesthesia typically used is termed nerve block. A local anesthetic is injected around the nerve trunk supplying the jaw where the root canal is to be performed.

11. An adult patient has signed an informed consent for surgery. One hour before surgery, the nurse offers the patient a preoperative medication, when the patient appears confused and asks the nurse "Why am I getting a preoperative medication?" The nurse should
    a. tell the patient that the medication will help her to relax before surgery
    b. explain the purpose of the medication and if confusion continues, notify the physician*
    c. cancel the patient's surgery until the physician can explain to the patient why surgery is necessary
    d. withhold the medication until the patient can explain why surgery is necessary

Reference: p. 643

Descriptors:

1. 29	2. 03	3. Application
4. IV-1	5. Nursing Process	6. Easy

Rationale: When the patient acts confused and questions the medication, it is the responsibility of the nurse to explain the purpose of the medication and, if the patient still appears confused, the surgeon should be notified immediately. The consent is not valid if the patient is in a confused state.

12. An adult patient is scheduled for outpatient surgery on her right arm in 2 days. The nurse determines that the patient needs further preoperative instructions when the patient says
    a. "I shouldn't wear any makeup or nail polish on the day of the surgery."
    b. "If possible, I should wear short sleeve clothes that button down the front."
    c. "I should have someone available to drive me to my home after the procedure."
    d. "It's acceptable to wear my watch and wedding rings as I usually do."*

Reference: p. 643

Descriptors:

1. 29	2. 01	3. Application
4. IV-1	5. Nursing Process	6. Moderate

Rationale: All jewelry and watches should be left at home and not worn during the surgery.

13. On admission to the preoperative area, the nurse should examine the patient's chart for the following legal document termed
    a. informed consent to surgery*
    b. durable power of attorney
    c. resuscitation status
    d. living will

Reference: p. 643

Descriptors:

1. 29	2. 02	3. Application
4. IV-1	5. Documentation	6. Moderate

Rationale: The nurse should first check for a signed informed consent on the patient's chart.

14. An adult patient with chronic obstructive pulmonary disease (COPD) is scheduled for surgery. Because of the patient's medical history, the nurse should assess the patient during the postoperative period for symptoms of
    a. thrombophlebitis
    b. hypotension
    c. prolonged healing
    d. pneumonia*

Reference: p. 646

Descriptors:

1. 29	2. 03	3. Application
4. IV-3	5. Nursing Process	6. Easy

Rationale: Because of the patient's impaired lung function, pneumonia may occur.

15. An adult patient with a history of chronic diabetes mellitus is scheduled for a total hip replacement. Following the surgery, the nurse should give priority for assessing the patient's
    a. degree of wound healing*
    b. serum calcium level
    c. degree of respiratory depression
    d. ability to consume a regular diet

Reference: p. 646

Descriptors:

1. 29	2. 03	3. Application
4. IV-3	5. Nursing Process	6. Moderate

Rationale: Wound healing can be especially difficult for patients with diabetes mellitus.

16. During a preoperative history taking by the nurse, the patient tells the nurse that he has been taking daily doses of aspirin for his arthritis. The nurse caring for the patient during the postoperative phase should pay particular attention to potential symptoms of
    a. cardiovascular collapse
    b. respiratory paralysis
    c. hemorrhage*
    d. paralytic ileus

Reference: p. 647

Descriptors:

1. 29	2. 03	3. Comprehensive
4. IV-3	5. Nursing Process	6. Moderate

Rationale: Aspirin can interfere with normal clotting, so hemorrhage may occur.

17. The nurse is caring for a patient on the first postoperative day following abdominal surgery. The patient has smoked one pack of cigarettes a day for 20 years. A priority assessment for the nurse to make is the patient's
    a. height and weight
    b. ability to ambulate
    c. nutritional status
    d. breath sounds*

Reference: p. 647

Descriptors:

1. 29   2. 03   3. Application
4. IV-3   5. Nursing Process   6. Easy

Rationale: Because of the patient's history of smoking, the nurse should assess the patient's breath sounds.

18. The nurse is caring for an obese adult patient in a home setting 1 week following hip replacement surgery. A priority nursing diagnosis for this patient is
    a. Risk for Infection related to patient's obesity*
    b. Altered Nutrition: More than Body Requirements related to surgical procedure
    c. Anxiety related to pain and immobility as a result of surgery
    d. Grief related to change in body image

Reference: p. 649

Descriptors:

1. 29   2. 03   3. Application
4. IV-3   5. Nursing Process   6. Moderate

Rationale: Because the patient is obese, the wound may not heal properly; therefore, the priority is Risk for Infection related to the patient's obesity.

19. An Asian American patient tells the nurse that she does not think she should ambulate to the chair on the first postoperative day following abdominal surgery. The nurse should
    a. ask the patient's family member to encourage the patient to ambulate
    b. tell the patient that the doctor has ordered her to get out of bed
    c. inform the patient that the nurse will return later and help her to the chair
    d. instruct the patient about the reasons for early ambulation during the postoperative period*

Reference: p. 648

Descriptors:

1. 29   2. 04   3. Application
4. IV-3   5. Nursing Process   6. Moderate

Rationale: In some cultures, the period following surgery is a time of bedrest. The nurse should explain to the patient and the family while ambulation is so important, for example, to prevent phlebitis.

20. An Asian American adult patient is scheduled to have a temporary colostomy to relieve a bowel obstruction. The patient tells the nurse that she wants the colostomy only if it is truly temporary. A priority nursing diagnosis for this patient is
    a. Risk for Infection related to extensive abdominal manipulation
    b. Risk for Spiritual Distress related to surgical outcome
    c. Anticipatory Grieving related to body image disturbance*
    d. Ineffective Individual Coping related to conflict between need for surgery and cultural beliefs

Reference: p. 649

Descriptors:

1. 29   2. 07   3. Application
4. IV-3   5. Culture   6. Moderate

Rationale: The priority diagnosis is Anticipatory Grieving related to body image disturbance because the patient is very concerned that the colostomy will only be temporary.

21. The nurse is caring for a patient who has smoked cigarettes for 10 years. The patient is scheduled for a bilateral mastectomy under general anesthesia. The nurse formulates which of the following nursing diagnoses as a priority?
    a. Risk for Ineffective Airway Clearance related to smoking and anesthesia*
    b. Impaired Mobility related to change in status and surgery
    c. Risk for Infection related to incision sites
    d. Risk for Ineffective Individual Coping related to smoking

Reference: pp. 647, 649

Descriptors:

1. 29   2. 03   3. Comprehensive
4. III-1   5. Nursing Process   6. Moderate

Rationale: A priority diagnosis is Risk for Ineffective Airway Clearance related to smoking and anesthesia because the anesthesia leads to pooling of secretions and thick mucus.

22. The nurse is assessing a patient during the postoperative period. All of the following assessments are important *except*
    a. temperature
    b. wound status
    c. level of consciousness
    d. type of insurance coverage*

Reference: p. 649

Descriptors:

1. 29	2. 03	3. Application
4. IV-3	5. Nursing Process	6. Moderate

Rationale: The type of insurance coverage that the patient has is not part of a postoperative assessment.

23. The nurse is providing preoperative teaching for a 6-year-old patient and his family. The child is scheduled for reconstructive surgery. To help alleviate the child's anxiety, the nurse plans to
    a. show the child an intravenous fluid kit and let him play with it
    b. demonstrate how the patient controlled analgesia machine is operated
    c. have the child meet with the surgeon who will perform the procedure
    d. take the child and family on a tour of the operating room*

Reference: p. 650

Descriptors:

1. 29	2. 05	3. Application
4. IV-3	5. Nursing Process	6. Easy

Rationale: A tour of the operating room prior to surgery can help to alleviate the child's anxiety.

24. The nurse's most important task preoperatively to ensure a beneficial postoperative outcome is
    a. vital signs
    b. preoperative teaching*
    c. safety prior to surgery
    d. oxygen saturation levels

Reference: p. 650

Descriptors:

1. 29	2. 06	3. Application
4. II-1	5. Nursing Process	6. Moderate

Rationale: To achieve the best outcome during the postoperative period, the most important aspect of care is preoperative teaching.

25. An adult patient is scheduled for back surgery to repair a herniated disk. An important preoperative teaching plan for the nurse to make for this patient should include
    a. nutritional needs following surgery
    b ambulation from the bed to the chair*
    c. methods to prevent hemorrhage
    d. use of intravenous fluid equipment

Reference: p. 651

Descriptors:

1. 29	2. 04	3. Application
4. IV-3	5. Teach/Learn	6. Moderate

Rationale: Back surgery can make ambulation difficult. The most important teaching aspect for this patient is ambulation from the bed to the chair.

26. A patient is scheduled for a coronary bypass procedure. Before the patient is taken to the surgical area, the nurse documents the patient's vital signs. The nurse should explain to the patient that this provides
    a. baseline data for comparison during and after the procedure*
    b. data to determine the type of pain medication needed during the postoperative period
    c. data that are useful for determining the type of anesthesia needed
    d. data that can be used to determine how to position the patient during the procedure

Reference: p. 652

Descriptors:

1. 29	2. 06	3. Application
4. IV-3	5. Teach/Learn	6. Moderate

Rationale: The patient's preoperative vital signs provide baseline data for comparison during and after the procedure. The position during the operation is dictated by the type of operative procedure.

27. Before surgery, the nurse has instructed a preoperative adult patient about the use of pain medication following surgery. The nurse determines that the patient needs further instructions when the patient says
    a. "I should ask for the pain medication before the pain gets too uncomfortable."
    b. "If I can't have any food or water on the first day, I'll get pain medicine by injection."
    c. "If I use relaxation and breathing techniques, the pain medication will be more effective."
    d. "I should wait until the pain becomes severe before requesting pain medication."*

Reference: p. 653

Descriptors:

1. 29	2. 05	3. Application
4. IV-1	5. Teach/Learn	6. Moderate

Rationale: The patient needs further instructions when he says "I should wait until the pain becomes severe before requesting pain medication." Waiting too long before receiving pain medication can make the medication less effective.

28. The nurse has taught a preoperative patient about the need for turning, coughing, and deep breathing during the postoperative period. The rationale for this teaching is to
    a. suppress the cough reflex
    b. prevent the incision from causing pain
    c. improve lung expansion*
    d. retain anesthetic effects

Reference: pp. 653–654

Descriptors:

1. 29	2. 07	3. Application
4. IV-3	5. Teach/Learn	6. Moderate

Rationale: Turning, coughing, and deep breathing aid lung expansion.

29. The nurse is planning to instruct a patient who will be undergoing abdominal surgery about postoperative deep-breathing techniques. Which of the following should be included in the nurse's teaching plan?
    a. The exercises will be done every 4 hours for the first 24 to 48 hours after surgery.
    b. During the exercise the patient should hold his breath and count to 10.
    c. The patient should be lying in a supine position for the most effectiveness.
    d. The patient should be in a semi-Fowler's position with the head and shoulders supported.*

Reference: p. 653

Descriptors:

1. 29	2. 05	3. Application
4. IV-3	5. Teach/Learn	6. Moderate

Rationale: The patient should be in a semi-Fowler's position with the head and shoulders supported for the most effective deep-breathing techniques.

30. The nurse is assisting a patient with coughing exercises on the first postoperative day after chest surgery. The nurse should
    a. offer the patient pain medication before the coughing exercises*
    b. have the patient repeat the exercise every 4 hours during the first 24 hours after surgery
    c. place the patient in a side-lying position with a supportive pillow
    d. instruct the patient to take a deep breath and hold it for 20 seconds

Reference: p. 654

Descriptors:

1. 29	2. 06	3. Application
4. IV-3	5. Teach/Learn	6. Moderate

Rationale: The patient should be offered pain medication about 30 minutes before the coughing exercises. The patient should also be taught how to splint the incision with a pillow.

31. The nurse has instructed a patient about incentive spirometry following abdominal surgery. The nurse determines that the patient understands the instructions when the patient says that incentive spirometry
    a. is used to help increase lung volume*
    b. should be done while flat in bed
    c. is performed once a day after surgery
    d. can be done immediately after mealtime

Reference: p. 654

Descriptors:

1. 29	2. 06	3. Application
4. IV-1	5. Nursing Process	6. Moderate

Rationale: Incentive spirometry is used to help increase lung volume. It is done three to four times per day and the patient should be in a semi-Fowler's or sitting position. It should be done between meal times.

32. The nurse is planning to instruct an adult patient who will be undergoing major surgery about leg exercises. The nurse should instruct the patient that leg exercises
    a. need to be performed at least once per day
    b. help promote venous return*
    c. are important to prevent contractures
    d. can improve urinary function

Reference: p. 654

Descriptors:

1. 29	2. 06	3. Application
4. IV-3	5. Nursing Process	6. Easy

Rationale: Leg exercises help promote venous return, improve circulation, and prevent thrombophlebitis.

33. An adult patient is scheduled for outpatient surgery to remove a mole on her back. The nurse should instruct the patient that prior to the surgery the
    a. back will be cleansed with betadine by the nurse and surgeon
    b. need for cleansing the back is not necessary
    c. skin around the area should be shaved 24 hours before surgery
    d. site should be cleansed with an antibacterial soap before surgery*

Reference: p. 655

Descriptors:

1. 29	2. 04	3. Application
4. IV-3	5. Nursing Process	6. Moderate

Rationale: To prevent infection, the site should be cleansed with an antibacterial soap before surgery is done.

34. An adult patient who has had preoperative barium diagnostic tests has an order for an enema prior to surgery. The nurse plans to instruct the patient that the purpose of the enema is to
    a. decrease diarrhea during the postoperative period
    b. prevent constipation during the postoperative period*
    c. cleanse the bowel of all bacteria and feces
    d. decrease the need for bowel elimination following surgery

Reference: p. 655

Descriptors:

1. 29	2. 06	3. Application
4. IV-3	5. Nursing Process	6. Moderate

Rationale: The nurse should explain that the purpose of the enema is to prevent constipation during the postoperative period, because the bowels are normally sluggish after surgery.

35. The nurse is caring for a 20-year-old patient with a hearing aid a few hours before scheduled surgery on his knee. The nurse completing the preoperative checklist should
    a. omit asking about dentures
    b. remove the patient's hearing aid
    c. place any jewelry in the bedside table
    d. leave the hearing aid in place*

Reference: p. 656

Descriptors:

1. 29	2. 04	3. Application
4. IV-1	5. Communication	6. Moderate

Rationale: Hearing aids should be left in place during surgery. The nurse should ask about and remove any dentures, regardless of age. Jewelry should be locked in a safe place.

36. The nurse has given a preoperative patient Demerol 50 mg IM an hour before surgery. The nurse plans to
    a. review the preoperative instructions one more time
    b. assist the patient to ambulate to the bathroom to void
    c. raise both side rails on the patient's bed*
    d. obtain the patient's signature on the surgical consent

Reference: p. 656

Descriptors:

1. 29	2. 05	3. Application
4. I-2	5. Nursing Process	6. Moderate

Rationale: After administering the narcotic Demerol, the nurse should not ambulate the patient because he may get dizzy. The side rails of the bed should be raised.

37. The operating room nurse has just received a patient in the holding area prior to surgery. A priority assessment for the nurse to make prior to surgery is to
    a. ask the patient about any allergies
    b. identify the patient by checking the identification band*
    c. determine who the support persons are for the patient
    d. discuss any spiritual concerns the patient may present

Reference: p. 658

Descriptors:

| 1. 29 | 2. 06 | 3. Application |
| 4. I-2 | 5. Nursing Process | 6. Moderate |

Rationale: A priority assessment for the nurse to make is to identify the patient by checking the identification band.

38. One of the primary responsibilities of the circulating nurse during the intraoperative phase is to ensure that the patient's
a. physical safety is maintained*
b. drapes are applied properly
c. surgical masks and gowns remain sterile
d. anesthesia level is appropriate

Reference: p. 658

Descriptors:

| 1. 29 | 2. 02 | 3. Application |
| 4. I-2 | 5. Nursing Process | 6. Moderate |

Rationale: One of the primary responsibilities of the circulating nurse during the intraoperative phase is to ensure that the patient's physical safety is maintained. The anesthesiologist is responsible for the level of anesthesia.

39. A patient is scheduled for a surgical procedure that requires that she be placed in a Trendelenburg position. Following the return of the patient to the supine position the nurse should assess the patient for
a. hypotension*
b. skin injuries
c. headache
d. back pain

Reference: p. 658

Descriptors:

| 1. 29 | 2. 02 | 3. Application |
| 4. I-2 | 5. Nursing Process | 6. Moderate |

Rationale: Following the return of the patient to the supine position from a Trendelenburg position, the nurse should assess the patient for hypotension from the position change.

40. One hour after abdominal surgery with general anesthesia the nurse observes that the patient's pulse has increased from 84 beats/min to 124 beats/min and the patient appears restless. The nurse should first
a. continue to monitor the patient every 15 minutes
b. decrease the intravenous fluid rate
c. assess the patient's skin temperature
d. notify the patient's physician of the change in status

Reference: p. 660

Descriptors:

| 1. 29 | 2. 06 | 3. Application |
| 4. IV-3 | 5. Nursing Process | 6. Moderate |

Rationale: The patient is demonstrating symptoms of shock. The nurse should notify the physician immediately.

41. Thirty minutes after abdominal surgery, the recovery room nurse determines that a patient's pulse has increased from 68 beats/min to 110 beats/min and the patient's skin is cool to the touch. The nurse notifies the patient's physician because these symptoms are indicative of
a. respiratory arrest
b. overmedication of anesthesia
c. cardiovascular shock*
d. dehydration

Reference: p. 660

Descriptors:

| 1. 29 | 2. 06 | 3. Comprehensive |
| 4. IV-3 | 5. Communication | 6. Moderate |

Rationale: Increased pulse and cool, clammy skin are symptoms of cardiovascular shock.

42. When assessing a postoperative patient for symptoms of pain, the most important guideline to follow is
a. administration of pain medication as ordered
b. assessment of the patient every 4 hours
c. pain is what the patient reports*
d. pain medications are used in greater doses for the elderly

Reference: p. 661

Descriptors:

| 1. 29 | 2. 07 | 3. Comprehensive |
| 4. IV-3 | 5. Nursing Process | 6. Moderate |

Rationale: The guideline for the nurse to follow is that everyone perceives pain differently and pain is what the patient reports.

43. During the recovery period following abdominal surgery the nurse determines that the patient is still not fully conscious. The nurse plans to position the patient in a
    a. prone position
    b. supine position
    c. semi-Fowler's position
    d. side-lying position*

    Reference: p. 662

    Descriptors:

1. 29	2. 06	3. Application
4. III-1	5. Nursing Process	6. Moderate

    Rationale: The side-lying position allows for drainage and secretions from the mouth, which helps to keep the airway clear.

44. The nurse is caring for a patient who has just been admitted to the hospital unit from the recovery room following surgery to remove a bullet from his left shoulder. The patient asks for pain medication, which has been ordered p.r.n. every 3 to 4 hours. Before administering the pain medication the nurse should
    a. ask the patient if he received any pain medication earlier
    b. determine if the medication is really needed
    c. evaluate the type of anesthesia that was given during surgery
    d. check the patient's record to verify if analgesia was administered earlier*

    Reference: p. 664

    Descriptors:

1. 29	2. 06	3. Application
4. IV-3	5. Nursing Process	6. Moderate

    Rationale: When a patient is transferred from one hospital unit to another, the nurse should check the patient's record to verify if and when analgesia may have already been administered to the patient.

45. An adult patient returns to her room following a 2-hour cholecystectomy. During the nurse's initial assessment, the patient complains of chest pain and dyspnea. The nurse observes that the patient's fingers and toes are cyanotic, with respirations at 32 breaths per minute and pulse 110 beats/min. These symptoms are indicative of
    a. hemorrhage
    b. pulmonary embolus*
    c. pneumonia
    d. atelectasis

    Reference: p. 666

    Descriptors:

1. 29	2. 07	3. Comprehensive
4. IV-2	5. Documentation	6. Moderate

    Rationale: These symptoms are indicative of pulmonary embolus and require prompt notification of the physician as well as administration of oxygen.

46. The nurse determines that a postoperative patient is experiencing hypovolemic shock. The nurse ensures that the patient has a patent airway and then
    a. contacts the patient's physician
    b. places the patient in Trendelenburg position
    c. obtains an order for a type and cross-match for blood
    d. elevates the patient's legs 45 degrees*

    Reference: p. 666

    Descriptors:

1. 29	2. 07	3. Application
4. IV-3	5. Nursing Process	6. Moderate

    Rationale: This is an emergency and elevation of the patient's legs 45 degrees will enhance blood return to the patient's brain and other vital organs.

47. The nurse has provided a postoperative patient with home care instructions before discharge. The nurse determines that the patient understands the instructions about his care when he says
    a. "If I have pain or redness in my calf, I should contact my physician."*
    b. "If thrombophlebitis develops, I will need to apply ice to the area."
    c. "I should change my antiembolic stockings before I go to bed."
    d. "If I develop a reddened area on my calf, massaging it will alleviate the pain."

    Reference: p. 666

    Descriptors:

1. 29	2. 07	3. Application
4. IV-3	5. Nursing Process	6. Moderate

    Rationale: The nurse determines that the patient understands the instructions about his care when he says, "If I have pain or redness in my calf, I should contact my physician." Ice will not be effective, and antiembolic stockings should be put on in the morning. The area should not be massaged because this may dislodge a clot.

48. While assessing a 78-year-old patient who had a total hip replacement 3 days ago, the nurse observes that the patient has a temperature of 100.6°, purulent sputum, and lung crackles. The nurse determines that the patient is most likely experiencing
    a. tuberculosis
    b. atelectasis
    c. pulmonary embolism
    d. pneumonia*

Reference: p. 667

Descriptors:

1. 29   2. 07   3. Comprehensive
4. IV-3   5. Teach/Learn   6. Moderate

Rationale: The elevated temperature, purulent sputum, and lung crackles are symptoms of pneumonia.

49. The nurse has auscultated the abdomen of a 3-day postoperative patient and has detected a high-pitched sound. The patient tells the nurse that he has "a lot of abdominal distention." The nurse determines that the patient is most likely experiencing
    a. paralytic ileus*
    b. peristalsis
    c. flatus
    d. diarrhea

Reference: p. 668

Descriptors:

1. 29   2. 07   3. Comprehensive
4. II-2   5. Nursing Process   6. Moderate

Rationale: A high-pitched abdominal auscultation and distention are associated with paralytic ileus.

50. The nurse visits a patient in the home on the fourth postoperative day. The patient tells the nurse she has had "a lot of hiccups and can't seem to get rid of them." The nurse should instruct the patient to
    a. chew some ice chips
    b. drink several glasses of water
    c. eat a teaspoon of salt
    d. rebreathe into a paper bag*

Reference: p. 669

Descriptors:

1. 29   2. 07   3. Application
4. IV-3   5. Nursing Process   6. Moderate

Rationale: Rebreathing into a paper bag can help to eliminate hiccups.

UNIT VII

Promoting Healthy Psychosocial Responses

CHAPTER 30

Self-Concept

1. The question, "Are you able to look at yourself in the mirror and like what you see?" is asking about which dimension of self-concept?
   a. self-evaluation*
   b. self-expectation
   c. self-orientation
   d. self-image
   Reference: p. 679
   Descriptors:

1. 30	2. 02	3. Application
4. III-1	5. Caring	6. Easy

   Rationale: Looking in the mirror at oneself is considered self-evaluation.

2. According to Coopersmith, one of the four bases of self-esteem is
   a. reorganization
   b. truth
   c. reliability
   d. significance*
   Reference: p. 679
   Descriptors:

1. 30	2. 02	3. Application
4. None	5. None	6. Moderate

   Rationale: According to Coopersmith, the four bases of self-concept are significance, competence, virtue, and power. Significance is feeling loved and approved of by others.

3. The first step in the formation of an individual's self-concept occurs when the
   a. child feels approval from peers
   b. infant feels love and affection from parents*
   c. child internalizes other people's attitudes toward self
   d. adult internalizes standards of society

   Reference: p. 679
   Descriptors:

1. 30	2. 03	3. Application
4. None	5. None	6. Moderate

   Rationale: The first step in the formation of an individual's self-concept occurs when the infant feels love and affection from parents and has basic needs met.

4. One variable that can influence a person's self-concept is
   a. developmental considerations*
   b. responses to peers
   c. achievement of goals
   d. use of counseling services
   Reference: p. 680
   Descriptors:

1. 30	2. 05	3. Knowledge
4. III-1	5. Nursing Process	6. Easy

   Rationale: Factors that can influence a person's self-concept include developmental considerations, culture, internal and external resources, history of success and failure, stressors, and aging, illness, and trauma.

5. While conducting a self-concept assessment of a hospitalized adult patient, the nurse should be aware of the limitations of
   a. behavior discrepancies
   b. self-assessment interview checklists
   c. self-reporting by the patient*
   d. stressors on the patient
   Reference: p. 680
   Descriptors:

1. 30	2. 04	3. Application
4. III-1	5. Nursing Process	6. Moderate

   Rationale: While conducting a self-concept assessment of a hospitalized adult patient, the nurse should be aware of self-reporting by the patient. The patient may tell the nurse what the patient thinks the nurse wants to hear.

6. A potential cause of disturbance of self-concept in a school-aged child is
   a. unreasonable role expectations
   b. multiple stressors related to growth and development
   c. failure to develop new goals
   d. dysfunctional family environment*

   Reference: p. 681

   Descriptors:

1. 30	2. 04	3. Knowledge
4. II-1	5. Nursing Process	6. Moderate

   Rationale: A potential cause of disturbance of self-concept in a school-aged child is a dysfunctional family environment and too much or too little structure.

7. The term "personal identity" is defined as an individual's
   a. description of his or her body and face
   b. conscious sense of who he or she is*
   c. how someone else would describe the person
   d. unconscious sense of how he or she is viewed in society

   Reference: p. 682

   Descriptors:

1. 30	2. 01	3. Knowledge
4. III-1	5. Nursing Process	6. Moderate

   Rationale: The term "personal identity" is defined as an individual's conscious sense of who he or she is. It is important for the nurse to determine if the individual is comfortable with his or her personal identity.

8. While conducting a self-concept assessment of an adult patient who is hospitalized, the nurse desires information about the patient's perceptions of his competence. An appropriate question by the nurse is
   a. "Do you have any close relationships?"
   b. "How do you let family members know you love them?"
   c. "How important is it for you to have control of your life?"
   d. "What are the things you need to do to feel important?"*

   Reference: p. 685

   Descriptors:

1. 30	2. 06	3. Application
4. III-1	5. Nursing Process	6. Moderate

   Rationale: To assess competence, an appropriate question by the nurse is "What are the things you need to do to feel important?"

9. A depressed patient is unable to describe himself in any positive way and accentuates his weaknesses associated with aging. A priority nursing diagnosis is
   a. Personal Identity Disturbance related to being depressed
   b. Self-Esteem Disturbance related to weaknesses associated with aging*
   c. Altered Role Performance related to the aging process
   d. Impaired Mobility related to altered thought processes

   Reference: p. 686

   Descriptors:

1. 30	2. 07	3. Application
4. III-2	5. Nursing Process	6. Moderate

   Rationale: A priority nursing diagnosis is Self-Esteem Disturbance related to weaknesses associated with aging. There is no evidence of Personal Identity Disturbance, Altered Role Performance, or Impaired Mobility.

10. A moderately overweight patient who recently lost 30 pounds just received news that she is pregnant with twins. When the nurse enters the room, the patient says, "I can't believe I am pregnant! Just when I've lost all that weight!" A priority nursing diagnosis is
    a. Chronic Low Self-Esteem related to obesity
    b. Chronic Body Image Disturbance related to impaired adjustment
    c. Situational Low Self-Esteem Disturbance related to pregnancy and weight gain*
    d. Personal Identity Disturbance related to pregnancy with twins and weight gain

    Reference: p. 686

    Descriptors:

1. 30	2. 06	3. Application
4. III-1	5. Nursing Process	6. Moderate

    Rationale: A priority nursing diagnosis is Situational Low Self-Esteem Disturbance related to pregnancy and weight gain.

11. The nurse is caring for a hospitalized patient who is about to undergo surgery to remove his foot because of gangrene. The most effective strategy to assist the patient in recognizing and using personal strength is to
    a. encourage the patient's self-identification of strengths*
    b. promote the patient's external thinking mechanisms
    c. provide advice to the patient about how to handle the loss of his foot
    d. assist the patient in maintaining an external locus of control

    Reference: p. 689

    Descriptors:

1. 30	2. 08	3. Application
4. III-2	5. Nursing Process	6. Moderate

    Rationale: The most effective strategy to assist the patient in recognizing and using personal strength is to encourage the patient's self-identification of strengths.

12. An appropriate strategy for the nurse to use in assisting a hospitalized patient to maintain a sense of self includes
    a. using the patient's first name or nickname when addressing him
    b. treating the patient with dignity and respect*
    c. explaining procedures only if the patient asks for information
    d. discouraging the use of personal items brought from home

    Reference: pp. 689–690

    Descriptors:

1. 30	2. 08	3. Application
4. IV-1	5. Caring	6. Moderate

    Rationale: An appropriate strategy for the nurse to use in assisting a hospitalized patient to maintain a sense of self includes treating the patient with dignity and respect.

13. The nurse is caring for an 84-year-old patient hospitalized with complications of diabetes. To promote the patient's self-esteem, the nurse should
    a. assist the patient to regain mastery if at all possible*
    b. make the difficult decisions for the patient
    c. assist the patient to identify negative traits of his personality
    d. give the patient advice about how to prevent problems in the future

    Reference: p. 692

    Descriptors:

1. 30	2. 08	3. Application
4. III-1	5. Caring	6. Moderate

    Rationale: To promote the patient's self-esteem, the nurse should assist the patient to regain mastery if at all possible. The patient should make the difficult decisions and the nurse should avoid negative traits and giving advice.

CHAPTER 31

Stress and Adaptation

1. The change that occurs in human beings as a response to a stressor is termed
   a. homeostasis
   b. reaction
   c. adaptation*
   d. reorganization
   Reference: p. 702
   Descriptors:

1. 31	2. 03	3. Knowledge
4. III-1	5. None	6. Easy

   Rationale: The change that occurs in human beings as a response to a stressor is termed adaptation, which is an ongoing process.

2. A patient states she is worried about the condition of her elderly mother while the patient is hospitalized. This is an example of a/an
   a. illness
   b. effect
   c. stressor*
   d. demand
   Reference: p. 702
   Descriptors:

1. 31	2. 01	3. Application
4. III-1	5. None	6. Moderate

   Rationale: The nurse must be able to identify stressors in a patient or patient's family to assist the patient or family to effect change and reduce the stress.

3. A 14-year-old girl voices anxiety over attending high school. Through the statements of anxiety related to attendance in a new school, she is attempting to
   a. adapt*
   b. evaluate
   c. change
   d. react
   Reference: p. 702
   Descriptors:

1. 31	2. 01	3. Application
4. III-1	5. None	6. Moderate

   Rationale: Adaptation is an ongoing process as a person strives to maintain balance in her external environment.

4. In human beings, homeostatic mechanisms are controlled by the
   a. autonomic nervous system*
   b. internal environment
   c. parasympathetic nervous system
   d. defense mechanisms
   Reference: p. 703
   Descriptors:

1. 31	2. 01	3. Knowledge
4. III-1	5. None	6. Easy

   Rationale: Homeostatic mechanisms are controlled by the autonomic nervous system and the endocrine system.

5. Physiologic mechanisms within the body respond to internal changes to maintain relative constancy in the internal environment, which is termed
   a. stress
   b. change
   c. adaptation
   d. homeostasis*
   Reference: p. 703
   Descriptors:

1. 31	2. 01	3. Knowledge
4. III-1	5. None	6. Easy

   Rationale: Various physiologic mechanisms within the body respond to internal changes to maintain relative constancy in the internal environment, called homeostasis.

6. A 20-year-old patient comes to the clinic with loss of weight and dysphagia. She states she is attending a new school and has moved away from home. This is an example of
   a. dysfunctional behavior
   b. mind–body interaction*
   c. acceptance of life change
   d. developmental crisis
   Reference: p. 704
   Descriptors:

1. 31	2. 05	3. Application
4. III-1	5. None	6. Difficult

   Rationale: This illustrates the relationship between psychological stressors and the physiologic stress response or the mind–body interaction.

7. Which of the following represents a homeostatic regulator of the body to stress?
   a. decreased heart rate
   b. constricted vessels
   c. decreased epinephrine
   d. elimination of waste*
   Reference: p. 704
   Descriptors:

1. 31	2. 02	3. Knowledge
4. III-1	5. None	6. Easy

   Rationale: To assist in maintenance of homeostasis the body eliminates waste products.

8. Physiologic indicators of stress are
   a. constricted pupils
   b. increased appetite
   c. insomnia*
   d. decreased urination
   Reference: p. 705
   Descriptors:

1. 31	2. 05	3. Knowledge
4. III-1	5. Nursing Process	6. Moderate

   Rationale: A physiologic indicator of stress is sleep disturbances, such as insomnia.

9. A patient has a wound on his buttocks with noted exudate; this is an example of which phase of the inflammatory response?
   a. first phase
   b. second phase*
   c. third phase
   d. fourth phase
   Reference: p. 705
   Descriptors:

1. 31	2. 05	3. Comprehensive
4. III-1	5. None	6. Moderate

   Rationale: The second stage of the inflammatory response elicits exudate to be released from the wound. The amount of exudate depends on the size, location, and severity of the wound.

10. In human beings, the fight-or-flight response is controlled by the
    a. pituitary gland
    b. adrenal gland
    c. voluntary nervous system
    d. autonomic nervous system*
    Reference: p. 706
    Descriptors:

1. 31	2. 02	3. Knowledge
4. III-1	5. None	6. Easy

    Rationale: In human beings, the fight-or-flight response is controlled by the autonomic nervous system, especially the sympathetic nervous system.

11. In the general adaptation syndrome (GAS), the phase in which the body has an increase in energy levels and increased cardiac output is the phase termed
    a. resistance
    b. exhaustion
    c. shock*
    d. reaction
    Reference: p. 706
    Descriptors:

1. 31	2. 05	3. Knowledge
4. III-1	5. None	6. Easy

    Rationale: In the general adaptation syndrome (GAS), the phase in which the body has an increase in energy levels and increased cardiac output is the shock phase.

12. In the general adaptation syndrome (GAS), the second phase in which the body perceives the threat and mobilizes the resources is the phase termed
    a. resistance*
    b. shock
    c. reaction
    d. exhaustion

Reference: p. 706

Descriptors:

1. 31	2. 05	3. Knowledge
4. III-1	5. None	6. Easy

Rationale: In the general adaptation syndrome (GAS), the second phase in which the body perceives the threat and mobilizes the resources is the phase termed resistance. The body attempts to regain homeostasis.

13. In the general adaptation syndrome, the autonomic nervous system initiates the
    a. psychological stress response
    b. exhaustion to stress response
    c. stage of resistance to stress
    d. fight-or-flight response*

Reference: p. 706

Descriptors:

1. 31	2. 05	3. Knowledge
4. III-1	5. Nursing Process	6. Easy

Rationale: The autonomic nervous system initiates the fight-or-flight response, and hormone levels rise to prepare the body to react.

14. A 42-year-old single mother states that she has feelings of apprehension about the responsibilities she has for her children and her career. This is an example of
    a. concern
    b. anxiety*
    c. grief
    d. panic

Reference: p. 706

Descriptors:

1. 31	2. 06	3. Application
4. III-1	5. Nursing Process	6. Moderate

Rationale: Anxiety is a vague, uneasy feeling of discomfort or dread accompanied by an autonomic response; the source is often nonspecific or unknown to the individual; a feeling of apprehension caused the anticipation of danger.

15. The school nurse notices an increase in student visits with complaints of nausea. She determines that the fourth grade class has begun oral presentations. These episodes could be related to
    a. mild anxiety
    b. moderate anxiety*
    c. severe anxiety
    d. panic

Reference: p. 707

Descriptors:

1. 31	2. 07	3. Application
4. III-1	5. Nursing Process	6. Difficult

Rationale: Moderate anxiety is manifested by a quivering voice, butterflies in the stomach, and slight increases in respirations and pulse.

16. A patient visiting the clinic states he has feelings of impending doom. He is suffering from
    a. mild anxiety
    b. moderate anxiety
    c. severe anxiety
    d. panic*

Reference: p. 707

Descriptors:

1. 31	2. 07	3. Application
4. III-2	5. Nursing Process	6. Moderate

Rationale: Panic causes the person to lose control and make statements of impending doom.

17. During a meeting, one member of the committee is very quiet after being verbally ridiculed by another committee member. This describes which defense mechanism?
    a. task-oriented reactions
    b. attack behavior
    c. withdrawal behavior*
    d. compromise behavior

Reference: p. 707

Descriptors:

1. 31	2. 07	3. Application
4. III-1	5. None	6. Difficult

Rationale: Withdrawal behavior involves physical withdrawal from the threat or emotional reactions such as admitting defeat, becoming apathetic, or feeling guilty or isolated.

18. Various forms of anxiety have different effects on human beings. The type of anxiety that increases motivation and facilitates problem solving is termed
    a. mild anxiety*
    b. moderate anxiety
    c. severe anxiety
    d. fearful anxiety

Reference: p. 707

Descriptors:

1. 31	2. 01	3. Knowledge
4. III-1	5. Nursing Process	6. Easy

Rationale: The type of anxiety that increases motivation and facilitates problem solving is termed mild anxiety.

19. A patient is seen in the emergency room after she was robbed and beaten by two men. The patient is incoherent and agitated, and is sweating. Her pulse rate is 110 beats/min. The nurse determines that the patient is demonstrating symptoms of
    a. severe anxiety
    b. moderate anxiety
    c. panic*
    d. bipolar disorder

Reference: p. 707

Descriptors:

1. 31	2. 01	3. Application
4. III-2	5. Nursing Process	6. Easy

Rationale: When the patient is incoherent, agitated, sweating, and has a pulse rate of 110 beats/min, the patient is demonstrating symptoms of panic.

20. Behaviors that indicate a moderate degree of anxiety in a patient include
    a. alertness, restlessness, irritability
    b. focus on details, physiologic complaints, feelings of dread
    c. Reduced ability to perceive, increased tension, selective inattention*
    d. incoherent, confused, disoriented

Reference: p. 707

Descriptors:

1. 31	2. 05	3. Comprehensive
4. III-2	5. Nursing Process	6. Moderate

Rationale: Symptoms of moderate anxiety are a decreased ability to perceive, increased tension, and selective inattention.

21. The wife of a hospitalized patient with terminal heart failure tells the nurse that she doesn't visit her husband very often because she just cannot deal with the fact that he is dying. The nurse determines that the patient's wife is demonstrating a behavior termed
    a. compromise
    b. repression
    c. withdrawal*
    d. suppression

Reference: p. 707

Descriptors:

1. 31	2. 05	3. Application
4. III-1	5. Nursing Process	6. Easy

Rationale: When the wife of a hospitalized patient with terminal heart failure tells the nurse that she doesn't visit her husband very often because she just cannot deal with the fact that he is dying, the patient's wife is demonstrating a behavior termed withdrawal.

22. After caring for an angry family member of a hospitalized patient, the nurse enters the nurse's station and throws the patient's chart onto the desk. The nurse is demonstrating a defense mechanism termed
    a. reaction formation
    b. displacement*
    c. repression
    d. compensation

Reference: p. 707

Descriptors:

1. 31	2. 05	3. Application
4. III-1	5. Caring	6. Moderate

Rationale: When the nurse enters the nurse's station and throws the patient's chart onto the desk, the nurse is demonstrating a defense mechanism termed displacement. This involves the transfer of emotions from one object or person to another object or person.

23. With a patient experiencing severe anxiety, an appropriate nursing intervention is to
    a. assist the patient to develop insight
    b. encourage the patient to problem solve
    c. make decisions for the patient regarding care*
    d. point out damaging defense mechanisms

Reference: p. 707

Descriptors

1. 31	2. 05	3. Comprehensive
4. III-2	5. Nursing Process	6. Moderate

Rationale: With severe anxiety, the patient is unable to problem solve. The nurse must take charge, particularly as it relates to the patient's care.

24. The nurse is caring for a 16-year-old postoperative patient. He tells the nurse, "I may not be good in math or history, but I can sure hit a baseball!" The nurse determines that the patient is expressing a defense mechanism termed
    a. displacement
    b. projection
    c. compensation*
    d. sublimation
    Reference: p. 707
    Descriptors:

1. 31	2. 05	3. Application
4. III-2	5. Nursing Process	6. Moderate

    Rationale: When the patient tells the nurse "I may not be good in math or history, but I can sure hit a baseball!" the patient is expressing a defense mechanism termed compensation. The patient is overcoming a perceived weakness by overachieving in another area (sports).

25. The nurse is caring for a neglected 5-year-old child hospitalized for parental abuse. When the child refuses to discuss his home life, the nurse determines that the child is demonstrating a defense mechanism termed
    a. regression
    b. repression*
    c. projection
    d. introjection
    Reference: p. 708
    Descriptors:

1. 31	2. 05	3. Application
4. III-2	5. Nursing Process	6. Easy

    Rationale: When the neglected child refuses to discuss his home life, the child is demonstrating a defense mechanism termed repression.

26. A preschooler is ill and refuses to drink from a cup, requiring a bottle. This is an example of which defense mechanism?
    a. displacement
    b. attack behavior
    c. compensation
    d. regression*
    Reference: p. 708
    Descriptors:

1. 31	2. 05	3. Application
4. III-2	5. Nursing Process	6. Moderate

    Rationale: Regression occurs when a person returns to an earlier method of behaving.

27. The nurse is counseling a couple with marital problems. The wife tells the nurse "Last night he told me how stupid I was. Then, today he brought me a bouquet of roses! I don't know how to act." The nurse determines that the husband is demonstrating a defense mechanism termed
    a. compensation
    b. sublimation
    c. rationalization
    d. undoing*
    Reference: p. 708
    Descriptors:

1. 31	2. 05	3. Application
4. III-2	5. Nursing Process	6. Moderate

    Rationale: Undoing is an act or communication that is used to negate a previous act or communication.

28. A nursing student fails a test, for which he did not study, and blames the instructor for his failure. This represents which defense mechanism?
    a. displacement*
    b. retrospection
    c. rationalization
    d. projection
    Reference: pp. 707–708
    Descriptors:

1. 31	2. 05	3. Application
4. III-1	5. Caring	6. Difficult

    Rationale: Displacement occurs when a person transfers an emotional reaction from one object or person to another object or person.

29. Following her divorce, a 28-year-old woman blames her parents for her failures. This stress affects which basic human need?
    a. physiologic
    b. love*
    c. security
    d. safety
    Reference: p. 708
    Descriptors:

1. 31	2. 06	3. Application
4. III-1	5. Nursing Process	6. Difficult

    Rationale: Blaming others for one's own faults threatens the basic human need of love and belonging.

30. A 55-year-old woman with a history of cardiovascular disease has just been told of the death of her 22-year-old son. What nursing assessment is primary in the woman's care?
    a. blood pressure*
    b. anxiety level
    c. religious affiliation
    d. coping strategy

    Reference: p. 709

    Descriptors:

1. 31	2. 06	3. Application
4. III-1	5. Nursing Process	6. Difficult

    Rationale: During situations of extreme stress, individuals experience an increase in blood pressure, respirations, and heart rate. It is the responsibility of the nurse to assess vital signs particularly when the nurse is aware of past history of cardiovascular disease.

31. Following the death of her husband due to cardiac arrest, an 80-year-old woman states, "My husband died because the hospital and doctor killed him." This statement reflects
    a. overprotection of family
    b. loss of companionship
    c. fear of the future
    d. condemnation of care*

    Reference: p. 709

    Descriptors:

1. 31	2. 06	3. Application
4. III-1	5. Nursing Process	6. Difficult

    Rationale: Family response to stress of illness and death can result in family members blaming healthcare providers or condemnation of care.

32. A middle-aged woman is the sole support for her ill mother following the death of her father. She is also working full-time, attending school, and raising two children. She tells the nurse "The stress in my life is becoming unbearable." She is experiencing
    a. physiologic stress
    b. maturational crisis
    c. situational stress*
    d. developmental stress

    Reference: p. 710

    Descriptors:

1. 31	2. 05	3. Application
4. III-1	5. Nursing Process	6. Difficult

    Rationale: Situational crisis occur when a life event disrupts a person's psychological equilibrium such as loss related to death.

33. A patient visits the clinic and the nurse determines that she is approximately 8 weeks pregnant. She tells the nurse that the pregnancy was not planned and "she doesn't know if her husband wants a baby right now." The nurse determines that the woman is experiencing
    a. developmental crisis
    b. anticipatory stress
    c. situational stress*
    d. moderate anxiety

    Reference: p. 710

    Descriptors:

1. 31	2. 06	3. Application
4. III-1	5. Nursing Process	6. Moderate

    Rationale: The reaction to the unplanned pregnancy is a situational stressor that should resolve over time.

34. The nurse is caring for a family in the community who is experiencing a stress related to the primary wage earner being laid off from his job. The wife tells the nurse that her husband hasn't been sleeping well at night. A priority nursing diagnosis for this family is
    a. Hopelessness related to inability to find work
    b. Defensive Coping related to loss of employment*
    c. Decisional Conflict related to anxiety
    d. Situational Distress related to financial concerns

    Reference: p. 711

    Descriptors:

1. 31	2. 05	3. Application
4. III-1	5. Nursing Process	6. Difficult

    Rationale: The priority nursing diagnosis is Defensive Coping related to loss of employment.

35. The nurse is caring for an obese 40-year-old patient who tells the nurse that she "has always been fat and hates diet foods, but she's tried every diet on the market." A priority nursing diagnosis for this patient is
    a. Individual Coping, potential for growth
    b. Denial related to being overweight
    c. Defensive Coping related to long-term obesity*
    d. Ineffective Denial related to poor nutritional status

Reference: p. 711

Descriptors:

1. 31	2. 05	3. Application
4. III-1	5. Nursing Process	6. Difficult

Rationale: A priority nursing diagnosis for this patient is Defensive Coping related to long-term obesity.

36. The nurse makes a home visit to a family where the adult male has advanced Alzheimer's disease. The patient's wife is the husband's primary caregiver and tells the nurse that she is worn out from caring for her deteriorating husband. The nurse determines that the wife is experiencing
    a. role exhaustion
    b. situational crisis
    c. caregiver denial
    d. caregiver burden*

Reference: p. 712

Descriptors:

1. 31	2. 06	3. Application
4. III-1	5. Nursing Process	6. Moderate

Rationale: The wife is experiencing caregiver burden. The nurse should refer the patient to a respite or a support group to prevent the wife from total burnout.

37. When a patient is exhibiting aggressive behavior because of a threatened self-concept, the *most* appropriate nursing action is to
    a. place patient in a secluded room
    b. provide an opportunity to express feelings*
    c. restrain the patient until the behavior subsides
    d. ignore the patient until he calms down

Reference: p. 713

Descriptors:

1. 31	2. 06	3. Application
4. III-1	5. Teach/Learn	6. Moderate

Rationale: When the self-concept is threatened, allowing the patient to express his feelings may decrease the aggressive behavior.

38. Since beginning a new job, a 28-year-old marketing executive is unable to sleep. How can the nurse assist this patient in reducing his stress?
    a. Instruct the patient on relaxation techniques.*
    b. Refer patient to a physician for care.
    c. Instruct on over-the-counter sleep aids.
    d. Refer the patient to a psychologist.

Reference: p. 713

Descriptors:

1. 31	2. 07	3. Application
4. III-1	5. Self Care	6. Moderate

Rationale: Relaxation techniques can be helpful in health and illness to facilitate rest and sleep.

39. A nursing student experiences test anxiety. Before taking the test, it is important that the student use
    a. memorization
    b. deep breathing*
    c. late night study
    d. projection

Reference: p. 715

Descriptors:

1. 31	2. 07	3. Application
4. III-1	5. Teach/Learn	6. Moderate

Rationale: Relaxation techniques such as deep breathing will assist in decreasing the student's anxiety and enhance learning and test success.

40. The nurse is caring for an expectant mother who expresses fears about labor, delivery, and parenting her newborn. The nurse should suggest a stress management technique termed
    a. meditation
    b. anticipatory guidance*
    c. crisis intervention
    d. progressive muscle relaxation

Reference: p. 715

Descriptors:

1. 31	2. 07	3. Application
4. III-2	5. Nursing Process	6. Moderate

Rationale: Anticipatory guidance focuses on preparing a person for an unfamiliar or painful event.

41. The nurse has been working with a family whose son was hospitalized after a severe automobile accident by using crisis intervention techniques. The nurse is concluding her care with the family and asks the family to complete the final step of the process by asking the family to
    a. identify alternatives
    b. choose from among the alternatives
    c. accept what they cannot change
    d. evaluate the outcomes*

Reference: p. 716

Descriptors:

1. 31	2. 07	3. Application
4. III-2	5. Nursing Process	6. Moderate

Rationale: The last step in crisis intervention is the evaluation of the outcome.

42. A nurse employed in a neonatal intensive care unit of a hospital finds that the job is very stressful. An appropriate stress management activity for the nurse to engage in is to
a. become involved in constructive change*
b. sleep 4 to 6 hours every night
c. exercise for 20 minutes once a week
d. eat high-carbohydrate foods daily

Reference: p. 716

Descriptors:

1. 31	2. 08	3. Application
4. III-2	5. Nursing Process	6. Moderate

Rationale: The nurse should become involved in constructive change, exercise often, eat minimal carbohydrates, and sleep 8 hours every night.

43. Which of the following coping measures would be most effective with stress and anxiety on a long-term basis?
a. pleading illness
b. problem solving*
c. eating snacks
d. exercising

Reference: p. 716

Descriptors:

1. 31	2. 07	3. Comprehensive
4. III-1	5. Teach/Learn	6. Moderate

Rationale: On a long-term basis, problem solving must be initiated with a patient as a method of coping to adapt. Exercise can help the patient cope temporarily.

44. A new graduate employed on the intensive care unit tells an experienced nurse that "she feels totally overwhelmed and is afraid she is so stressed that she may experience burnout." The experienced nurse offers some stress relief suggestions to the novice. The nurse determines that the new graduate needs further instructions when she says
a. "I should try to learn something new and challenging."
b. "I need to take some time for myself each day."
c. "High-fat foods can help me cope with the stress."*
d. "It's important that I take my dinner break off the unit."

Reference: p. 717

Descriptors:

1. 31	2. 08	3. Application
4. III-1	5. None	6. Moderate

Rationale: The nurse determines that the new graduate needs further instructions when she says "High-fat foods can help me cope with the stress." The novice nurse should maintain a healthy diet and follow the Food Guide Pyramid with low-fat foods.

CHAPTER 32

Loss, Grief, and Dying

1. The daughter of a hospitalized patient who has died has been crying outside of her father's room. The nurse determines that the daughter is experiencing a/an
   a. actual loss*
   b. perceived loss
   c. reflective loss
   d. anticipatory loss

   Reference: p. 726

   Descriptors:

1. 32	2. 02	3. Application
4. III-1	5. Nursing Process	6. Easy

   Rationale: The daughter is expressing actual loss. This occurs when the person displays grief behaviors for a loss that has occurred.

2. An 84-year-old patient tells the nurse that she hasn't been eating very well since the loss of her husband 2 days ago. The nurse determines that the patient is in a state of
   a. shock*
   b. mourning
   c. bereavement
   d. denial

   Reference: pp. 726–727

   Descriptors:

1. 32	2. 03	3. Application
4. III-1	5. Nursing Process	6. Moderate

   Rationale: The patient is in a state of shock, which is the first phase of grieving for the person experiencing the loss.

3. Following the death of the patient's spouse the nurse notes that the patient has been eating a nutritionally deficient diet and having abdominal discomfort. This patient is experiencing
   a. bereavement*
   b. mourning
   c. grief
   d. despair

   Reference: p. 726

   Descriptors:

1. 32	2. 02	3. Application
4. III-1	5. Nursing Process	6. Moderate

   Rationale: Bereavement may have profound health consequences that require additional care.

4. A young mother has a 10-year-old mentally disabled child with severe congenital cardiac anomalies. She states, "I know the end of his life is coming and it is already difficult." The mother's statement reflects
   a. physical loss
   b. perceived loss
   c. anticipatory loss*
   d. psychological loss

   Reference: p. 726

   Descriptors:

1. 32	2. 02	3. Application
4. III-2	5. Nursing Process	6. Moderate

   Rationale: Anticipatory loss is loss that has not yet occurred.

5. A hospitalized patient has just been informed that he has terminal cancer and less than 6 months to live. He says to the nurse "There must be some mistake in the diagnosis." The nurse determines that the patient is demonstrating which of the following?
   a. denial*
   b. anger
   c. bargaining
   d. acceptance

   Reference: pp. 727, 730

   Descriptors:

1. 32	2. 04	3. Application
4. III-1	5. Nursing Process	6. Easy

   Rationale: When the patient refuses to admit that the diagnosis is correct, the patient is expressing denial.

6. The nurse is caring for a 40-year-old patient with end-stage breast cancer. The patient says to the nurse, "At least God let me live to see my daughter's college graduation. I am at peace now." The nurse determines that the patient is in the Kübler-Ross stage of grief termed
a. shock
b. restitution
c. bargaining
d. acceptance*

Reference: p. 727

Descriptors:

| 1. 32 | 2. 04 | 3. Application |
| 4. III-2 | 5. Nursing Process | 6. Easy |

Rationale: When the patient tries to barter for more time, the patient is in the bargaining stage of grief according to Kübler-Ross.

7. During the death of a family member the family requests a clergyman. According to Engel this represents
a. shock and disbelief
b. developing awareness
c. restitution*
d. resolving the loss

Reference: p. 727

Descriptors:

| 1. 32 | 2. 03 | 3. Comprehensive |
| 4. III-2 | 5. None | 6. Moderate |

Rationale: Restitution involves the rituals surrounding loss and death.

8. A 55-year-old patient with terminal cancer states that he hopes he lives to see his daughter graduate from law school. He states, "If I live to see that happen, I will be ready to die." According to Kübler-Ross this statement reflects
a. anger
b. bargaining*
c. depression
d. acceptance

Reference: pp. 727, 730

Descriptors:

| 1. 32 | 2. 03 | 3. Comprehensive |
| 4. III-2 | 5. Nursing Process | 6. Moderate |

Rationale: Bargaining is a stage in which the patient desires to live to participate in one of life's events.

9. A nurse caring for a 15-year-old patient with terminal cancer has assessed that the patient is very quiet and has not expressed his feelings. The nurse will need to implement
a. referrals for bereavement resources to enhance care
b. interventions for patient isolation and inner thought
c. assessment skills to determine fear and anxiety
d. therapeutic skills to enhance communication*

Reference: p. 728

Descriptors:

| 1. 32 | 2. 09 | 3. Application |
| 4. III-1 | 5. Nursing Process | 6. Difficult |

Rationale: Interventions, which enhance anticipatory grieving, should include commitment to the patient's well-being through communication.

10. The nurse is caring for a patient who is dying of terminal cancer. While assessing the patient for signs of impending death, the nurse should observe the patient for
a. elevated blood pressure
b. Cheyne-Stokes respirations*
c. elevated pulse rate
d. flushed skin

Reference: p. 727

Descriptors:

| 1. 32 | 2. 11 | 3. Application |
| 4. III-2 | 5. Caring | 6. Moderate |

Rationale: One sign of impending death is Cheyne-Stokes (noisy) respiration. Other signs include lowered blood pressure, cool and clammy skin, and elevated temperature.

11. A terminal patient's husband does not want to cry or voice his fears in front of his wife. The patient states, "I don't think my husband is upset that I am dying." It is important for the nurse to
a. encourage the couple to voice their feelings*
b. encourage the patient to accept what she feels
c. provide the patient and husband quiet time
d. determine the patient's awareness of dying

Reference: p. 728

Descriptors:

| 1. 32 | 2. 09 | 3. Application |
| 4. III-2 | 5. Nursing Process | 6. Difficult |

Rationale: The nurse must assist the patient and family in their progression through the stages of death and dying.

12. A patient who is undergoing an amputation in the morning will require interventions that enhance self-concept. The most appropriate intervention is
   a. patient education on rehabilitation
   b. time periods of verbal expression*
   c. knowledge of stress relief activity
   d. interaction with an another amputee

   Reference: p. 728

   Descriptors:

1. 32	2. 09	3. Application
4. III-1	5. Nursing Process	6. Moderate

   Rationale: A patient who is experience the loss of a limb will require time to voice concerns and fears regarding physical loss. This activity will enhance the patient's self-concept.

13. In the United States, there are several definitions of death currently being used. The definition that uses apnea testing and pupillary responses to light is termed
   a. whole brain death*
   b. heart–lung death
   c. circulatory death
   d. higher brain death

   Reference: p. 729

   Descriptors:

1. 32	2. 05	3. Knowledge
4. None	5. None	6. Moderate

   Rationale: The definition that uses apnea testing and pupillary responses to light is termed whole brain death.

14. A legal document that appoints a person to make decisions in the event of the appointing person's subsequent incapacity is a/an
   a. living will
   b. durable power of attorney*
   c. do-not-resuscitate order
   d. informed consent

   Reference: pp. 731–733

   Descriptors:

1. 32	2. 06	3. Knowledge
4. None	5. Documentation	6. Easy

   Rationale: A durable power of attorney is a legal document that appoints a person to make decisions in the event of the appointing person's subsequent incapacity.

15. A newborn infant is diagnosed with severe mental disability and will likely die in a few days. The parents appear to be unaware of the severity of the infant's illness. It is important that the parents are informed by a/an
   a. clergyman and nurse
   b. grief counselor and nurse
   c. physician and nurse*
   d. social worker and nurse

   Reference: p. 730

   Descriptors:

1. 32	2. 06	3. Application
4. III-1	5. Nursing Process	6. Easy

   Rationale: The physician and nurse should provide the patient and family with information regarding terminal illness.

16. A patient who has ovarian cancer with metastasis to the liver complains of increased pain and dysphagia. A physician orders a barium enema. The patient states, "I don't want this test. What should I do?" The nurse should
   a. inform her to refuse the test
   b. inform the physician of her statements*
   c. educate her on the test's benefits
   d. educate her on the procedure

   Reference: p. 731

   Descriptors:

1. 32	2. 06	3. Application
4. I-1	5. Communication	6. Moderate

   Rationale: The nurse must be an advocate for the terminally ill patient.

17. Specific information regarding the type of healthcare patients require when they are unable to speak for themselves is contained in a/an
   a. living will*
   b. durable power of attorney
   c. do-not-resuscitate order
   d. informed consent

   Reference: p. 731

   Descriptors:

1. 32	2. 06	3. Knowledge
4. None	5. Documentation	6. Easy

   Rationale: Living wills provide specific instructions about the kind of healthcare that should be provided or forgone in particular situations.

18. The nurse is caring for a patient who is unresponsive from a cerebrovascular accident (stroke); the patient requires a ventilator. When the healthcare team interviews the son, who is the durable power of attorney, it is determined that he is undecided about the patient's future treatment. The most appropriate nursing diagnosis is
    a. Ineffective Individual Coping related to impending loss
    b. Anxiety related to impending loss
    c. Ineffective Family Coping related to impending loss
    d. Decisional Conflict related to impending loss*

    Reference: p. 732

    Descriptors:

1. 32	2. 09	3. Application
4. IV-1	5. Nursing Process	6. Difficult

    Rationale: Decisional Conflict is the state of uncertainty about the cause of action to be taken when choice exists among competing risks and loss or challenges to personal life values.

19. The nurse is caring for a dying patient who has persistently requested that the nurse "help her to die and be in peace. Give me an overdose of morphine." According to the Code for Nurses, the nurse should
    a. ask the patient if she has signed the advance directives document
    b. tell the patient that the nurse will ask another nurse to care for the patient
    c. instruct the patient that only a physician can legally assist a suicide in this state
    d. try to make the patient as comfortable as possible but refuse to assist in the death*

    Reference: pp. 733, 746

    Descriptors:

1. 32	2. 10	3. Application
4. IV-1	5. Caring	6. Moderate

    Rationale: According to the Code for Nurses, the nurse should try to make the patient as comfortable as possible but refuse to assist in the death. Nurses cannot ethically assist patients to die by giving them an overdose.

20. The nurse is caring for a terminally ill patient when the physician tells the nurse that if necessary, only a "slow code" should be initiated for the patient. The nurse should
    a. ask the physician to write do-not-resuscitate orders for the patient*
    b. ask the family if this is the patient's desire according to the advance directives
    c. instruct the cardiopulmonary resuscitation team that a "slow code" has been ordered
    d. tell the patient that his life will not be prolonged indefinitely

    Reference: p. 736

    Descriptors:

1. 32	2. 06	3. Application
4. IV-1	5. Documentation	6. Moderate

    Rationale: Slow codes are inappropriate and many institutions do not allow these to be performed. The nurse should ask the physician to write a do-not-resuscitate order for the patient.

21. The nurse is caring for a 91-year-old dying patient who has a desire for comfort measures only and a dignified death. If the patient experiences respiratory arrest,
    a. cardiopulmonary resuscitation efforts will be initiated
    b. comfort measures only will be provided*
    c. slow-code efforts will begin
    d. only respiratory resuscitation will be initiated

    Reference: p. 737

    Descriptors:

1. 32	2. 06	3. Application
4. IV-1	5. Caring	6. Moderate

    Rationale: If the patient experiences respiratory arrest, comfort measures only are provided.

22. A physician writes orders for a patient who has experienced brain death to have terminal weaning. The nurse plans to support the family members by
    a. informing them that this will result in inevitable death
    b. providing the family members with analgesia during the process if necessary
    c. describing what to expect during the process by providing information*
    d. helping them to make funeral arrangements for the dying patient

Reference: p. 737

Descriptors:

1. 32	2. 08	3. Application
4. III-1	5. Caring	6. Moderate

Rationale: The nurse plans to support the family members by describing what to expect during the process by providing information. Terminal weaning does not always result in death.

23. A 39-year-old patient who is apparently dead is brought to the hospital by ambulance. A concerned neighbor found the patient alone in his apartment in this condition. The tentative cause of death is suicide. Even though the family has refused an autopsy, an autopsy can be ordered by the
   a. family's physician
   b. county court
   c. city police department
   d. county coroner*

Reference: p. 738

Descriptors:

1. 32	2. 12	3. Knowledge
4. None	5. None	6. Moderate

Rationale: Even though the family has refused an autopsy, an autopsy can be ordered by the county coroner in cases of mysterious death, suicide, or homicide.

24. A nurse caring for an 80-year-old patient who has end-stage renal disease has been told by her family that she is a very religious woman. It is important for the nurse to
   a. ascertain her current religious needs
   b. encourage her past religious practices*
   c. call her clergyman to visit her daily
   d. pray with her when she requests it

Reference: p. 738

Descriptors:

1. 32	2. 12	3. Application
4. IV-1	5. Caring	6. Difficult

Rationale: The implementation of the patient's past religious practices will increase her self-concept and assist her in a peaceful death.

25. According to developmental theory, the death of a parent
   a. prepares a middle-aged adult for death*
   b. allows a child to understand death
   c. brings families closer together
   d. provides for the realization of death

Reference: p. 738

Descriptors:

1. 32	2. 13	3. Comprehensive
4. II-1	5. Nursing Process	6. Moderate

Rationale: The death of a parent allows the middle-aged adult time to prepare for loss of a significant other and accept his own death.

26. To assist the patient and family in the process of grief, the nurse must
   a. have taken care of patients who have died
   b. understand the process of prolonging life
   c. identify personal losses in his or her own life*
   d. care for the neediest family members

Reference: p. 739

Descriptors:

1. 32	2. 13	3. Application
4. I-1	5. Caring	6. Difficult

Rationale: Nurses caring for patients experiencing loss or grief must identify personal losses that are influencing current state of well-being and identify and use effective coping strategies.

27. The nurse is caring for a 4½-year-old patient in the clinic when the mother expresses concerns about the child's toilet training. The child was toilet trained completely but suffered the loss of his father in an auto accident 2 months ago. The nurse should explain to the mother that the child's behavior indicates a
   a. normal grief response*
   b. dysfunctional grief response
   c. need for psychological counseling
   d. fear of his own death

Reference: p. 738

Descriptors:

1. 32	2. 07	3. Application
4. III-1	5. Nursing Process	6. Moderate

Rationale: The nurse should explain to the mother that the child's behavior indicates a normal grief response. Regression is a common manifestation of grief in children.

28. The nurse is caring for a 70-year-old patient who is receiving chemotherapy for cancer. The patient requests pain medication every 2 hours. A priority nursing diagnosis for this patient is
    a. Anxiety related to fear of dying
    b. Altered Comfort related to effects of chemotherapy*
    c. Fatigue related to heavy sedation
    d. Knowledge Deficit related to effects of medications

Reference: p. 740

Descriptors:

1. 32	2. 09	3. Application
4. IV-1	5. Nursing Process	6. Moderate

Rationale: When the patient requests pain medication every 2 hours, a priority nursing diagnosis for the patient is Altered Comfort related to effects of chemotherapy.

29. The nurse has informed the family of a terminally ill comatose patient about the loss of various senses during imminent death. The nurse determines that the family understands the instructions when one of the family members says that it is believed that the last sense to leave the body is the sense of
    a. sight
    b. touch
    c. smell
    d. hearing*

Reference: p. 742

Descriptors:

1. 32	2. 08	3. Application
4. IV-1	5. Teach/Learn	6. Moderate

Rationale: The nurse determines that the family understands the instructions when one of the family members says that it is believed that the last sense to leave the body is the sense of hearing.

30. The hospice nurse is visiting a terminally ill patient and his family. The wife begins to cry and states, "I don't know how much longer I can hold up. He needs constant care and I am about to collapse." The most appropriate nursing diagnosis is
    a. Ineffective Coping related to care of husband
    b. Caregiver Role overload related to terminal illness
    c. Anxiety related to terminal illness of husband
    d. Caregiver Role Strain related to care of husband*

Reference: p. 740

Descriptors:

1. 32	2. 09	3. Application
4. III-1	5. Caring	6. Difficult

Rationale: Many families experience caregiver role strain due to stress of providing nursing care and the patient's impending death.

31. A young mother whose child died of cancer states, "I can't go on anymore. I have no one who understands how I feel." The most appropriate nursing intervention is to
    a. refer her to pastoral care
    b. refer her to a support group*
    c. call the physician
    d. assess her medical needs

Reference: p. 742

Descriptors:

1. 32	2. 09	3. Application
4. I-1	5. Nursing Process	6. Moderate

Rationale: A grief support group is an excellent resource for families. It allows the family to express their grief to other individuals in similar situations.

32. The nurse in the emergency room observes several family members behaving in a stunned manner after the physician has informed the family that their 4-month-old child is dead and the cause is most likely sudden infant death syndrome. The nurse should
    a. ask the family to make funeral arrangements
    b. determine if the family is willing to make an organ donation
    c. urge the family members to return home
    d. provide a quiet place for the family to grieve*

Reference: p. 746

Descriptors:

1. 32	2. 13	3. Application
4. IV-1	5. Caring	6. Moderate

Rationale: The nurse should provide a quiet place for the family to grieve. The family should be allowed to stay with the child as long as they desire.

33. The nurse is caring for a competent 78-year-old patient who is diagnosed with a terminal illness. After planning care with the patient, an appropriate outcome is that the patient will
    a. demonstrate all phases of the grief process
    b. determine who will be with the patient during the time of death
    c. share concerns with significant others and seek needed help*
    d. formulate plans for legal arrangements following the death

Reference: p. 742

Descriptors:

1. 32　　　2. 08　　　　　　　3. Application
4. III-2　　5. Caring　　　　　　6. Moderate

Rationale: After planning care with the patient, an appropriate outcome is that the patient will share concerns with significant others and seek needed help.

34. A 70-year-old woman has been rehospitalized and is dying of cancer. Her husband tells the nurse, "I just didn't know it would be this hard...taking care of her all the time." The husband has dark circles under his eyes and looks exhausted. A priority nursing diagnosis is
    a. Decisional Conflict related to who will care for dying wife
    b. Anticipatory Grieving related to inevitability of wife's death
    c. Hopelessness related to providing care for wife
    d. Caregiver Role Strain related to providing care for dying wife*

Reference: p. 743

Descriptors:

1. 32　　2. 13　　　　　　3. Application
4. III-1　5. Nursing Process　6. Moderate

Rationale: A priority nursing diagnosis is Caregiver Role Strain related to providing care for dying wife.

35. The nurse is counseling a couple who are likely to be divorced. Two years ago, the wife delivered a preterm infant who died 2 days after birth. The couple has failed to come to peace over the neonate's death. The wife has gained 20 pounds and the husband stays out every night. A priority nursing diagnosis for this couple is
    a. Dysfunctional Grieving related to inability to accept infant's death*
    b. Continued Grieving related to death of a preterm infant
    c. Ineffective Denial related to inability to cope with infant's death
    d. Hopelessness related to probable divorce due to infant's death

Reference: p. 743

Descriptors:

1. 32　　2. 13　　　　　　3. Application
4. III-1　5. Nursing Process　6. Moderate

Rationale: A priority nursing diagnosis for this couple is Dysfunctional Grieving related to inability to accept infant's death. Continued Grieving is not a diagnosis. The couple is not in denial nor do they exhibit hopelessness.

36. The nurse is caring for a terminally ill patient on a hospice unit of the institution. The nurse should explain to the patient's family that a primary concern for the dying patient is fear of
    a. loss of control
    b. accidental bed wetting
    c. isolation*
    d. pain

Reference: p. 745

Descriptors:

1. 32　　2. 13　　　　　　3. Application
4. III-1　5. Nursing Process　6. Moderate

Rationale: A primary concern for the dying patient is fear of isolation or dying alone.

37. A 70-year-old male patient is comatose after a cerebrovascular accident. The family is at the bedside. It is important for the nurse to
    a. allow the patient adequate time to rest
    b. sedate the patient to prevent anxiety
    c. inform the family he can probably still hear*
    d. administer oral fluids to the patient

Reference: p. 745

Descriptors:

1. 32	2. 09	3. Application
4. III-2	5. Teach/Learn	6. Moderate

Rationale: It is important that the family understand that the comatose patient can hear almost to the moment of death.

38. A young child with terminal cancer has difficulty communicating his feelings. It is important to
   a. allow frequent visits with social workers
   b. provide quiet time for inner reflection
   c. limit visits with family and friends
   d. encourage the use of art therapy*

Reference: p. 745

Descriptors:

1. 32	2. 09	3. Application
4. III-1	5. Nursing Process	6. Moderate

Rationale: Art therapy for terminally ill children enhances the expression of the child's feelings regarding the future and impending death.

39. Following the death of a patient the nurse is
   a. legally responsible for placing identification on the body*
   b. required to send the body immediately to the morgue
   c. responsible for the cleaning of the patient's room
   d. legally bound to inform the family of an autopsy

Reference: p. 746

Descriptors:

1. 32	2. 12	3. Comprehensive
4. IV-1	5. Nursing Process	6. Easy

Rationale: The nurse is legally responsible for placing identification tags on both the shroud or garment the body is clothed in and on the ankle to ensure that the body can be identified even if it is separated from the shroud.

CHAPTER 33

Sensory Stimulation

1. The ability of a patient to sit upright in a chair is due in part to which of the following types of sensory perception?
   a. kinesthetic*
   b. gustatory
   c. stereognosis
   d. visual

   Reference: p. 756

   Descriptors:

   1. 33   2. 01   3. Application
   4. None   5. None   6. Moderate

   Rationale: Kinesthesia refers to awareness of positioning of body parts and movements. Stereognosis is the sense that perceives the solidity of objects.

2. The primary purpose of the reticular activating system (RAS) in the sensory experience is to
   a. maintain a steady sense of balance
   b. mediate arousal through a poorly defined network*
   c. force the body to pay attention to external stimuli
   d. alter states of the body's consciousness

   Reference: p. 757

   Descriptors:

   1. 33   2. 03   3. Application
   4. None   5. None   6. Moderate

   Rationale: Through a poorly defined network, the RAS in the sensory experience mediates arousal. It monitors and directs incoming stimuli.

3. Which of the following patients is most likely to experience sensory overload? A patient who
   a. has a slight hearing impairment
   b. is in solitary confinement for violent behavior
   c. has had brain damage from an auto accident
   d. is admitted to a step-down unit after treatment in the intensive care unit*

   Reference: p. 758

   Descriptors:

   1. 33   2. 01, 04   3. Comprehensive
   4. IV-1   5. Nursing Process   6. Moderate

   Rationale: The patient who is most likely to experience sensory overload is the patient admitted to a step-down unit after treatment in intensive care unit.

4. While assessing a patient's need for sensory stimulation, which data would be most important for the nurse to collect?
   a. weight
   b. memory
   c. gender
   d. culture*

   Reference: pp. 758, 761

   Descriptors:

   1. 33   2. 05   3. Application
   4. IV-1   5. Cultural   6. Moderate

   Rationale: The patient's cultural affiliation is an important factor to obtain data to prevent cultural care deprivation.

5. A priority nursing diagnosis for a patient who experiencing depression and boredom from recent blindness is
   a. Diversional Activity Deficit related to impaired vision*
   b. Ineffective Coping, Individual, related to depression
   c. Chronic Low Self-Esteem related to blindness
   d. Activity Intolerance related to depression and boredom

   Reference: p. 765

   Descriptors:

   1. 33   2. 06   3. Application
   4. III-1   5. Nursing Process   6. Moderate

   Rationale: The priority nursing diagnosis is Diversional Activity Deficit related to impaired vision because of the patient's boredom and depression.

6. An effective nonpharmacologic method of providing relaxation for mechanically ventilated patients in an intensive care unit is
   a. silence during care
   b. quiet, soothing music*
   c. keeping the lights dim
   d. maintaining privacy by curtains

   Reference: p. 768
   Descriptors:
   1. 33   2. 07   3. Application
   4. III-2   5. Caring   6. Moderate

   Rationale: An effective nonpharmacologic method of providing relaxation for mechanically ventilated patients in an intensive care unit is quiet, soothing music.

7. In caring for a hospitalized patient who is deaf and blind, when the nurse enters the room, the nurse should first
   a. identify herself by name*
   b. tell the patient the reason for entering the room
   c. provide diversions using other senses
   d. provide guidance to the patient about the procedure

   Reference: p. 768
   Descriptors:
   1. 33   2. 07   3. Application
   4. IV-1   5. Nursing Process 6. Moderate

   Rationale: In caring for a hospitalized patient who is deaf and blind, when the nurse enters the room, she should first identify herself by name. Next is to explain the purpose for touching the patient.

8. Which of the following would not be an appropriate nursing strategy when caring for elderly patients who are hospitalized?
   a. Determine the patient's need for glasses or a hearing aid.
   b. Offer prescription eyedrops to keep the patient's eyes moist.*
   c. Note the fit and condition of the patient's dentures.
   d. Provide large print books and magazines.

   Reference: p. 768
   Descriptors:
   1. 33   2. 07   3. Application
   4. IV-1   5. Nursing Process 6. Moderate

   Rationale: Offering prescription eyedrops to keep the patient's eyes moist should not be done unless the physician has ordered the drops for the patient.

9. While caring for a male patient who is unconscious, the nurse should explain to the family members who are visiting the patient to
   a. keep environmental noises at a relatively loud level
   b. talk to the patient in a subdued tone of voice
   c. assume that the patient can hear the person who is speaking*
   d. touch the patient before speaking to him

   Reference: p. 771
   Descriptors:
   1. 33   2. 08   3. Application
   4. IV-1   5. Nursing Process 6. Moderate

   Rationale: The nurse should explain to the family members who are visiting the patient to assume that the patient can hear the person who is speaking. It is believed that the sense of hearing is the last sense to be lost.

10. Successful resolution of the nursing diagnosis of Sleep Pattern Disturbance related to sensory overload has been achieved when the patient
    a. received a hypnotic medication
    b. maintained a darkened environment
    c. performed bedtime rituals
    d. stated that a nap was restful*

    Reference: p. 771
    Descriptors:
    1. 33   2. 07, 08   3. Application
    4. IV-1   5. Nursing Process 6. Moderate

    Rationale: Successful resolution of the nursing diagnosis of Sleep Pattern Disturbance related to sensory overload has been achieved when the patient stated that a nap was restful.

CHAPTER 34

Sexuality

1. A person's inner sense of being male or female is referred to as
   a. biologic sex
   b. gender identity*
   c. emotional health
   d. gender role

   Reference: p. 780

   Descriptors:

1. 34	2. 01	3. Knowledge
4. None	5. None	6. Easy

   Rationale: Gender identity is the inner sense a person has of being male or female, which may be the same as or different from biologic gender.

2. A 32-year-old man portrays himself with great masculinity. This action denotes his
   a. gender role*
   b. gender identity
   c. biologic sex
   d. inner prowess

   Reference: p. 780

   Descriptors:

1. 34	2. 01	3. Comprehensive
4. None	5. None	6. Moderate

   Rationale: Gender role behavior is the behavior a person conveys about being male or female, which may or may not be the same as biologic gender or gender identity.

3. A male patient admitted to the hospital for cardiac symptoms states that he has sexual relationships with male and female partners. In the sexual history the nurse documents that he is a
   a. transvestite
   b. heterosexual
   c. bisexual*
   d. transsexual

   Reference: p. 781

   Descriptors:

1. 34	2. 04	3. Comprehensive
4. II-1	5. Nursing Process	6. Difficult

   Rationale: A bisexual is a person who finds pleasure with both the opposite-sex and same-sex partners.

4. A man who wears women's clothing is identified as a
   a. transvestite*
   b. bisexual
   c. transsexual
   d. heterosexual

   Reference: p. 781

   Descriptors:

1. 34	2. 04	3. Comprehensive
4. II-1	5. Nursing Process	6. Easy

   Rationale: A transvestite is an individual who desires to take on the role or wear the clothes of the opposite sex.

5. A female patient states to the nurse, "I know I should be a man. I feel like a man. I have never felt like a woman." The patient is expressing to the nurse that she is a
   a. transvestite
   b. bisexual
   c. transsexual*
   d. homosexual

   Reference: p. 781

   Descriptors:

1. 34	2. 04	3. Comprehensive
4. II-1	5. Nursing Process	6. Difficult

   Rationale: The patient is expressing that she is a transsexual when she wishes she were a man.

6. During a woman's hospitalization to deliver a baby, she and her husband hold hands and hug frequently. They are displaying their
   a. sexual fulfillment*
   b. negative feelings
   c. diminished bonding
   d. decreased adaptation

   Reference: p. 781

   Descriptors:

1. 34	2. 04	3. Application
4. II-1	5. Communication	6. Moderate

   Rationale: The couple is displaying sexual fulfillment when they hold hands and hug during the woman's labor and delivery process.

7. During sexual intercourse the labia minora become
   a. pale pink
   b. dark red*
   c. dusky white
   d. light blue

   Reference: p. 781

   Descriptors:

1. 34	2. 03	3. Knowledge
4. None	5. None	6. Easy

   Rationale: When stimulated by touch, the labia minora may turn dark pink or even red owing to the increase in blood vessels.

8. Fertilization of the ova occurs in which female structure?
   a. vagina
   b. uterus
   c. fallopian tube*
   d. ovary

   Reference: p. 781

   Descriptors:

1. 34	2. 03	3. Knowledge
4. None	5. None	6. Easy

   Rationale: Fertilization of the ovum by the sperm normally occurs in the fallopian tube.

9. The cessation of a woman's menstrual activity is referred to as
   a. menarche
   b. menses
   c. menopause*
   d. ovulation

   Reference: p. 782

   Descriptors:

1. 34	2. 03	3. Knowledge
4. None	5. None	6. Easy

   Rationale: The cessation of a woman's menstrual activity is referred to as menopause and usually occurs at age 45 to 55 years.

10. Pain, located over the ovulating ovary, and occurring in the middle of the menstrual cycle, is called
    a. ovarian discomfort
    b. endometriosis
    c. dysmenorrhea
    d. mittelschmerz*

    Reference: p. 782

    Descriptors:

1. 34	2. 02	3. Comprehensive
4. None	5. None	6. Moderate

    Rationale: Pain, located over the ovulating ovary, and occurring in the middle of the menstrual cycle, is called mittelschmerz or middle pain.

11. During the menstrual cycle, disintegration of the endothelial lining is known as the
    a. endomorphic phase
    b. secretory phase*
    c. fertilization phase
    d. proliferative phase

    Reference: p. 782

    Descriptors:

1. 34	2. 02	3. Knowledge
4. None	5. None	6. Easy

    Rationale: During the luteal phase in the ovaries the uterus undergoes changes. This phase is called the secretory phase.

12. Normal blood loss during menstruation is
    a. 10 to 20 mL
    b. 20 to 25 mL
    c. 30 to 80 mL*
    d. 80 mL

    Reference: p. 782

    Descriptors:

1. 34	2. 02	3. Knowledge
4. None	5. None	6. Easy

    Rationale: The nurse must assess menstrual discharge to determine whether the amount exceeds the normal output. Normal blood loss is 30 to 80 mL.

13. Irritability that occurs several days before the onset of menses is referred to as
    a. hormone insufficiency
    b. a psychotic disorder
    c. female neurosis
    d. premenstrual syndrome*

    Reference: p. 783

    Descriptors:

1. 34	2. 02	3. Knowledge
4. None	5. None	6. Moderate

    Rationale: Menstrual cycle-related distress, commonly known at premenstrual syndrome, reportedly occurs in 50% to 90% of the female population.

14. A young couple visiting the obstetrical clinic state they have been trying to become pregnant for approximately 6 months. During the interview the nurse notes that the male is wearing extremely tight-fitting denim jeans. What test should the nurse practitioner order for the couple?
    a. sperm count*
    b. pregnancy test
    c. progesterone level
    d. testosterone level

    Reference: p. 783

    Descriptors:

1. 34	2. 02	3. Application
4. II-1	5. Nursing Process	6. Difficult

    Rationale: Tight-fitting jeans will increase the scrotal temperature and cause sperm death.

15. Male sperm is produced in the
    a. testes*
    b. vas deferens
    c. epididymus
    d. ejaculatory duct

    Reference: p. 782

    Descriptors:

1. 34	2. 02	3. Knowledge
4. None	5. None	6. Easy

    Rationale: The testes produce the sperm and hormones necessary for maintenance of the male sex characteristics.

16. During a bed bath, the male patient may experience an
    a. ejaculation
    b. erection*
    c. emission
    d. orgasm

    Reference: pp. 782–783

    Descriptors:

1. 34	2. 03	3. Application
4. II-1	5. Nursing Process	6. Moderate

    Rationale: An erection is a normal physiologic response and not something the man can voluntarily control.

17. During a bed bath a male patient develops an erection. The nurse's best response is to
    a. inform the patient that this behavior is inappropriate
    b. proceed with the bath, washing the patient's back*
    c. abruptly leave the patient's room without commenting
    d. continue with the patient's bath on the lower anterior side

    Reference: pp. 782–783

    Descriptors:

1. 34	2. 09	3. Application
4. II-1	5. Nursing Process	6. Difficult

    Rationale: An erection is a normal physiologic response and not something the man can voluntarily control. Focus nursing care posteriorly to prevent the patient's embarrassment.

18. The female clitoris is comparable to which male reproductive organ?
    a. testes
    b. scrotum
    c. penis*
    d. glans

    Reference: p. 781

    Descriptors:

1. 34	2. 01; 02	3. Knowledge
4. None	5. None	6. Moderate

    Rationale: The female clitoris is comparable to the male penis because it can be stimulated to achieve an orgasm.

19. One of the major differences in the male and female sexual responses is that the
    a. male has a heightened excitement phase
    b. females experience no refractory period*
    c. males have many more erogenous zones
    d. females experience a less intense orgasmic phase

Reference: p. 785

Descriptors:

1. 34   2. 03   3. Knowledge
4. None   5. None   6. Moderate

Rationale: Females experience no refractory periods and can have multiple orgasms.

20. The first obvious sign of arousal in men is
    a. ejaculation
    b. sex flush
    c. contractions
    d. erection*

Reference: p. 785

Descriptors:

1. 34   2. 03   3. Comprehensive
4. None   5. None   6. Easy

Rationale: The first obvious sign of arousal in the man is an erection of the penis caused by increased penile congestion of blood.

21. For which of the following hospitalized patients is obtaining a sexual history most important for the nurse to assess? A patient with
    a. hypertension controlled by medication*
    b. diabetes controlled with diet
    c. a previous history of tuberculosis
    d. bronchial pneumonia

Reference: pp. 789, 792

Descriptors:

1. 34   2. 04   3. Application
4. IV-1   5. Nursing Process   6. Moderate

Rationale: A sexual history would be most important for the patient with hypertension controlled by medication because these medications can lead to changes in the sexual functioning.

22. A couple in a senior citizen complex visit the nurse stating, "We still desire to have sexual relations, but due to arthritic pain it is difficult and painful." The best statement a nurse can make to this couple is that
    a. sexual desire can be attained through the use of alternate positions*
    b. sexual activity is inappropriate for the senior citizen population
    c. sexual dysfunction can result from pain and will limit sexual pleasure
    d. other couples have experienced this and a referral will be made

Reference: p. 789

Descriptors:

1. 34   2. 07   3. Application
4. II-1   5. Communication   6. Difficult

Rationale: Altered or modified positions for coitus are sometimes necessary. The provision of this information is within the practice of the nurse to provide a totality of patient care.

23. Following a mastectomy the patient will experience anxiety and fear related to
    a. ideal self
    b. self-concept
    c. perceived self
    d. body image*

Reference: p. 789

Descriptors:

1. 34   2. 07   3. Application
4. II-1   5. Nursing Process   6. Moderate

Rationale: Mastectomy has a great effect on the woman's image of her body.

24. An 18-year-old man visits the clinic with a complaint of pain on urination and urethral soreness. The nurse suspects infection with
    a. *Gardnerella*
    b. *Neisseria gonorrhoeae*
    c. *Chlamydia**
    d. cytomegalovirus

Reference: pp. 789–791

Descriptors:

1. 34   2. 06   3. Application
4. II-2   5. Nursing Process   6. Moderate

Rationale: The most prevalent sexually transmitted disease is chlamydia. Women are usually asymptomatic, whereas men will experience pain on urination and have urethral soreness and dysuria.

25. The nurse must inform an individual who is diagnosed with a sexually transmitted disease that she must
    a. remain sexually inactive for 6 months
    b. inform any sexual partners that they need to be checked*
    c. take medications until asymptomatic
    d. monitor intake and output

Reference: pp. 789–791

Descriptors:

1. 34	2. 06	3. Application
4. II-2	5. Nursing Process	6. Difficult

Rationale: Sexually transmitted diseases are hard to control because the partner or partners also need treatment.

26. For the nurse to be able to counsel and assist patients with sexual issues, the nurse must
   a. develop one's own sexual self-awareness*
   b. have or have had a sexual relationship
   c. have experienced sexual intimacy
   d. use intimidation with patients who have sexually transmitted diseases

Reference: p. 790

Descriptors:

1. 34	2. 08	3. Application
4. I-1	5. Communication	6. Difficult

Rationale: The nurse must be able to develop self-awareness regarding sexual topics.

27. The development of pelvic inflammatory disease in women can lead to
   a. dysuria
   b. angina
   c. dysmenorrhea
   d. infertility*

Reference: p. 790

Descriptors:

1. 34	2. 06	3. Comprehensive
4. II-2	5. Nursing Process	6. Easy

Rationale: The development of pelvic inflammatory disease can lead to infertility in women.

28. A patient tells the nurse he has the desire to have a sexual relationship with her. The nurse's best response is to
   a. tell the patient that a relationship would be appropriate after the patient's discharge
   b. ignore the patient's request and inform the patient of care needed
   c. look the patient in the eye and state that a relationship is inappropriate*
   d. inform the patient you will sue for sexual harassment and prosecute

Reference: p. 790

Descriptors:

1. 34	2. 08	3. Application
4. II-1	5. Communication	6. Difficult

Rationale: The nurse in this scenario should use confrontation. The nurse should look the harasser in the eye and state that such a relationship is inappropriate.

29. A woman is experiencing a foul-smelling, thin, grayish white vaginal discharge. The nurse suspects that she may be infected with
   a. *Chlamydia*
   b. *Gardnerella vaginalis**
   c. *Neisseria gonorrhea*
   d. *Trichomonas vaginalis*

Reference: p. 791–792

Descriptors:

1. 34	2. 06	3. Application
4. II-2	5. Nursing Process	6. Difficult

Rationale: A woman experiencing a foul-smelling, thin, grayish white vaginal discharge possesses the symptoms of *Gardnerella vaginalis* infection.

30. A new male medical student has made inappropriate comments to the nurse on the hospital unit and frequently asks her for a date, even though he knows she is married. The nurse should first
   a. contact the nursing supervisor
   b. notify the Equal Employment Opportunity Commission
   c. look him in the eye and tell him to stop*
   d. put details of the incident in a written, registered letter

Reference: p. 791

Descriptors:

1. 34	2. 01	3. Application
4. I-1	5. Communication	6. Moderate

Rationale: The nurse should first look him in the eye and tell him to stop. The next step, if the harassment continues, is to document the events in writing.

31. A 57-year-old male patient is being discharged following cardiac bypass surgery. While counseling the patient about postoperative sexuality, the nurse should start the conversation with
    a. "I am wondering about your feelings related to sexuality."
    b. "Have you and your partner discussed your sexuality after surgery?"
    c. "Do you think your surgery will cause problems with your sexuality?"
    d. "Many people feel anxious about their sexuality after this type of surgery."*

    Reference: p. 792

    Descriptors:

1. 34	2. 05	3. Application
4. III-1	5. Communication	6. Moderate

    Rationale: While counseling the patient about postoperative sexuality, the nurse should start the conversation with "Many people feel anxious about their sexuality after this type of surgery." This opening statement helps the patient to know that he is not alone in the way he feels.

32. Small amounts of which of the following medications can be found in semen?
    a. antipsychotics*
    b. methyldopa
    c. lithium
    d. narcotics

    Reference: p. 793 ·

    Descriptors:

1. 34	2. 09	3. Application
4. IV-2	5. Nursing Process	6. Moderate

    Rationale: Antipsychotic medications have been detected in semen.

33. Of the following, which anticonvulsant medication reduces sexual response?
    a. phenobarbital
    b. Depakote
    c. Tegretol
    d. Dilantin*

    Reference: p. 793

    Descriptors:

1. 34	2. 09	3. Application
4. IV-1	5. Nursing Process	6. Moderate

    Rationale: Dilantin has sedative effects, which may decrease desire and reduce sexual response.

34. What is the most appropriate nursing diagnosis for a patient with erectile dysfunction?
    a. Sexual Dysfunction*
    b. Altered Body Image
    c. Altered Sexual Patterns
    d. Impaired Self-Esteem

    Reference: p. 799

    Descriptors:

1. 34	2. 07	3. Application
4. II-1	5. Nursing Process	6. Moderate

    Rationale: Sexual Dysfunction is the appropriate nursing diagnosis.

35. To assist a patient with sexual dysfunction the nurse must
    a. develop a trusting relationship*
    b. explain sexual dysfunction
    c. determine past sexuality history
    d. perform a physical assessment

    Reference: p. 799

    Descriptors:

1. 34	2. 09	3. Application
4. II-1	5. Caring	6. Moderate

    Rationale: For the nurse to best assist the patient who is experiencing sexual dysfunction a trusting relationship must be formed.

CHAPTER 35

Spirituality

1. A person's relationship with a nonmaterial life force or higher power is termed
   a. spirituality*
   b. religion
   c. meditation
   d. faith
   Reference: p. 818
   Descriptors:

1. 35	2. 01	3. Comprehensive
4. None	5. None	6. Easy

   Rationale: Spirituality is anything that pertains to a person's relationship with a nonmaterial life force or higher power.

2. Catholicism is referred to as a
   a. prayer
   b. religion*
   c. scripture
   d. practice
   Reference: p. 818
   Descriptors:

1. 35	2. 01	3. Comprehensive
4. None	5. None	6. Easy

   Rationale: Religion refers to an organized system of beliefs about a higher power.

3. One of the universal spiritual needs for human beings is
   a. forgiveness*
   b. God's permission
   c. actualization
   d. trust
   Reference: p. 818
   Descriptors:

1. 35	2. 01, 02	3. Knowledge
4. None	5. None	6. Easy

   Rationale: The three universal spiritual needs for human beings are meaning and purpose, love and relatedness, and forgiveness.

4. The difference between spirituality and religion is that spirituality is a/an
   a. belief about a higher power
   b. organized weekly worship
   c. individual's relationship with a higher power*
   d. belief in an afterlife
   Reference: p. 818
   Descriptors:

1. 35	2. 02, 03	3. Knowledge
4. None	5. None	6. Easy

   Rationale: With spirituality there is a belief about an individual's relationship with a higher power.

5. Spirituality affects a person's life in all of the following areas *except*
   a. nutritional intake
   b. sexual expression
   c. coping abilities
   d. genetic makeup*
   Reference: p. 818
   Descriptors:

1. 35	2. 03	3. Knowledge
4. None	5. None	6. Easy

   Rationale: Genetic makeup is not related to an individual's spirituality.

6. A dying patient states to the nurse, "I don't care if I die—there is no higher power or God. We developed through evolution." This statement reflects that he is a/an
   a. atheist*
   b. Buddhist
   c. unifier
   d. witness
   Reference: p. 819
   Descriptors:

1. 35	2. 01	3. Application
4. III-1.	5. Communication	6. Moderate

   Rationale: An atheist is a person who denies the existence of God.

7. A patient in the hospital wishes to say his daily prayers prior to his morning care. This practice enhances the patient's
   a. healthcare
   b. living habits
   c. spiritual beliefs*
   d. radical expression

Reference: p. 819

Descriptors:

1. 35	2. 02	3. Application
4. III-1.	5. Caring	6. Difficult

Rationale: Spiritual beliefs and practices are associated with all aspects of a person's life, including health and illness.

8. Which of the following is an example of a religious belief that is a life-denying experience?
   a. Roman Catholic/sacrament of the sick
   b. Islam/restriction on sterilization*
   c. Jewish/Kosher foods
   d. Middle East/yoga and biofeedback

Reference: p. 819

Descriptors:

1. 35	2. 04, 05	3. Knowledge
4. None	5. None	6. Easy

Rationale: An example of a religious belief that is a life-denying experience is Islam's restriction on sterilization.

9. A 32-year-old woman has just delivered a baby and has begun to hemorrhage. Blood transfusions have been ordered. The nurse should determine if the patient is a/an
   a. Buddhist
   b. Jehovah's Witness*
   c. Orthodox Jew
   d. Hindu

Reference: p. 820

Descriptors:

1. 35	2. 06	3. Application
4. IV-4	5. Nursing Process	6. Moderate

Rationale: In this scenario the woman may require a blood transfusion. According the teachings of the Jehovah's Witness, blood transfusions may not be administered.

10. The nurse is caring for a child who is an Adventist. When providing the patient with nutritional interventions, the nurse should provide
    a. pork and potatoes
    b. beans and beef
    c. garden burgers*
    d. pepperoni pizza

Reference: p. 821

Descriptors:

1. 35	2. 10	3. Application
4. III-1	5. Nursing Process	6. Moderate

Rationale: When caring for patients who practice the Adventist faith, it is important to determine if they are vegetarians.

11. Life practices to enhance self-esteem are tenets of the faith of
    a. Mormons
    b. Protestants
    c. Buddhists
    d. Muslims*

Reference: p. 821

Descriptors:

1. 35	2. 05	3. Comprehensive
4. None	5. None	6. Moderate

Rationale: Muslims accept the Koran as their sacred scripture, and educate to build self-esteem.

12. A 50-year-old woman has broken her hip but refuses to have surgery to set the bone due to her religious beliefs. What religion does this woman most likely practice?
    a. Adventist
    b. Christian Scientist*
    c. Baha'i International
    d. Unification Church

Reference: p. 821

Descriptors:

1. 35	2. 05	3. Comprehensive
4. III-1	5. Nursing Process	6. Moderate

Rationale: Christian Scientists will use orthopedic services to set a bone (eg, fracture) but decline drugs and surgical procedures.

13. On Fridays during the time of Lent many Christian faiths abstain from
    a. meat*
    b. fish
    c. vegetables
    d. milk

Reference: p. 823

Descriptors:

1. 35	2. 05	3. Comprehensive
4. III-1	5. Nursing Process	6. Moderate

Rationale: Christian faiths abstain from meat on Fridays during Lent.

14. Children learn most of their religious beliefs from their
    a. teachers
    b. preschool teachers
    c. clerics or ministers
    d. parents*

Reference: p. 825

Descriptors:

1. 35	2. 06	3. Comprehensive
4. II-1	5. Nursing Process	6. Easy

Rationale: A child's parent plays a key role in the development of the child's spirituality.

15. While assessing a patient's spirituality needs, an appropriate question for the nurse to ask is
    a. "How can I help you better your relationship with God?"
    b. "Do you have any spiritual needs that may affect your care?"*
    c. "What church or mosque do you attend?"
    d. "Are you angry that God allowed you to become ill?"

Reference: p. 826

Descriptors:

1. 35	2. 07	3. Application
4. III-1	5. Nursing Process	6. Easy

Rationale: Asking the patient if he has any spiritual needs that may affect care is an appropriate question to ask while assessing the patient's spirituality needs. The patient is more likely to discuss his needs with the nurse.

16. A newly delivered mother expresses her spiritual anger to God for allowing her premature neonate to die. A priority nursing diagnosis for this mother is
    a. Dysfunctional Grieving related to anger at God
    b. Hopelessness related to state of grief
    c. Spiritual Distress, Anger, related to death of neonate*
    d. Knowledge Deficit related to cause of neonatal death

Reference: p. 827

Descriptors:

1. 35	2. 08	3. Application
4. III-1	5. Nursing Process	6. Moderate

Rationale: The priority diagnosis is Spiritual Distress, Anger, related to death of neonate.

17. A patient's daughter states that her father is a very religious man and has never been away from church. He is admitted to a public hospital without immediate clergy support. The nurse should
    a. call a clergyman
    b. sit with the patient
    c. assess his spiritual needs*
    d. pray with the patient

Reference: p. 827

Descriptors:

1. 35	2. 10	3. Application
4. III-1	5. Nursing Process	6. Difficult

Rationale: In this scenario it is important for the nurse to assess the patient's spiritual needs so that appropriate interventions can be implemented.

18. A patient's family member states, "I know why this accident happened. It's because we don't go to church enough." The most appropriate nursing diagnosis is
    a. Spiritual Distress related to decreased religious affiliation*
    b. Spiritual Insufficiency related to accident and hospitalization
    c. Powerless related to lack of religious attendance and support
    d. Dysfunctional Grieving related to powerless feelings and guilt

Reference: p. 827

Descriptors:

1. 35	2. 08	3. Application
4. III-1	5. Nursing Process	6. Difficult

Rationale: Spiritual distress may be related to guilt over past religious practices and decreased religious affiliation.

19. A goal for a patient is to "Develop and maintain positive spiritual practices." An appropriate nursing strategy would be to
    a. note the patient's request to wear a medal while in surgery
    b. encourage the patient to discuss his wishes after death
    c. document the patient's religious affiliation
    d. encourage visitation by the minister while hospitalized*

    Reference: p. 829

    Descriptors:

1. 35	2. 09	3. Application
4. III-1	5. Nursing Process	6. Moderate

    Rationale: An appropriate strategy by the nurse is to encourage visitation by the minister while the patient is hospitalized.

20. When a nurse is uncomfortable in meeting the spiritual needs of the patient, it is appropriate to notify the
    a. medical doctor
    b. nurse practitioner
    c. social worker
    d. spiritual counselor*

    Reference: p. 831

    Descriptors:

1. 35	2. 10	3. Application
4. III-1	5. Nursing Process	6. Moderate

    Rationale: Not every nurse feels comfortable in the role of spiritual counselor. The nurse may suggest that the patient talk to a spiritual counselor.

21. A successful resolution for a patient with a nursing diagnosis of Spiritual Distress, Anger, related to loss of spouse occurs when the patient
    a. asks to visit the hospital's chapel
    b. receives communion from the minister or priest
    c. confesses to his daughter that he is angry
    d. reconciles his anger with the higher power*

    Reference: p. 832

    Descriptors:

1. 35	2. 10	3. Application
4. III-1	5. Nursing Process	6. Moderate

    Rationale: Successful resolution occurs when the patient reconciles his anger with the higher power.

UNIT VIII

Promoting Healthy Physiologic Responses

CHAPTER 36

Hygiene

1. While bathing an adult patient, the nurse observes slight discoloration and bruising on the patient's knee. The nurse plans to document this assessment of the patient's integumentary system as
   a. sebaceous epidermis
   b. ecchymosis of the dermis*
   c. subcutaneous bruise
   d. epidermal abrasion

   Reference: p. 844

   Descriptors:

1. 36	2. 01	3. Application
4. IV-3	5. Nursing Process	6. Moderate

   Rationale: An abrasion of the dermis with slight discoloration is termed ecchymosis of the dermis.

2. The nurse has presented a class on hygiene and skin care to a group of high school students. The nurse determines that one of the students needs further instructions when the student says that one of the primary functions of the skin is to
   a. store calcium*
   b. protect the body
   c. excrete waste products
   c. absorb vitamin D

   Reference: p. 846

   Descriptors:

1. 36	2. 02	3. Application
4. II-2	5. Nursing Process	6. Moderate

   Rationale: The primary functions of the skin are to protect the body, excrete waste products, and absorb vitamin D. The skin also regulates body temperature, acts as a sense organ, and maintains water and electrolyte balance.

3. The nurse is planning a presentation about hygiene and skin care to a group of adolescents. Which of the following would be important to include in the teaching plan?
   a. Average-sized individuals tend to be more susceptible to skin irritation as compared to obese individuals.
   b. Dehydration makes the skin in the elderly appear taut and shiny.
   c. Adolescents tend to have skin that is dry and rough due to excessive outdoor exposure.
   d. Adolescents are predisposed to acne due to enlarged sebaceous glands caused by hormonal changes in the body.*

   Reference: p. 846

   Descriptors:

1. 36	2. 02	3. Application
4. II-2	5. Nursing Process	6. Moderate

   Rationale: Adolescents are predisposed to acne due to enlarged sebaceous glands and glandular secretions caused by hormonal changes in the body. Obese people are more susceptible to irritation. Dehydration makes the skin appear loose. Adolescents tend to have oily skin, not dry and rough skin.

4. A 75-year-old patient in the clinic asks the nurse what she can do to get rid of the brown spots on her hands and arms. The nurse should explain to the patient that
   a. she should avoid exposure to wind and sun to prevent more brown spots*
   b. special handcreams are available by prescription to remove the spots
   c. the physician should be notified because these may indicate liver disease
   d. brown spots occur due to biliary blockage, so high-fat foods should be avoided

Reference: p. 846

Descriptors:

1. 36	2. 02	3. Application
4. IV-3	5. Teach/Learn	6. Moderate

Rationale: Brown spots are often called "liver spots" and appear after age 35 years. They are unrelated to the liver and are caused by excessive exposure to wind and sun.

5. An adult patient from South America is hospitalized following abdominal surgery. On the second postoperative day, the patient refuses a complete bath by the nurse. The nurse should
   a. tell the patient that it is hospital policy that postoperative patients receive a daily bath
   b. ask another nurse to assist in giving the patient a complete bath
   c. negotiate with the patient for a partial bath because his culture may influence his hygiene practices*
   d. contact the patient's family and ask for advice on how to accomplish the bath with this patient

Reference: p. 846

Descriptors:

1. 36	2. 03	3. Application
4. II-2	5. Documentation	6. Moderate

Rationale: Many people in North America place a high value on daily bathing. In some cultures, a daily bath is not part of their routine. The nurse should negotiate and try to find a compromise with the patient for a partial bath.

6. The nurse is caring for an 80-year-old patient who is seen in the clinic because of dry, scaly skin. An appropriate question for the nurse to ask during the assessment of this patient is
   a. "Does the area cause itching?"*
   b. "Do you find that you have more bruising?"
   c. "Is your skin cool to the touch?"
   d. "Have you noticed any brown spots on your skin?"

Reference: p. 847

Descriptors:

1. 36	2. 03	3. Application
4. IV-3	5. Nursing Process	6. Moderate

Rationale: The nurse should ask the patient how long the problem has persisted and whether or not there is any itching, which can be uncomfortable and may be treatable.

7. An adult patient had bilateral bunionectomy surgery 2 days ago and is using crutches. She has had difficulty maintaining her normal bathing routine. A priority diagnosis for this patient is
   a. Body Image Disturbance related to surgery
   b. Impaired Skin Integrity related to postoperative course
   c. Ineffective Individual Coping related to immobility
   d. Bathing/Hygiene Self-Care Deficit related to immobility*

Reference: pp. 848–849

Descriptors:

1. 36	2. 05	3. Comprehensive
4. IV-3	5. Nursing Process	6. Moderate

Rationale: The priority nursing diagnosis is Bathing/Hygiene Self-Care Deficit related to immobility. The nurse should suggest that the patient cover her feet with plastic and get a chair to sit in the shower for bathing.

8. The nurse observes a small nodule on an adult patient's left foot while assisting the patient with a bath. The nurse should first
   a. palpate the nodule with a firm indentation
   b. compare the right foot with the left foot*
   c. report the finding to the patient's physician
   d. ask the patient if the nodule is painful

Reference: p. 848

Descriptors:

1. 36	2. 04	3. Application
4. IV-3	5. Teach/Learn	6. Moderate

Rationale: The nurse should compare bilateral parts for symmetry by looking at both feet to determine if the nodule is on one foot or both feet. It should then be documented in the patient's record related to skin assessment.

9. The nurse is caring for a hospitalized patient who is receiving intravenous chemotherapy. During every shift, the nurse should examine the patient's
   a. pressure points
   b. buccal mucosa
   c. infusion site*
   d. skin temperature

Reference: p. 851

Descriptors:

1. 36	2. 09	3. Application
4. IV-1	5. Caring	6. Moderate

Rationale: Phlebitis can occur with intravenous chemotherapy; therefore, the infusion site should be checked at least once per shift.

10. During morning report, the night nurse tells the oncoming nurse that an adult postoperative patient is able to have a partial bed bath. The nurse plans to assist the patient with bathing the
   a. ears
   b. arms
   c. chest
   d. back*

   Reference: p. 852

   Descriptors:

   1. 36   2. 06   3. Application
   4. IV-3   5. Nursing Process   6. Easy

   Rationale: The nurse should assist the patient who is having a partial bed bath with areas of the body that the patient cannot reach, such as the back.

11. The nurse is caring for a patient who has been diaphoretic for the past 4 hours. The nurse plans to
   a. offer the patient the bedpan q 3 hours
   b. keep the emesis basin near the bedside
   c. change the bed linens frequently*
   d. offer oral care q 2 hours

   Reference: p. 852

   Descriptors:

   1. 36   2. 06   3. Application
   4. IV-1   5. Document   6. Moderate

   Rationale: A patient who is diaphoretic or sweating profusely should have the bed linens changed several times per shift for the patient's comfort.

12. After completing the patient's H.S. care, the nurse plans to
   a. ask the patient if he needs the side rails up
   b. elevate the bed to the highest position for comfort
   c. keep the patient's chair near the side of the bed
   d. be certain that the nurse's call light is within reach*

   Reference: p. 852

   Descriptors:

   1. 36   2. 08   3. Application
   4. II-2   5. Nursing Process   6. Moderate

   Rationale: After completing H.S. care, the nurse should ask the patient if he needs anything, and then be certain that the nurse's call light is within the patient's reach. The bed should be lowered to the lowest position, in case the patient needs to ambulate at night.

13. On the third postoperative day, a 78-year-old patient who is weak requests that he be allowed to take a shower. Before the patient takes a shower, the nurse should
   a. place a nonskid mat on the shower floor
   b. instruct the patient to take a bed bath with help
   c. be certain there is a lock on the shower room door
   d. place a commode chair with the pan removed in the shower*

   Reference: p. 852

   Descriptors:

   1. 36   2. 06   3. Application
   4. II-2   5. Nursing Process   6. Moderate

   Rationale: If the physician has written an order for the patient to shower, the nurse should stay nearby while the patient showers and place a commode chair with the pan removed in the shower in case the patient gets dizzy or has symptoms of fainting.

14. A female adult patient is to have a complete bed bath. Before beginning the bath, the nurse should
   a. offer the patient the bedpan*
   b. lower the patient's bed to the lowest position
   c. assist the patient to brush her dentures
   d. cover the patient with a large bath towel

   Reference: p. 855

   Descriptors:

   1. 36   2. 08   3. Application
   4. IV-3   5. Nursing Process   6. Moderate

   Rationale: Before beginning the complete bed bath, the nurse should offer the patient a bedpan to prevent interruption of the bath. Warm bath water may stimulate the urge to void or defecate.

15. The nurse is bathing a patient who has an intravenous solution connected to her right forearm. The nurse should
   a. discontinue the intravenous infusion until the bath is completed
   b. place the clean gown on the affected arm first
   c. check the intravenous drip rate after the gown is changed*
   d. remove both arms of the gown at the same time

   Reference: p. 855

   Descriptors:

   1. 36   2. 08   3. Application
   4. II-2   5. Nursing Process   6. Moderate

   Rationale: The nurse should remove the gown from the other arm first and once the gown is removed, the intravenous drip rate should be rechecked.

16. The nurse is preparing to give a "bag bath" to a 70-year-old hospitalized patient. The nurse plans to
    a. towel dry the skin briefly after cleansing
    b. microwave the bag containing moistened washcloths*
    c. check the patient's gown to be certain it is tied in back
    d. use the towel in the bag to cleanse the entire body

Reference: pp. 854–855

Descriptors:

| 1. 36 | 2. 08 | 3. Application |
| 4. II-2 | 5. Nursing Process | 6. Moderate |

Rationale: For a "bag bath," the nurse should microwave 8 to 10 moistened washcloths for 1 to 2 minutes.

17. A physician has ordered antiembolic stockings for an adult patient. The patient is sitting in a chair in the room when the nurse prepares to apply the stockings. The nurse should first
    a. give the patient a partial bath before application
    b. ask the patient if he wants the antiembolic stockings on at this time
    c. massage the legs in brief, short strokes after the stockings are in place
    d. ask the patient to lie in bed with legs elevated for 15 minutes before application*

Reference: p. 854

Descriptors:

| 1. 36 | 2. 09 | 3. Application |
| 4. IV-3 | 5. Teach/Learn | 6. Moderate |

Rationale: Because the patient's legs have been in a dependent position, the nurse should first ask the patient to lie in bed with the legs elevated for 15 minutes before application of the stockings.

18. After removing a patient's antiembolic stockings, the nurse observes a positive Homans' sign in the patient's left leg. The nurse plans to
    a. ask another nurse to confirm the findings
    b. massage the leg with long, smooth strokes
    c. check the patient's right leg for a positive Homans' sign
    d. contact the patient's physician immediately*

Reference: pp. 854, 862

Descriptors:

| 1. 36 | 2. 04 | 3. Application |
| 4. IV-1 | 5. Nursing Process | 6. Moderate |

Rationale: After determining that the patient has a positive Homans' sign, the nurse should notify the patient's physician immediately, because this can be indicative of thrombophlebitis. If a clot is present and dislodged, the patient can experience pulmonary embolism.

19. The nurse is preparing to provide evening care and a backrub to a 70-year-old patient who has been on bed rest. An appropriate statement for the nurse to make before beginning the care is
    a. "Would you care for a backrub?"
    b. "Can you sit up for a backrub?"
    c. "Now it is time for your backrub."*
    d. "If you would like, I'll scrub your back and rub it."

Reference: p. 860

Descriptors:

| 1. 36 | 2. 07 | 3. Application |
| 4. IV-3 | 5. Communication | 6. Moderate |

Rationale: The most appropriate statement for the nurse to make is, "Now it is time for a backrub." Providing a backrub for a patient on bed rest allows the nurse to make a skin assessment and generally is very soothing for the patient.

20. The nurse is preparing to make an occupied bed for a patient who is receiving oxygen by nasal cannula for dyspnea. The nurse plans to
    a. discontinue the oxygen temporarily while making the bed
    b. keep the head of the bed elevated during the procedure*
    c. lower both the of the side rails for easy access to the patient
    d. adjust the patient's bed to the lowest position before beginning

Reference: pp. 868–869

Descriptors:

| 1. 36 | 2. 08 | 3. Application |
| 4. IV-1 | 5. Teach/Learn | 6. Moderate |

Rationale: The nurse should keep the head of the bed elevated, which allows the patient to breathe more easily. Continuous oxygen should never be discontinued, and the bed should be in the highest position to prevent back strain on the nurse.

21. At 1 AM, a hospitalized patient in a semiprivate room awakens and complains of severe itching of his forearms and abdomen. The nurse caring for this patient should
    a. use a small flashlight to observe the site of itching
    b. turn on the bathroom light to observe the site of the itching
    c. turn on the ceiling light in the room for adequate lighting
    d. turn on the lights above the bed to observe the site of itching*

    Reference: p. 868

    Descriptors:

    1. 36   2. 08   3. Application

    4. IV-3   5. Teach/Learn   6. Moderate

    Rationale: The nurse needs adequate lighting to observe the patient's rash. The nurse should turn on the bright lights above the patient's bed to observe the site of the itching. The overhead ceiling lights are not necessary and could disturb the patient in the next bed.

22. A 64-year-old, thin patient with rheumatoid arthritis has been admitted to the hospital following an automobile accident. To aid the patient's comfort in bed, the nurse plans to
    a. provide the patient with a sheepskin*
    b. use a rubberized mattress with a thin sheet
    c. cover the bottom sheet with a wool blanket
    d. place a comforter on top of the sheet

    Reference: p. 868

    Descriptors:

    1. 36   2. 10   3. Application

    4. IV-1   5. Teach/Learn   6. Moderate

    Rationale: The patient who is thin and has arthritis should be provided with a sheepskin, a soft blanket, or a flannelette blanket to provide extra warmth and comfort.

23. A nurse has instructed a 76-year-old patient in how to care for her very dry skin. The nurse determines that the patient needs further instructions when the patient says
    a. "Bubble baths should be infrequent."
    b. "I should use emollient creams after bathing."
    c. "Wool clothing provides the least skin irritation."*
    d. "I should try to increase my fluid intake."

    Reference: p. 874

    Descriptors:

    1. 36   2. 09   3. Application

    4. IV-1   5. Self-Care   6. Moderate

    Rationale: The patient needs further instruction when she says wool clothing provides the least irritation to the skin. Wool is very irritating to some patients and can make the itching worse. Baths should be taken less frequently and emollient creams can be soothing.

24. The most appropriate nursing intervention to correct skin dryness is to
    a. avoid bathing until the condition is remedied and notify the physician
    b. ask the physician to refer the patient to a dermatologist
    c. consult the dietitian to increase the fat intake
    d. increase the fluid intake, use nonirritating soap, and apply lotion*

    Reference: p. 874

    Descriptors:

    1. 36   2. 01   3. Application

    4. IV-1   5. Nursing Process 6. Moderate

    Rationale: To correct dry skin, increase the fluid intake, use a nondrying soap, and apply lotion.

25. An adolescent patient has been instructed how to care for her skin, which is prone to acne. The nurse determines that the patient has understood the instructions when the patient says
    a. "I shouldn't squeeze or pick at the infected area."*
    b. "I can use an emollient on my face over the area."
    c. "I can use an ultraviolet lamp daily to control the acne."
    d. "Wearing makeup will control the acne breakouts."

    Reference: p. 874

    Descriptors:

    1. 36   2. 09   3. Application

    4. IV-1   5. Self-Care   6. Moderate

    Rationale: Squeezing or picking at the infected area can make the acne worse. The patient should not use makeup or emollient creams, which can worsen the condition. Ultraviolet lamps are not recommended.

26. A 14-year-old patient has received treatment for her acne, which has resulted in erythema and some peeling of her skin. The nurse should advise the patient to
    a. refrain from washing her skin more than twice a day
    b. use an ultraviolet lamp once a day to aid the healing
    c. avoid sun exposure, because sunburn could result*
    d. use heavy makeup to hide the red skin tissue

Reference: p. 874

Descriptors:

1. 36	2. 10	3. Application
4. IV-1	5. Self Care	6. Moderate

Rationale: Frequent skin washing can keep the area clean. Ultraviolet lamps are not recommended. Sun exposure can be dangerous and should be avoided. Makeup can block the sebaceous ducts.

27. An adult patient visits the clinic and complains of a dry, itching rash that developed after working in the garden. After providing the patient with instructions about care of the rash, the nurse determines that the patient understands the instructions when the patient says
    a. "Cool or cold baths can help alleviate the itching."
    b. "After washing the area, I should leave the soap on for a few minutes."
    c. "Medicated powders will help dry the area and stop the itching."
    d. "Caladryl or hydrocortisone lotion may provide some relief."*

Reference: p. 874

Descriptors:

1. 36	2. 10	3. Application
4. IV-1	5. Teach/Learn	6. Moderate

Rationale: Tepid baths may relieve the itching. Caladryl or hydrocortisone lotion may provide some relief. Soap can be more irritating and should not be left on the skin. Medicated powders are useful for a wet rash.

28. A priority nursing action when administering oral care to a dependent patient is to
    a. assist the patient to a prone position
    b. wear disposable gloves*
    c. use a firm toothbrush to clean teeth and gums
    d. irrigate forcefully with hydrogen peroxide

Reference: p. 877

Descriptors:

1. 36	2. 07	3. Application
4. IV-1	5. Nursing Process	6. Moderate

Rationale: Disposable gloves must be worn when exposed to any blood or body fluids (Standard Precautions).

29. An adult patient with apparently poor hygiene has been admitted to the hospital following an automobile accident. The nurse collaborates with the patient and formulates a goal with the patient to perform a complete bath with assistance while hospitalized. The nurse evaluates progress toward accomplishing this goal by
    a. bathing the patient daily to be certain the goal is reached
    b. instructing the patient why cleanliness is so important
    c. observing the patient while he is performing morning care*
    d. asking the patient if he has completed his daily bath

Reference: p. 878

Descriptors:

1. 36	2. 10	3. Application
4. IV-1	5. Self Care	6. Moderate

Rationale: By observing the patient performing his morning care, the nurse can evaluate whether or not the goal has been achieved.

30. A patient refuses to bathe, saying, "I'm not dirty." A nurse's therapeutic response might be to say to the patient
    a. "This is a daily hospital routine and everyone must comply."
    b. "The doctor and my supervisor expect me to help you bathe today."
    c. "If you don't have a bath now, I'm not sure if I'll have time to do it later."
    d. "The bath will stimulate your circulation and relax and refresh you."*

Reference: p. 852

Descriptors:

1. 36	2. 01	3. Comprehensive
4. IV-1	5. Communication	6. Moderate

Rationale: The purpose of a bath is stimulate circulation of the body and increase self-concept/esteem. By telling the patient that the bath will stimulate circulation and relax and refresh the patient, the patient is much more likely to cooperate.

31. While working in an emergency room, an adult patient with poor oral hygiene tells the nurse that he has severe bleeding gums and several loose teeth. The nurse determines that the patient is most likely experiencing
    a. dental caries
    b. halitosis
    c. gingivitis
    d. pyorrhea*

Reference: p. 875

Descriptors:

1. 36   2. 10   3. Application
4. IV-1   5. Nursing Process   6. Moderate

Rationale: Severe bleeding gums and loose teeth are typically associated with pyorrhea or periodontal disease.

32. A thin adult patient receiving chemotherapy tells the nurse he has had difficulty eating and has developed a sore and reddened mouth. The nurse should explain to the patient that this is a result of
    a. vitamin B deficiencies
    b. analgesic medications
    c. decreased fluid intake
    d. chemotherapy medications*

Reference: pp. 875; 880

Descriptors:

1. 36   2. 10   3. Application
4. IV-4   5. Nursing Process   6. Moderate

Rationale: One of the side effects of some chemotherapy medications is an inflammation of the oral mucosa, which makes eating difficult.

33. The nurse is planning to provide oral care to an unconscious patient in the critical care unit. To perform oral care, the nurse plans to use
    a. a regular toothbrush and toothpaste*
    b. soft paper towels moistened with mouthwash
    c. swabs moistened with normal saline
    d. a small bulb syringe containing diluted hydrogen peroxide

Reference: p. 879

Descriptors:

1. 36   2. 10   3. Application
4. IV-1   5. Nursing Process   6. Moderate

Rationale: For providing oral care to a dependent patient, the nurse should plan to use a regular toothbrush with toothpaste.

34. The nurse is preparing to clean the dentures of an immobile homebound patient. The nurse plans to
    a. wear sterile gloves
    b. use diluted hydrogen peroxide
    c. clean the dentures with hot water
    d. rinse well after cleansing*

Reference: p. 876

Descriptors:

1. 36   2. 10   3. Application
4. IV-1   5. Nursing Process   6. Moderate

Rationale: Clean gloves should be worn. Plain tap water with a denture paste or powder can be used and the dentures should be rinsed well after cleaning. The sink should be protected with a towel in case the dentures are dropped.

35. The nurse has instructed an 8-year-old patient how to floss his teeth for good oral hygiene. The nurse determines that the patient needs further instructions when the patient says
    a. "I should move the floss in an up and down motion."
    b. "It's important that I rinse my mouth well after flossing."
    c. "If I have to, I should force the floss into the gumline."*
    d. "I should keep about 1 to 1½ inches of floss taut."

Reference: pp. 880–881

Descriptors:

1. 36   2. 08   3. Application
4. IV-1   5. Teach/Learn   6. Moderate

Rationale: The patient needs further instructions when he says he should force the floss into the gumline. This can lead to gum injury.

36. The nurse plans to provide oral care to a dependent patient. To remove the water from the patient's oral cavity, the nurse plans to use a/an
    a. irrigating syringe*
    b. gravity and slow drainage
    c. 10-mL syringe
    d. dry washcloth

Reference: p. 881

Descriptors:

1. 36   2. 10   3. Application
4. IV-1   5. Nursing Process   6. Moderate

Rationale: An irrigating syringe should be used to remove the water from the patient's oral cavity.

37. A 74-year-old patient is scheduled for outpatient surgery to correct bilateral cataracts. The patient tells the nurse that she is scared, but that her daughter is with her. A priority nursing diagnosis for this patient is
   a. Anticipatory Grieving related to surgery
   b. Risk for Injury related to visual impairment
   c. Sensory Alteration due to impaired sight
   d. Fear related to impending surgery*

Reference: p. 882

Descriptors:

1. 36	2. 10	3. Application
4. III-1	5. Nursing Process	6. Moderate

Rationale: The priority diagnosis based on the patient's statement of "scared" is Fear related to impending surgery.

38. The nurse is assisting a weak postoperative patient with morning care. To cleanse the patient's eyes, the nurse should
   a. use mild soap and water around the edges of the eyes
   b. clean from the outer canthus to the inner canthus of the eyes
   c. clean from the inner canthus to the outer canthus of the eyes*
   d. use cool wet cotton balls to cleanse crustations

Reference: p. 882

Descriptors:

1. 36	2. 08	3. Application
4. IV-1	5. Nursing Process	6. Moderate

Rationale: To cleanse the eyes, the nurse should use plain water and cleanse from the inner canthus to the outer canthus of the eyes.

39. The nurse is caring for a comatose patient in a rehabilitation center. To care for the patient's eyes, the nurse plans to
   a. use artificial tear solution in the eyes q. 4 hours*
   b. place wet washcloths over the eyes q. 2 hours
   c. keep moistened cotton balls near the bedside to moisten the eyes
   d. instill normal saline drops into the eyes at least once every 8 hours

Reference: p. 883

Descriptors:

1. 36	2. 08	3. Application
4. IV-1	5. Nursing Process	6. Moderate

Rationale: Artificial tear solution should be instilled every 4 hours to keep the eyes moistened.

40. The nurse prepares to clean a patient's prescription eyeglasses. The nurse plans to dry the lenses with a
   a. sheet of toilet tissue
   b. soft cloth*
   c. sheet of paper towel
   d. special washcloth

Reference: p. 883

Descriptors:

1. 36	2. 08	3. Application
4. IV-1	5. Nursing Process	6. Moderate

Rationale: A soft cloth should be used on prescription glasses to prevent scratching of the lenses.

41. The nurse is caring for a patient in the clinic who is wearing extended-wear contact lenses. The nurse should instruct the patient that these types of contact lenses should be
   a. removed at least every other day
   b. removed before sleeping
   c. cleansed at least once per week*
   d. replaced daily to prevent infection

Reference: p. 883

Descriptors:

1. 36	2. 08	3. Application
4. IV-3	5. Teach/Learn	6. Moderate

Rationale: Extended wear contact lenses should be cleansed at least once per week.

42. An alert adult patient tells the nurse that the "dry air in the hospital" has made his nose very stuffy. The nurse should
   a. use an irrigating syringe to suction the patient's nose
   b. introduce a moistened cotton-tipped applicator into the patient's nose
   c. irrigate both nares with normal saline solution
   d. ask the patient to blow gently into a soft tissue*

Reference: p. 885

Descriptors:

1. 36	2. 08	3. Application
4. IV-1	5. Self Care	6. Moderate

Rationale: Asking the patient to blow gently into the soft tissues will usually clear up the stuffiness of the nose.

43. An adult patient is seen in the emergency room in an unconscious state following an automobile accident. The patient is wearing hard contact lenses and has suffered head and facial injuries. The nurse plans to
    a. remove the lenses with gentle suctioning
    b. use gentle pressure to center the lens on the cornea
    c. grasp the lens near the lower edge of the eye
    d. leave the lenses in place, because injury may be present*

Reference: p. 883

Descriptors:

1. 36	2. 08	3. Application
4. IV-3	5. Nursing Process	6. Moderate

Rationale: Because the patient has suffered head and facial injuries, the contact lenses should be left in place.

44. The camp nurse has explained to a 10-year-old child why he must be inspected for ticks after spending the afternoon in the camp's wooded area. The nurse determines that the child understands the instructions when the child says that ticks can result in
    a. Lyme disease*
    b. pediculosis
    c. bulimia
    d. fungal disease

Reference: p. 886

Descriptors:

1. 36	2. 04	3. Application
4. II-2	5. Teach/Learn	6. Moderate

Rationale: Ticks can spread Lyme disease and Rocky Mountain spotted fever if not removed from the body.

45. To assist an adult male with a facial shave using a razor, the nurse should
    a. use firm, long strokes with gentle pressure
    b. wear gloves, because contact with blood is possible*
    c. shave in the opposite direction of hair growth
    d. rinse the face with an alcohol solution before beginning

Reference: p. 888

Descriptors:

1. 36	2. 08	3. Application
4. IV-1	5. Nursing Process	6. Moderate

Rationale: The nurse should follow Universal Precautions and wear clean gloves before shaving a patient. Firm, short strokes and following the hair growth should be used. Alcohol is drying to the skin and should be avoided.

46. The nurse has instructed an adult patient with diabetes about proper foot care. The nurse determines that the patient understands the instructions when the nurse observes the patient
    a. cutting the toenails at the corners
    b. trimming the toenails with scissors
    c. using a file to trim the toenails*
    d. walking barefoot in the hospital room

Reference: p. 889

Descriptors:

1. 36	2. 08	3. Application
4. IV-3	5. Teach/Learn	6. Moderate

Rationale: The patient is performing the procedure properly when the patient uses a file to trim the toenails.

47. A sexually active adult female patient asks the nurse about douching. The nurse instructs the patient that vaginal douches
    a. should be done after every sexual contact
    b. are needed prior to a vaginal examination
    c. should be used with a vaginal deodorant
    d. are not usually necessary for adult females*

Reference: p. 892

Descriptors:

1. 36	2. 10	3. Application
4. IV-3	5. Self Care	6. Moderate

Rationale: Vaginal douches are usually not necessary for adult females.

48. Which of the following statements is true about aging skin? The skin
    a. becomes thinner, less elastic, dry and often scaly*
    b. has enlarged sebaceous glands with increased secretions
    c. becomes increasingly resistant to injury and infection
    d. is supple with a smooth, soft texture

Reference: p. 847

Descriptors:

| 1. 36 | 2. 02 | 3. Comprehensive |
| 4. None | 5. None | 6. Moderate |

Rationale: In old age, skin has decreased secretions from sebaceous glands meaning less natural oil on the skin.

49. The nurse notes a heavy, brownish, oily substance in the external ears of a patient. Which of the following explains this? It is
    a. sebum from the sebaceous glands
    b. perspiration from the sweat glands
    c. a discharge from the mucous membranes
    d. cerumen from the ceruminal glands*

Reference: p. 845

Descriptors:

| 1. 36 | 2. 03 | 3. Knowledge |
| 4. IV-1 | 5. Nursing Process | 6. Easy |

Rationale: Cerumen is a brownish substance secreted from the ceruminal gland of the ear.

50. An elderly patient's skin should be assessed for
    a. temperature, moisture, turgor*
    b. mobility, turgor, integrity
    c. vascularity, evidence of bleeding, edema
    d. edema, bleeding, mobility

Reference: p. 848

Descriptors:

| 1. 36 | 2. 03 | 3. Comprehensive |
| 4. IV-1 | 5. Nursing Process | 6. Moderate |

Rationale: Assessing the temperature of the skin, moisture (wet or dry), and turgor in an elderly patient can help to determine the hydration status.

CHAPTER 37

Skin Integrity and Wound Care

1. The nurse is caring for a postoperative patient following abdominal surgery when the nurse observes that the wound has dehisced. The nurse notifies the patient's physician and then should
   a. cover the patient with a clean blanket
   b. tell the patient that the wound is infected and needs repair
   c. cover the wound with sterile towels moistened with normal saline*
   d. provide the patient with an analgesic for the discomfort

   Reference: p. 903

   Descriptors:

   1. 37   2. 01   3. Application
   4. IV-3   5. Nursing Process 6. Moderate

   Rationale: After notifying the physician of the dehiscence, the nurse should cover the wound with sterile towels moistened with normal saline solution to keep the area moist.

2. While assessing a bedridden patient at home for the presence of pressure ulcers, the nurse plans to inspect the patient's
   a. buttocks
   b. forearm
   c. thigh
   d. coccyx*

   Reference: p. 929

   Descriptors:

   1. 37   2. 08   3. Application
   4. IV-3   5. Nursing Process 6. Moderate

   Rationale: Most pressure ulcers form over the sacrum and coccyx, followed by the trochanter and heel.

3. While assessing a patient in bed at home, the nurse inspects the patient's environment for potential sources of friction that may lead to skin abrasions. The nurse should inspect the patient's
   a. bed sheets*
   b. blankets
   c. bedside chair
   d. bath linens

   Reference: p. 929

   Descriptors:

   1. 37   2. 01   3. Application
   4. IV-3   5. Nursing Process 6. Moderate

   Rationale: Most sources of friction in a patient's bed occur from bed sheets.

4. The nurse has instructed a group of nursing assistants about prevention of pressure ulcers due to shearing forces. The nurse determines that one of the nursing assistants needs further instructions when he says that shearing forces can be decreased when patients are
   a. lifted when moved up in bed
   b. assisted by a bed trapeze during movement
   c. transferred to a stretcher using bed linens
   d. pulled when they need to be moved up in bed*

   Reference: p. 929

   Descriptors:

   1. 37   2. 10   3. Application
   4. I-1   5. None   6. Moderate

   Rationale: One of the nursing assistants needs further instruction when he says that shearing forces can be decreased when patients are pulled when they need to be moved up in bed. Patients should be lifted to decrease shearing force.

5. After turning a bedridden patient from her side to her back, the nurse observes the area over the trochanter appears reddened. The nurse should document this observation as
   a. stage I ulcer
   b. ischemia
   c. eschar
   d. hyperemia*

   Reference: p. 931

   Descriptors:

   1. 37   2. 01   3. Comprehensive
   4. IV-3   5. Documentation   6. Moderate

   Rationale: A reddened area is termed hyperemia. Eschar is a scab.

6. A 75-year-old disoriented patient is admitted to the hospital for surgery. The nurse observes damage to the patient's subcutaneous tissue around the patient's coccyx. The nurse determines that this stage of a pressure ulcer is stage
   a. I
   b. II
   c. III*
   d. IV

   Reference: p. 932

   Descriptors:

1. 37	2. 09	3. Comprehensive
4. IV-3	5. Nursing Process	6. Moderate

   Rationale: Damage to the patient's subcutaneous tissue is evidence of a stage III ulcer.

7. The nurse makes a home visit to a 70-year-old patient with limited mobility. The patient's daughter has been caring for the patient following a total hip replacement. The nurse instructs the daughter that she should encourage the patient to consume foods that are high in
   a. vitamin D
   b. fats
   c. riboflavin
   d. protein*

   Reference: pp. 921, 933

   Descriptors:

1. 37	2. 08	3. Application
4. IV-3	5. Teach/Learn	6. Moderate

   Rationale: Foods that are high in protein help with wound healing.

8. The nurse has instructed a caregiver of a bedridden incontinent patient about care of the patient to prevent pressure ulcers. The nurse determines that the caregiver understands the instructions when the caregiver says
   a. "Ammonia in the urine can increase the risk of ulcers."
   b. "I should change the linens at least every day."
   c. "I should try to get an order for a catheter."
   d. "Moisture associated with incontinence is a risk factor."*

   Reference: p. 930

   Descriptors:

1. 37	2. 07	3. Application
4. IV-3	5. Teach/Learn	6. Moderate

   Rationale: Moisture associated with incontinence is a risk factor for pressure ulcers. The patient should be kept clean and dry.

9. The nurse is caring for an incoherent patient with a pressure ulcer and begins to change the patient's dressing. When the patient grimaces and starts to cry the nurse should
   a. try to calm the patient with soothing words
   b. provide comfort and pain relief*
   c. perform the dressing change as quickly as possible
   d. delay the dressing change until the patient is asleep

   Reference: p. 937

   Descriptors:

1. 37	2. 11	3. Application
4. IV-1	5. Caring	6. Moderate

   Rationale: A grimace and cry are indications of discomfort. The nurse should provide the patient with comfort and pain relief.

10. The nurse is caring for a group of patients in a nursing home. The nurse plans to inspect the at-risk patients for skin breakdown at least every
    a. 4 hours
    b. 8 hours
    c. 16 hours
    d. 24 hours*

    Reference: p. 933

    Descriptors:

1. 37	2. 08	3. Application
4. IV-3	5. Nursing Process	6. Moderate

    Rationale: At-risk patients should be assessed every 24 hours to identify potential areas of skin breakdown.

11. While inspecting a pressure ulcer on a 90-year-old patient, the nurse observes new tissue growth around the area, which is pinkish red in color. The nurse documents the presence of
    a. epithelialization
    b. necrotic tissue
    c. granulation tissue*
    d. reactive hyperemia

    Reference: p. 901

    Descriptors:

1. 37	2. 01	3. Application
4. IV-1	5. Documentation	6. Moderate

    Rationale: New tissue growth around the area that is pinkish red in color is termed granulation.

12. The nurse determines that the patient who is at risk for developing a pressure ulcer is the patient who has a/an
    a. albumin level of 2.5 mg/dL*
    b. lymphocyte level of $2400/mm^3$
    c. hematocrit of 36 mg/dL
    d. hemoglobin of 14 mg/dL

    Reference: p. 933

    Descriptors:

    1. 37   2. 08   3. Application
    4. IV-3   5. Nursing Process   6. Moderate

    Rationale: Normal albumin levels should be 3.5 to 5 mg/dL. Decreased albumin levels place the patient at greater risk for skin breakdown.

13. The nurse is using the Norton scale to assess a newly admitted 78-year-old patient. An important assessment for the nurse to make using the Norton scale is
    a. sensory deprivation
    b. presence of moisture
    c. friction and shear forces
    d. activity level*

    Reference: p. 936

    Descriptors:

    1. 37   2. 09   3. Application
    4. IV-1   5. Nursing Process   6. Moderate

    Rationale: The Norton scale uses activity levels as part of the assessment.

14. The nurse admits an 80-year-old patient from the hospital to the rehabilitation center following knee replacement surgery. The patient has had difficulty ambulating since the surgery. The nurse observes a stage III pressure ulcer on the patient's heel. The priority nursing diagnosis for this patient is
    a. Impaired Mobility related to postoperative complications
    b. Impaired Tissue Integrity related to prolonged bed rest*
    c. Pain related to stage III pressure ulcer
    d. Impaired Skin Integrity related to advanced age

    Reference: p. 934

    Descriptors:

    1. 37   2. 10   3. Application
    4. IV-3   5. Nursing Process   6. Moderate

    Rationale: The priority diagnosis is Impaired Tissue Integrity related to prolonged bed rest.

15. The nurse is assessing an 85-year-old patient using the Braden scale for predicting pressure sores. An important aspect for the nurse to assess while using the Braden scale is
    a. patient's knowledge level
    b. dependence on caregivers
    c. friction and shear potential*
    d. physical condition

    Reference: p. 936

    Descriptors:

    1. 37   2. 08   3. Application
    4. IV-3   5. Nursing Process   6. Moderate

    Rationale: The Braden scale uses friction and shear potential as part of the assessment.

16. Using the Braden scale for assessing a patient for potential pressure ulcers, the nurse observes that the patient eats over half of most meals and has at least 4 servings of protein daily. The nurse determines that the patient's nutritional state is
    a. very poor
    b. probably inadequate
    c. probably adequate*
    d. excellent

    Reference: p. 936

    Descriptors:

    1. 37   2. 08   3. Application
    4. IV-3   5. Nursing Process   6. Moderate

    Rationale: When a patient eats over half of most meals and gets at least 4 servings of protein per day, the patient's nutritional state is considered probably adequate.

17. The nurse visits a 76-year-old patient who is bedridden at home following abdominal surgery. The nurse observes that the patient has a donut-type device under her buttocks. The nurse should instruct the patient's caregiver that donut-type devices
    a. prevent shearing forces that lead to abrasions
    b. cause increased venous pressure and shouldn't be used*
    c. need to be readjusted every 2 to 4 hours
    d. should have a pillowcase over them to reduce moisture

    Reference: p. 935

    Descriptors:

    1. 37   2. 07   3. Application
    4. IV-3   5. Teach/Learn   6. Moderate

    Rationale: Donut-type devices cause increased venous pressure and should never be used.

18. The nurse is preparing to cleanse a pressure ulcer of a 91-year-old patient. To accomplish the procedure, the nurse plans to obtain
    a. warm, wet washcloths
    b. normal saline solution*
    c. hydrogen peroxide
    d. povidine solution
    Reference: p. 937
    Descriptors:

1. 37	2. 11	3. Application
4. IV-1	5. Nursing Process	6. Moderate

    Rationale: To cleanse a pressure ulcer, the nurse should use normal saline solution.

19. While cleaning a pressure ulcer of a newly admitted 74-year-old patient, the nurse observes a thick white exudate and necrotic tissue. The nurse should
    a. perform a wet-to-dry dressing
    b. obtain an irrigating device for suction
    c. collect a specimen of the tissue for laboratory analysis
    d. notify the patient's physician as soon as possible*
    Reference: p. 938
    Descriptors:

1. 37	2. 11	3. Application
4. IV-3	5. Nursing Process	6. Moderate

    Rationale: The physician should be notified as soon as possible. The presence of necrosis may need whirlpool therapy or surgical excision.

20. The nurse has instructed a caregiver of a 77-year-old patient how to perform dressing changes on the patient's pressure ulcer. The nurse determines that the caregiver understands the instructions when the caregiver says
    a. "I should pack the gauze tightly into the wound."
    b. "It's important that the skin be kept moist."
    c. "I should use a moisture barrier ointment on the skin."*
    d. "Wet-to-dry dressings are used for pressure ulcers."
    Reference: p. 939
    Descriptors:

1. 37	2. 07	3. Application
4. IV-1	5. Teach/Learn	6. Moderate

    Rationale: A dressing should absorb exudate but still maintain a moist environment that promotes healing.

21. A student nurse is caring for a hospitalized patient who is on a static flotation mattress for prevention of pressure ulcers. The nurse plans to explain to the student that one of the disadvantages of this type of mattress is that this mattress has
    a. high moisture retention*
    b. high costs per day of use
    c. low pressure reduction
    d. low shear forces
    Reference: p. 936
    Descriptors:

1. 37	2. 10	3. Application
4. IV-3	5. None	6. Moderate

    Rationale: Static flotation mattresses have a disadvantage of high moisture retention.

22. During a return demonstration of the "no-touch" technique of dressing change, the nurse determines that a patient's caregiver understands the procedure when the nurse observes the caregiver
    a. don sterile gloves before beginning
    b. clean the wound from the outer edges to the middle
    c. touch the front center of the sterile gauze
    d. use clean gloves to pour the normal saline into a basin*
    Reference: p. 937
    Descriptors:

1. 37	2. 07	3. Application
4. IV-3	5. Teach/Learn	6. Moderate

    Rationale: The "no-touch" technique is being followed when the caregiver uses clean gloves to pour the normal saline into a basin.

CHAPTER 38

Activity

1. A patient has partial left-sided paralysis due to a stroke. The nurse performs passive range-of-motion (PROM) exercises to his affected side because
   a. the patient complains of pain when he moves his left side
   b. the patient is not able to move his left side by himself*
   c. there is not enough time to perform active ROM exercises
   d. PROM exercises are best for recovery of the patient

   Reference: p. 977
   Descriptors:

1. 38	2. 09	3. Application
4. IV-1	5. Nursing Process	6. Moderate

   Rationale: PROM exercise is provided when the patient is unable to move body parts on his own.

2. The nurse is caring for a postoperative patient when he asks the nurse why he needs to walk so much. Your response is based on the knowledge that the stress and strain of weight-bearing activity stimulates
   a. bone destruction
   b. loss of bone calcium
   c. increased flexibility
   d. bone formation*

   Reference: p. 961
   Descriptors:

1. 38	2. 05	3. Comprehensive
4. II-2	5. Teach/Learn	6. Moderate

   Rationale: Bone formation is stimulated by exercise and activity.

3. A patient who has atelectasis is suffering from which of the following?
   a. decreased coordination
   b. hypostatic pneumonia
   c. bronchitis
   d. a collapsed lung*

   Reference: p. 961
   Descriptors:

1. 38	2. 05	3. Knowledge
4. None	5. None	6. Easy

   Rationale: A collapsed lung is termed atelectasis.

4. What position is best to assess the extension of the hip joint?
   a. dorsal recumbent
   b. lithotomy
   c. prone*
   d. supine

   Reference: p. 982
   Descriptors:

1. 38	2. 09	3. Comprehensive
4. IV-1	5. Nursing Process	6. Moderate

   Rationale: When lying face down (prone), the extension of the hip joint can be best evaluated.

5. When positioning a patient, the *most* important principle of body mechanics is to
   a. elevate the arms on pillows
   b. make the patient comfortable
   c. maintain functional alignment*
   d. keep the head higher than the heart

   Reference: p. 972
   Descriptors:

1. 38	2. 06	3. Comprehensive
4. IV-1	5. Nursing Process	6. Moderate

   Rationale: Body mechanics are directly related to the functional alignment of the musculoskeletal system.

6. When the nurse performs dorsiflexion and plantar flexion on the patient, these maneuvers are associated with which one of the following joints?
   a. hip
   b. ankle*
   c. shoulder
   d. knee

Reference: p. 983

Descriptors:

1. 38	2. 09	3. Application
4. IV-1	5. Nursing Process	6. Easy

Rationale: Range of motion of the ankle is dorsiflexion and plantar flexion.

7. The *most* important reason for the nurse to maintain a patient in good body alignment while he is in the supine position would be to
   a. increase the strain on joints, muscles, tendons, and ligaments
   b. promote proper body function of the musculoskeletal structures*
   c. decrease the amount of energy required to maintain balance
   d. enhance the amount of muscular effort by patient and nurse

Reference: p. 972

Descriptors:

1. 38	2. 08	3. Application
4. IV-3	5. Nursing Process	6. Moderate

Rationale: Proper body functioning of the musculoskeletal system depends on proper body alignment.

8. Which of the following best describes shearing force? Shearing force is
   a. layers of tissue moving on each other*
   b. the skin becoming pale and blanching
   c. blood rushing to an area after pressure is removed
   d. the breaking down of skin in the area under pressure

Reference: p. 984

Descriptors:

1. 38	2. 05	3. Knowledge
4. None	5. None	6. Moderate

Rationale: Shearing force is layers of tissue moving on each other, for example, moving a patient up in bed.

9. The nurse should assess the patient who has been immobile for the potential for
   a. hemophilia
   b. increased muscle mass
   c. muscle cramping
   d. orthostatic hypotension*

Reference: p. 992

Descriptors:

1. 38	2. 05	3. Comprehensive
4. IV-3	5. Nursing Process	6. Moderate

Rationale: Orthostatic hypotension is a drop in blood pressure after a patient has been lying down immobile for a period of time.

10. The nurse should explain to an immobile patient that the purpose of antiembolic stockings is to
    a. increase the arterial blood flow to the legs
    b. provide movement to the legs
    c. help force blood from superficial veins to deeper veins and prevent stagnation*
    d. force blood out of the arteries and prevent blood from clotting

Reference: pp. 958, 961

Descriptors:

1. 38	2. 05	3. Comprehensive
4. IV-3	5. Teach/Learn	6. Moderate

Rationale: Antiembolic stockings help force the blood from the veins in the legs and aid in circulation.

11. The type of joint in which the oval head of one bone fits into a shallow cavity of another, such as the wrist, is termed
    a. ball-and-socket
    b. gliding
    c. condyloid*
    d. saddle

Reference: p. 949

Descriptors:

1. 38	2. 01	3. Knowledge
4. None	5. None	6. Easy

Rationale: The condyloid joint is type of joint in which the oval head of one bone fits into a shallow cavity of another, such as the wrist.

12. When the nurse assists a bedridden patient to perform range-of-motion exercises with the shoulders, the nurse should explain to the patient that this type of joint is termed
    a. condyloid
    b. hinge
    c. pivot
    d. ball-and-socket*

Reference: p. 949

Descriptors:

1. 38	2. 01	3. Knowledge
4. IV-3	5. Teach/Learn	6. Easy

Rationale: The nurse should explain to the patient that this type of joint is termed ball-and-socket.

13. To assist a 73-year-old patient to perform adduction, the nurse plans to move the patient's
    a. outstretched arm to a position along side the body*
    b. leg inward with toes pointing toward the midline
    c. neck and head upward toward the ceiling
    d. right and left leg in a circular motion

Reference: p. 949

Descriptors:

1. 38	2. 01	3. Knowledge
4. IV-3	5. Nursing Process	6. Moderate

Rationale: Adduction is performed when the nurse moves the patient's outstretched arms to a position along side the body.

14. While assessing a comatose patient, the nurse observes that the patient's foot is rotated inward at the ankle. The nurse documents this as
    a. eversion
    b. inversion*
    c. pronation
    d. dorsiflexion

Reference: p. 949

Descriptors:

1. 38	2. 01	3. Application
4. IV-1	5. Documentation	6. Easy

Rationale: When the nurse observes that the patient's foot is rotated inward at the ankle, the nurse should document this as inversion.

15. A 16-year-old patient visits the emergency room after an automobile accident in which he fractured his nose. The nurse determines that the patient has sustained an injury to his
    a. ligament
    b. joint
    c. tendon
    d. cartilage*

Reference: p. 950

Descriptors:

1. 38	2. 02	3. Knowledge
4. IV-1	5. Nursing Process	6. Easy

Rationale: An injury or fracture of the nose is damage to cartilage.

16. Maintenance of posture, heat production, and motion are functions performed by the
    a. central nervous system
    b. neurons
    c. muscle contractions*
    d. extensor reflexes

Reference: p. 950

Descriptors:

1. 38	2. 02	3. Knowledge
4. None	5. None	6. Easy

Rationale: Maintenance of posture, heat production, and motion are functions performed by the muscle contractions.

17. A family member of a hospitalized patient who has been on prolonged bed rest asks the nurse why range-of-motion exercises are being performed on his 75-year-old mother. The nurse should explain that prolonged bed rest can result in
    a. decreased muscle tonus*
    b. decreased body mechanics
    c. increased muscle spasms
    d. increased skeletal pain

Reference: p. 951

Descriptors:

1. 38	2. 02	3. Application
4. IV-3	5. Teach/Learn	6. Moderate

Rationale: Prolonged bed rest can lead to decreased muscle tonus. Range-of-motion exercises are beneficial in increasing muscle tone.

18. The nurse is preparing to assist an adult patient to move from the bed to a chair. To increase balance and stability, the nurse should
    a. use minor muscle groups to their fullest advantage
    b. increase the base of support and lower the center of gravity*
    c. rock forward and help push the patient to the chair
    d. alter the patient's center of gravity by raising his arms

Reference: p. 951

Descriptors:

1. 38	2. 08	3. Application
4. IV-3	5. Nursing Process	6. Moderate

Rationale: To increase balance and stability, the nurse should increase the base of support and lower the center of gravity.

19. A 6-year-old patient visits the clinic and is diagnosed with an ear infection. He tells the mother and the nurse that he feels "dizzy." The nurse should explain to the patient and his mother that the ear infection has affected a postural reflex termed
    a. proprioceptor sense
    b. kinesthetic sense
    c. gravitational sense
    d. labyrinthine sense*

Reference: p. 952

Descriptors:

1. 38	2. 03	3. Application
4. IV-1	5. Teach/Learn	6. Moderate

Rationale: Feeling dizzy indicates that the patient's labyrinthine sense has been affected.

20. The nurse makes a home visit to a 70-year-old postoperative patient who is being cared for by his daughter. After instructing the caregiver about proper body mechanics, the nurse determines that the caregiver understands the instructions when the nurse observes the caregiver
    a. place her feet apart and flex at the knees when bending down*
    b. bend over at the waist while keeping her knees straight
    c. reach out far in front of her to move the patient to the bed
    d. lift the patient from the chair to the bend while bending over

Reference: p. 952

Descriptors:

1. 38	2. 08	3. Application
4. IV-3	5. Teach/Learn	6. Moderate

Rationale: The nurse determines that the caregiver understands the instructions when the nurse observes the caregiver place her feet apart and flex at the knees when bending down.

21. The nurse visits a patient in the home who is recovering from a stroke that left her partially paralyzed on her right side. After observing the patient move successfully from the bed to the chair, the nurse should reinforce the patient by
    a. encouraging the patient to use caution when ambulating
    b. congratulating the patient on moving successfully*
    c. showing the patient how to perform isometric exercises
    d. demonstrating to the patient how to stand in an erect position

Reference: p. 954

Descriptors:

1. 38	2. 03	3. Application
4. IV-1	5. Nursing Process	6. Moderate

Rationale: The nurse should reinforce the patient's movement by congratulating the patient on moving successfully. A paralyzed patient will have difficulty ambulating.

22. The nurse is caring for a patient with a diagnosis of achondroplasia. The nurse should assess the patient for symptoms of
    a. dwarfism*
    b. brittle bones
    c. bone deformities
    d. giantism

Reference: p. 954

Descriptors:

1. 38	2. 03	3. Application
4. II-2	5. Nursing Process	6. Moderate

Rationale: The nurse should assess the patient for symptoms of dwarfism, which is associated with achondroplasia.

23. An adolescent patient visits the emergency room after falling while playing soccer. The injury has resulted in a partial tear to the ligaments around the ankle, known as a
    a. spur
    b. dislocation
    c. sprain*
    d. strain

Reference: p. 956

Descriptors:

1. 38	2. 03	3. Application
4. IV-1	5. Nursing Process	6. Moderate

Rationale: Partial tear of the ligaments is termed a sprain.

24. The nurse is performing a developmental assessment on a 3-year-old child. The nurse determines that the child needs further assessment when the nurse observes that the child cannot
   a. work a simple puzzle*
   b. hop on one foot
   c. climb stairs without a hand rail
   d. use a jump rope

Reference: p. 955

Descriptors:

1. 38	2. 03	3. Application
4. II-1	5. Nursing Process	6. Moderate

Rationale: Most 3-year-old children are capable of working a simple puzzle.

25. The nurse assesses a 3-month-old infant and determines that the infant is developing at a normal rate when the nurse observes the infant in a prone position
   a. creep on all fours without assistance
   b. pull herself up in the crib
   c. roll over adeptly
   d. raise her head from floor*

Reference: p. 955

Descriptors:

1. 38	2. 03	3. Application
4. II-1	5. Nursing Process	6. Moderate

Rationale: A 3-month-old infant in a prone position should be able to raise her head from the floor.

26. The nurse is caring for an adult patient with multiple fractures and traction that requires prolonged bed rest. A priority nursing diagnosis for the patient is
   a. Risk for Ineffective Individual Coping related to injuries
   b. Hypovolemia related to multiple trauma injuries
   c. Risk for Altered Tissue Perfusion related to immobility*
   d. Risk for Social Isolation related to prolonged bed rest

Reference: p. 967

Descriptors:

1. 38	2. 07	3. Application
4. IV-3	5. Nursing Process	6. Moderate

Rationale: The priority nursing diagnosis is Risk for Altered Tissue Perfusion related to immobility.

27. The nurse is caring for an adult patient diagnosed with HIV disease who has a poor appetite and has limited mobility because of the disease. A priority nursing diagnosis for the patient is
   a. Impaired Gas Exchange related to decreased exercise
   b. Altered Nutrition: Less than Body Requirements related to disease state*
   c. Risk for Activity Intolerance related to decreased endurance
   d. Fluid Volume Excess related to dependent edema

Reference: p. 968

Descriptors:

1. 38	2. 07	3. Application
4. IV-3	5. Nursing Process	6. Moderate

Rationale: A priority nursing diagnosis for the patient is Altered Nutrition: Less than Body Requirements related to disease state.

28. A 75-year-old patient tells the nurse that she has been constipated. After giving the patient instructions about how to decrease the constipation, the nurse determines that the patient needs further instructions when the patient says
   a. "I should eat more vegetables and whole grain products."
   b. "It is important that I drink plenty of fluids throughout the day."
   c. "It is OK if I take a laxative every night before I go to bed."*
   d. "Having a bedside commode might be helpful."

Reference: p. 968

Descriptors:

1. 38	2. 10	3. Application
4. IV-3	5. Teach/Learn	6. Moderate

Rationale: The patient needs further instructions when she says it is OK to take a laxative every night before she goes to bed. This can lead to dependence on laxatives.

29. An adult patient visits the clinic and tells the nurse that he is undergoing a great deal of stress on his new job and doesn't have time to exercise. The nurse should instruct the patient that
   a. when the stressors at work are decreased, he'll have more time to exercise
   b. fatigue from stress can contribute to the need for more rest
   c. regular exercise can be energizing and decrease the effects of stress*
   d. a regular program of strenuous exercise can be started when the stressors are relieved

Reference: p. 969

Descriptors:

| 1. 38 | 2. 10 | 3. Application |
| 4. III-1 | 5. Teach/Learn | 6. Moderate |

Rationale: The nurse should instruct the patient that regular exercise can be energizing and decrease the effects of stress.

30. A patient tells the nurse that she has joined a local club and is able to swim three times a week. The nurse should instruct the patient that swimming is an
a. isometric exercise that can improve muscle mass
b. isotonic exercise that can improve cardiovascular function*
c. isokinetic exercise that can improve respiratory function
d. isometric exercise that strengthens the quadriceps muscles

Reference: p. 959

Descriptors:

| 1. 38 | 2. 04 | 3. Application |
| 4. II-2 | 5. Teach/Learn | 6. Moderate |

Rationale: Swimming is an isotonic exercise that can improve cardiovascular function.

31. An adolescent patient asks the nurse about exercises to increase his muscle mass and endurance. An appropriate exercise program for the nurse to suggest to the patient is
a. aerobics
b. stretching
c. isotonic
d. strength*

Reference: p. 960

Descriptors:

| 1. 38 | 2. 05 | 3. Application |
| 4. II-1 | 5. Teach/Learn | 6. Easy |

Rationale: The patient should do strength training exercises to increase his muscle mass.

32. A 75-year-old patient who has been on bed rest for 5 days asks the nurse why she needs to exercise when she doesn't feel like doing so. The nurse explains to the patient the reasons for the exercises and determines that the patient understands the instructions when the patient says that prolonged bed rest can lead to
a. increased cardiac workload*
b. decreased heart rate
c. increased blood pressure
d. decreased cardiac stroke volume

References: p. 960

Descriptors:

| 1. 38 | 2. 05 | 3. Application |
| 4. IV-3 | 5. Teach/Learn | 6. Moderate |

Rationale: Prolonged bed rest can result in increased cardiac workload.

33. A 76-year-old patient has been on bed rest for 3 days after abdominal surgery. The patient has been receiving morphine. The nurse caring for this patient plans to assess the patient for
a. contractures
b. ankylosis
c. pneumonia*
d. atrophy

Reference: p. 961

Descriptors:

| 1. 38 | 2. 05 | 3. Application |
| 4. IV-3 | 5. Nursing Process | 6. Moderate |

Rationale: For an elderly patient who has been on bed rest for 3 days after abdominal surgery, the nurse should assess the patient for pneumonia.

34. After several days of prolonged bed rest, the nurse ambulates the patient for the first time from the bed to the chair. The patient tells the nurse he is surprised how weak his legs have become. The nurse should explain to the patient that prolonged bed rest can result in
a. contractures
b. ankylosis
c. osteoporosis
d. atrophy*

Reference: p. 961

Descriptors:

| 1. 38 | 2. 05 | 3. Application |
| 4. IV-3 | 5. Teach/Learn | 6. Moderate |

Rationale: Prolonged bed rest can lead to atrophy or wasting of the tissues.

35. After a period of prolonged bed rest, the physician tells the patient that she has developed brittle bones. The nurse should explain to the patient that the prolonged bed rest has resulted in
a. osteoporosis*
b. contractures
c. fractures
d. atrophy

Reference: p. 961

Descriptors:

1. 38   2. 05   3. Application
4. IV-1   5. Teach/Learn 6. Moderate

Rationale: Osteoporosis can result from prolonged bed rest.

36. The nurse is planning to discuss osteoporosis with a group of perimenopausal women. Which of the following substances would be important for the nurse to include in the teaching plan to prevent or delay osteoporosis?
a. vitamin B_{12}
b. calcium*
c. β-carotene
d. vitamin C

Reference: p. 961

Descriptors:

1. 38   2. 05   3. Application
4. II-2   5. Teach/Learn 6. Moderate

Rationale: Calcium is an important mineral for the prevention of osteoporosis.

37. While caring for a patient on prolonged bed rest, the nurse can help prevent the formation of renal calculi by
a. decreasing the patient's calcium intake
b. improving urinary alkalinity
c. monitoring intake and output*
d. encouraging Kegel's exercises

Reference: p. 962

Descriptors:

1. 38   2. 10   3. Application
4. IV-3   5. Nursing Process 6. Moderate

Rationale: Adequate hydration and monitoring of I&O can prevent the formation of renal calculi.

38. The nurse makes a home visit to a 70-year-old patient who lives alone in a rural area. The patient has limited mobility and limited financial resources and has recently been widowed after 40 years of marriage. A priority nursing diagnosis for the patient is
a. Ineffective Individual Coping related to limited finances
b. Powerlessness related to inability to perform self-care activities
c. Risk for Infection related to limited mobility
d. Social Isolation related to immobility and loss of spouse*

Reference: p. 969

Descriptors:

1. 38   2. 07   3. Application
4. III-1   5. Nursing Process 6. Moderate

Rationale: The priority nursing diagnosis is Social Isolation related to immobility and loss of spouse.

39. A 40-year-old sedentary patient who is overweight asks the nurse if he should begin a jogging program. The nurse should instruct the patient that before beginning an exercise program, he should
a. have a preexercise medical examination*
b. lose 10 pounds
c. have his cholesterol levels evaluated
d. wear the appropriate footwear to avoid injury

Reference: p. 963

Descriptors:

1. 38   2. 09   3. Application
4. II-2   5. Nursing Process 6. Moderate

Rationale: Before a sedentary, overweight patient begins an exercise program, he should have a preexercise medical examination.

40. After several weeks of jogging, a patient visits the clinic and complains of foot pain. The physician diagnoses the patient with a torn tendon. The nurse should instruct the patient to
a. apply heat to the injured area
b. continue with his jogging routine
c. keep the foot in a dependent position
d. apply a compression bandage to the foot*

References: p. 964

Descriptors:

1. 38   2. 10   3. Application
4. IV-3   5. Teach/Learn 6. Moderate

Rationale: A torn tendon should be treated with a compression bandage on the foot.

41. The nurse who wishes to serve as a role model for others and keep physically fit while preventing back injuries should
    a. lift a bedridden patient when the nurse is fatigued
    b. perform work activities even though shortness of breath occurs
    c. perform weekly exercises for 30 minutes three times per week*
    d. keep weight to below normal for height

References: p. 951

Descriptors:

| 1. 38 | 2. 05 | 3. Application |
| 4. I-1 | 5. Self Care | 6. Moderate |

Rationale: Weekly exercises should be performed for 30 minutes three times per week.

42. A 10-year-old patient with cerebral palsy visits the clinic. The nurse observes the patient sitting quietly but as the child reaches for a sucker on the counter the patient's hand begins to shake. The nurse determines that the patient has
    a. intentional tremors*
    b. postural tremors
    c. athetosis
    d. dystonia

Reference: p. 957

Descriptors:

| 1. 38 | 2. 06 | 3. Application |
| 4. IV-1 | 5. Nursing Process | 6. Moderate |

Rationale: The child is exhibiting intentional tremors, which are associated with cerebral palsy.

43. The nurse assesses a 75-year-old patient and observes that the patient is demonstrating brief, rapid, and jerky unpredictable movements. The nurse determines that the patient is exhibiting
    a. crepitation
    b. dystonia
    c. fasciculations
    d. chorea*

Reference: p. 966

Descriptors:

| 1. 38 | 2. 06 | 3. Application |
| 4. IV-1 | 5. Nursing Process | 6. Moderate |

Rationale: Brief, rapid, jerky, unpredictable movements are associated with chorea.

44. The nurse is caring for an adult patient who demonstrates a grotesque and twisted posture while sitting in a chair. The nurse determines that the patient is exhibiting symptoms of
    a. chorea
    b. dystonia*
    c. myoclonus
    d. athetosis

Reference: p. 966

Descriptors:

| 1. 38 | 2. 06 | 3. Application |
| 4. IV-1 | 5. Nursing Process | 6. Moderate |

Rationale: The patient is exhibiting symptoms of dystonia.

45. While assisting a 80-year-old patient with range-of-motion exercises, the nurse hears a crunching sound while abducting the patient's leg. The nurse documents this finding as
    a. subluxation
    b. asymmetry
    c. crepitation*
    d. athetosis

Reference: pp. 966; 969

Descriptors:

| 1. 38 | 2. 06 | 3. Application |
| 4. II-2 | 5. Documentation | 6. Moderate |

Rationale: A "crunching sound" is associated with crepitation.

46. A patient with cancer tells the nurse that he has decreased muscle mass in both legs. The nurse verifies the finding by measuring both legs and documents this finding as muscle
    a. flaccidity
    b. hypertrophy
    c. hemiplegia
    d. atrophy*

Reference: pp. 961; 966

Descriptors:

| 1. 38 | 2. 06 | 3. Application |
| 4. II-1 | 5. Documentation | 6. Moderate |

Rationale: Decreased muscle mass is termed atrophy.

47. The nurse is preparing to examine an adult patient with hemiparesis following a stroke. The nurse anticipates that the patient will have
    a. weakness over one half of the body*
    b. paralysis over one half of the body
    c. paralysis of both legs
    d. spasticity of both arms

Reference: p. 966

Descriptors:

1. 38	2. 06	3. Application
4. IV-1	5. Nursing Process	6. Moderate

Rationale: Hemiparesis is the term for weakness over one half of the body.

48. The nurse is caring for an adult patient on the third postoperative day and assesses the patient's endurance by observing the patient
   a. push the foot against the chair
   b. pull himself up in bed
   c. turn himself in bed*
   d. push the nurse's palms apart

Reference: p. 970

Descriptors:

1. 38	2. 06	3. Application
4. IV-1	5. Nursing Process	6. Moderate

Rationale: A patient's endurance can be tested by observing the patient turn himself in the bed.

49. A 63-year-old patient with advanced osteoarthritis and limited mobility tells the nurse that she "feels badly because she cannot even cook a simple meal for her family because of her arthritis." A priority nursing diagnosis is
   a. Ineffective Family Coping related to the need for assistance
   b. Self-Esteem Disturbance related to inability to meet role expectations*
   c. Knowledge Deficit related to appropriate exercise programs
   d. Risk for Injury related to falls secondary to immobility

Reference: p. 971

Descriptors:

1. 38	2. 07	3. Application
4. III-1	5. Nursing Process	6. Moderate

Rationale: The priority nursing diagnosis is Self-Esteem Disturbance related to inability to meet role expectations.

50. After his annual physical examination, the physician encourages an adult patient to start a regular exercise program. The nurse plans goals with the patient and an appropriate goal for this patient is: In 3 days, the patient will
   a. document the need for an exercise program
   b. maintain full joint range of motion
   c. be exercising daily for 30 minutes
   d. list support systems to reinforce exercise efforts*

Reference: p. 972

Descriptors:

1. 38	2. 10	3. Application
4. II-2	5. Nursing Process	6. Moderate

Rationale: An appropriate goal is that in 3 days the patient will list his support systems to reinforce the exercise efforts.

51. The physician has ordered the bed of an adult patient to be in the high Fowler's position. The nurse plans to elevate the head of the patient's bed
   a. 15 degrees
   b. 30 degrees
   c. 45 degrees
   d. 90 degrees*

Reference: p. 974

Descriptors:

1. 38	2. 10	3. Application
4. IV-1	5. Nursing Process	6. Moderate

Rationale: High Fowler's indicates that the bed needs to be elevated 90 degrees.

52. While caring for a patient who is bedridden in a semi-Fowler's position, an important assessment for the nurse to make is an assessment of the patient's
   a. sacrum*
   b. forearms
   c. calves
   d. neck

Reference: p. 974

Descriptors:

1. 38	2. 06	3. Application
4. IV-3	5. Nursing Process	6. Moderate

Rationale: Because the patient is in a semi-Fowler's position, the nurse should make an assessment of the patient's coccyx because a pressure ulcer may be forming.

53. The nurse plans to turn an unconscious bedridden patient to the Sims' position. The nurse should plan to
   a. place a pillow under the patient's neck for support
   b. ensure that the two shoulders are in line with the hips*
   c. adduct the shoulder slightly in a flexed position
   d. place a foam pillow next to the patient's ribcage

Reference: p. 976

Descriptors:

1. 38   2. 08   3. Application
4. IV-3   5. Nursing Process   6. Moderate

Rationale: Ensuring that the two shoulders are in line with the hips will aid in proper body alignment.

54. The nurse has instructed a nursing student how to perform passive range-of-motion exercises on an adult patient. The nurse determines that the student needs further instructions when the student says
    a. "It's important to cup my hand under the elbow to support it."
    b. "I should start gradually and work slowly until completed."
    c. "If the patient experiences pain, I should stop the exercises."
    d. "The patient's neck should be hyperextended toward the ceiling."*

Reference: p. 977

Descriptors:

1. 38   2. 10   3. Application
4. IV-3   5. Teach/Learn   6. Moderate

Rationale: The student needs further instructions when the student says that the patient's neck should be hyperextended toward the ceiling.

55. The nurse is planning to move an obese patient from a stretcher to the bed. Before transferring the patient the nurse should plan to use a
    a. transfer board*
    b. drawsheet
    c. three-carrier lift
    d. trapeze

Reference: p. 985

Descriptors:

1. 38   2. 08   3. Application
4. IV-3   5. Nursing Process   6. Moderate

Rationale: For an obese patient and for safety reasons, the nurse should use a transfer board.

56. The nurse is preparing to transfer an adult patient with left-sided weakness from the bed to a chair. The nurse should
    a. raise the bed to the highest level with head elevated
    b. lower the head of the bed to the lowest position
    c. stand behind the patient while holding his waist
    d. position the chair facing the head or foot of the bed*

Reference: p. 990

Descriptors:

1. 38   2. 08   3. Application
4. IV-3   5. Nursing Process   6. Moderate

Rationale: The nurse should position the chair facing the head or foot of the bed to transfer a patient with left-sided weakness.

57. The nurse is caring for a patient who has limited mobility in her left leg and who uses a walker. The nurse determines that the patient is using the walker correctly when the nurse observes the patient
    a. adjust the legs of the walker to a height of the patient's diaphragm
    b. move the walker and the right leg forward 6 to 8 inches before the left leg
    c. move the walker and the left leg forward 6 to 8 inches before the right leg*
    d. use the walker for support when rising from a sitting to a standing position

Reference: p. 998

Descriptors:

1. 38   2. 08   3. Application
4. IV-3   5. Nursing Process   6. Moderate

Rationale: The affected leg (left) should be moved before the right leg.

58. The nurse is planning to instruct a patient how to walk with assistance of a cane. Which of the following should be included in the teaching plan? The patient should
    a. lean forward while walking with the cane
    b. hold the tip of the cane about 6 inches to the side of the foot
    c. start with a single-ended cane and move to a three-prong cane
    d. hold the cane with elbows flexed on the unaffected side*

Reference: p. 998

Descriptors:

1. 38   2. 10   3. Application
4. IV-1   5. Teach/Learn   6. Moderate

Rationale: The patient should hold the cane with elbows flexed on the unaffected side.

59. The nurse is caring for an adult patient who will be using axillary crutches because of a fractured foot. The nurse should
    a. measure the distance of the patient's axillary fold and add 2 inches*
    b. instruct the patient that support should come primarily from the axilla
    c. adjust the handgrips while the patient keeps his elbows straight
    d. instruct the patient to ambulate upstairs with the affected leg first

    Reference: p. 998

    Descriptors:

    1. 38   2. 10   3. Application
    4. IV-1   5. Nursing Process   6. Moderate

    Rationale: The nurse should measure the distance of the patient's axillary fold and add 2 inches for crutches.

60. After a normal annual physical examination, a patient tells the nurse she wishes to develop a personal exercise program. The nurse should *first*
    a. identify support persons for the patient
    b. explore feasible exercise activities with the patient*
    c. discuss potential threats to the patient's exercise program
    d. ask the patient if she is really motivated to exercise

    Reference: p. 1002

    Descriptors:

    1. 38   2. 09   3. Application
    4. II-2   5. Nursing Process   6. Moderate

    Rationale: The nurse should first explore feasible exercise activities with the patient.

61. The nurse is caring for a patient with rheumatoid arthritis and impaired physical mobility. An appropriate goal for the patient is that the patient will
    a. identify four reasons why a daily exercise program is necessary
    b. demonstrate methods to conserve energy while exercising
    c. perform activities of daily living with the greatest degree of independence possible*
    d. maintain a pain-free status while exercising by using analgesic agents

    Reference: p. 992

    Descriptors:

    1. 38   2. 10   3. Application
    4. IV-1   5. Nursing Process   6. Moderate

    Rationale: An appropriate goal for the patient with arthritis is that the patient will perform activities of daily living with the greatest degree of independence possible.

CHAPTER 39

Rest and Sleep

1. The nurse provides the postoperative patient with a backrub and an analgesic medication and then darkens the room before the patient goes to sleep for the night. The nurse's actions
   a. help decrease the patient's circadian rhythm
   b. stimulate hormonal changes in the brain
   c. decrease stimuli from the cerebral cortex*
   d. alert the hypothalamus in the brain

   Reference: p. 1028

   Descriptors:

   1. 39   2. 08   3. Knowledge
   4. IV-1   5. Caring   6. Easy

   Rationale: The nurse's actions help to decrease stimuli from the cerebral cortex.

2. Following an automobile accident that caused a head injury to an adult patient, the nurse observes that the patient sleeps for long periods. The nurse determines that the patient has experienced injury to the
   a. hypothalamus*
   b. thalamus
   c. cortex
   d. medulla

   Reference: p. 1015

   Descriptors:

   1. 39   2. 02   3. Application
   4. IV-1   5. Nursing Process   6. Moderate

   Rationale: The patient has most likely suffered an injury to the hypothalamus, which controls sleep.

3. A hospitalized adult patient who routinely works from midnight until 8 AM has a temperature of 99.1°F at 4 AM. The nurse determines that this is most likely due to
   a. delta sleep
   b. slow brain waves
   c. bronchitis
   d. circadian rhythm*

   Reference: p. 1015

   Descriptors:

   1. 39   2. 01   3. Application
   4. IV-1   5. Nursing Process   6. Moderate

   Rationale: Temperature fluctuations are due to the patient's circadian rhythm.

4. The nurse empties a Foley catheter bag for a patient who appears to be asleep. The patient is easily aroused when the nurse is near the patient's bedside. The nurse determines that the patient was most likely in the non-REM sleep stage
   a. I
   b. II*
   c. III
   d. IV

   Reference: p. 1016

   Descriptors:

   1. 39   2. 01   3. Application
   4. IV-1   5. Nursing Process   6. Moderate

   Rationale: When the patient is easily aroused after appearing to be asleep, the patient is most likely in non-REM stage II of sleep.

4. In human beings, rhythmic phenomena that recur every 24 hours are called
   a. biorhythms
   b. ultradian rhythms
   c. infradian rhythms
   d. circadian rhythms*

   Reference: p. 1015

   Descriptors:

   1. 39   2. 04   3. Knowledge
   4. IV-1   5. Nursing Process   6. Easy

   Rationale: Circadian rhythms complete a full cycle every 24 hours.

5. The rapid eye movement (REM) stage of sleep is characterized by
   a. decreased blood pressure and pulse
   b. muscle twitching and leg movements
   c. increased blood pressure and pulse*
   d. perceptions of drifting off to sleep

   Reference: pp. 1015–1016

   Descriptors:

1. 39	2. 04	3. Comprehensive
4. None	5. None	6. Moderate

   Rationale: REM sleep plays a role in memory, dreams, and adaptation, causing an increase in blood pressure and pulse.

6. The time it takes to complete an average sleep cycle is approximately
   a. 30 minutes
   b. 45 minutes
   c. 90 minutes*
   d. 2 hours

   Reference: p. 1016

   Descriptors:

1. 39	2. 04	3. Knowledge
4. None	5. None	6. Easy

   Rationale: Each sleep cycle lasts approximately 90 to 100 minutes.

7. A hospitalized adult patient appears to be asleep when the nurse assesses the patient's blood pressure. The nurse observes that the patient's respirations are irregular and there is a 5-second period of apnea between respirations. The nurse determines that the patient is experiencing
   a. non-REM sleep
   b. REM sleep*
   c. narcolepsy
   d. sleep apnea

   Reference: p. 1016

   Descriptors:

1. 39	2. 05	3. Application
4. None	5. None	6. Moderate

   Rationale: When the nurse observes that the patient's respirations are irregular and a 5-second period of apnea is present, the patient is most likely in REM sleep.

8. The nurse is caring for a patient who has just delivered a healthy newborn boy when the patient asks the nurse about newborn sleep patterns. The nurse should instruct the patient that for the first 3 weeks newborns generally
   a. have less REM sleep than older children
   b. demonstrate alert inactivity with eyes open
   c. sleep about 16 hours per day*
   d. need one nap per day

   Reference: p. 1018

   Descriptors:

1. 39	2. 04	3. Application
4. IV-4	5. Nursing Process	6. Moderate

   Rationale: Most newborns less than 3 weeks of age sleep an average of 16 hours per day.

9. When discussing newborn sleep patterns with a first-time mother, the patient asks "When will my baby sleep through the night?" The best response by the nurse is to instruct the patient that newborns generally sleep through the night by
   a. 1 month of age
   b. 2 to 4 months of age*
   c. 5 to 6 months of age
   d. 7 to 8 months of age

   Reference: p. 1018

   Descriptors:

1. 39	2. 04	3. Application
4. II-1	5. Teach/Learn	6. Moderate

   Rationale: Newborns generally sleep through the night when they are 2 to 4 months of age.

10. A patient who smokes one pack of cigarettes every day tells the nurse that he has had trouble falling asleep for the past few nights because he is worried about possible loss of his job. The nurse instructs the patient to
    a. decrease or stop smoking during the day*
    b. practice relaxation techniques during the day
    c. exercise for 30 minutes before bedtime
    d. try to fall asleep even if not sleepy

    Reference: p. 1019

    Descriptors:

1. 39	2. 03	3. Application
4. II-1	5. Teach/Learn	6. Moderate

    Rationale: Smoking and nicotine can cause sleeplessness, so the nurse should tell the patient to stop or decrease smoking.

11. While discussing sleep patterns of school-aged children with a group of parents, which of the following would be appropriate for the nurse to include in the teaching plan? School-aged children
    a. often have difficulty sleeping through the night
    b. may require less sleep during growth spurts
    c. generally sleep 8 to 10 hours each night*
    d. usually require a nap after school

    Reference: p. 1018

    Descriptors:

1. 39	2. 04	3. Application
4. III-1	5. Teach/Learn	6. Moderate

    Rationale: The nurse should instruct the parents that school-aged children generally sleep 8 to 10 hours per night and they usually do not require a nap.

12. The nurse is planning a presentation about sleep for a group of adults aged 65 or older. Which of the following should be included in the teaching plan?
    a. Sleep–wakefulness patterns are often altered as one ages.*
    b. The amount of REM sleep increases as one ages.
    c. Some adults have no stage I sleep after the age of 60 years.
    d. Over the age of 60 years, patients are less likely to be disturbed by noise.

    Reference: p. 1019

    Descriptors:

1. 39	2. 04	3. Application
4. II-1	5. Teach/Learn	6. Moderate

    Rationale: Sleep–wakefulness patterns are often altered as one ages. Noise can be particularly disturbing to older patients.

13. A patient tells the nurse that she has been suffering from chronic fatigue even though she has been getting 10 to 12 hours of sleep each night. The nurse should assess the patient for
    a. dietary deficiencies
    b. somnambulism
    c. symptoms of illness*
    d. parasomnia

    Reference: p. 1020

    Descriptors:

1. 39	2. 03	3. Application
4. II-1	5. Teach/Learn	6. Moderate

    Rationale: The nurse should assess the patient for symptoms of excessive stress, depression, or other illness.

14. A patient tells the nurse that he has been experiencing insomnia the past few days. The nurse should suggest to the patient that an appropriate snack before bedtime to aid the sleep process is
    a. an orange
    b. crackers*
    c. hot tea
    d. a carbonated beverage

    Reference: p. 1029

    Descriptors:

1. 39	2. 08	3. Application
4. II-2	5. Nursing Process	6. Moderate

    Rationale: A light carbohydrate such as soda crackers can aid in sleep. Tea and carbonated beverages may contain caffeine.

15. A nurse works the day/night rotation on a general nursing unit. When she switches from the day to the night shift, she has difficulty sleeping. An alteration in her biologic sleep cycle
    a. will occur immediately if she is healthy
    b. often takes several weeks before the body will adjust*
    c. has little influence on her actual physiologic function
    d. is unrelated to the environmental temperature or light

    Reference: p. 1015

    Descriptors:

1. 39	2. 03	3. Comprehensive
4. IV-1	5. Teach/Learn	6. Moderate

    Rationale: Alterations in an individual's sleep–wake cycle take time to adjust when the circadian rhythm is disrupted.

16. The nurse looking for behaviors reflecting sleep deprivation in patients unaware of their sleep problems should note
    a. irritability, fatigue, and lethargy*
    b. daytime sleepiness and snoring
    c. depression and slurred speech
    d. sleepwalking and nocturnal enuresis

    Reference: p. 1025

    Descriptors:

1. 39	2. 06	3. Comprehensive
4. I-1	5. Self Care	6. Moderate

    Rationale: Reports of irritability, fatigue, and lethargy are associated with insomnia.

17. A 78-year-old patient has suffered the loss of her husband of 45 years about 2 months ago. While visiting the patient in her home, the patient tells the nurse that she has been sleeping 14 to 16 hours a day and has no energy. The nurse determines that the patient is most likely experiencing
    a. chronic illness
    b. hypersomnia*
    c. sleep apnea
    d. narcolepsy
    Reference: p. 1021
    Descriptors:

1. 39	2. 06	3. Application
4. II-2	5. Nursing Process	6. Moderate

    Rationale: The patient is grieving and suffering from hypersomnia.

18. Narcolepsy is a type of sleep disturbance that results in a/an
    a. uncontrollable urge to sleep*
    b. sleep walking
    c. insomnia
    d. emotional stress
    Reference: p. 1021
    Descriptors:

1. 39	2. 06	3. Knowledge
4. III-1	5. Nursing Process	6. Easy

    Rationale: Narcolepsy is a sleep disorder that results in an uncontrollable urge to sleep.

19. A patient visits the clinic and tells the nurse that he has recently taken a new job and has had difficulty falling asleep for the past few days. The nurse determines that the patient is most likely experiencing
    a. transitional insomnia
    b. sleep deprivation
    c. parasomnia
    d. transient insomnia*
    Reference: p. 1021
    Descriptors:

1. 39	2. 06	3. Application
4. None	5. None	6. Moderate

    Rationale: The patient is experiencing transient insomnia.

20. A patient has been diagnosed with narcolepsy and given a prescription for an agrypnotic medication (Ritalin). The nurse should instruct the patient that he should
    a. take the medications faithfully each day*
    b. discontinue leisure activities for at least 2 weeks
    c. reduce carbohydrate intake before bedtime
    d. discontinue the medications when sleep patterns return to normal
    Reference: p. 1022
    Descriptors:

1. 39	2. 09	3. Application
4. III-1	5. Nursing Process	6. Moderate

    Rationale: A patient with narcolepsy should take the medication faithfully each day.

21. While caring for an adult male patient, the nurse observes that the patient is snoring while sleeping and stops breathing for 20 seconds between the snoring. The nurse determines that the patient is most likely experiencing
    a. narcolepsy
    b. hypersomnia
    c. parasomnia
    d. sleep apnea*
    Reference: p. 1022
    Descriptors:

1. 39	2. 06	3. Application
4. IV-2	5. Teach/Learn	6. Moderate

    Rationale: The patient's symptoms of apnea lasting 20 seconds are associated with sleep apnea.

22. A 78-year-old patient who has had chronic insomnia most of her adult life tells the nurse that sometimes she wakes up because "her legs feel like there is something crawling on them." The nurse determines that the patient is most likely experiencing
    a. vitamin D deficiency
    b. restless leg syndrome*
    c. nocturnal apnea
    d. nocturnal clonus
    Reference: p. 1022
    Descriptors:

1. 39	2. 06	3. Application
4. IV-1	5. Nursing Process	6. Moderate

    Rationale: The patient's symptoms are associated with restless leg syndrome.

23. The nurse is caring for a 45-year-old obese male patient who is being treated for sleep apnea syndrome. The nurse instructs the patient that sleep apnea syndrome is associated with
    a. cardiac arrhythmias*
    b. hypotension
    c. chronic lung congestion
    d. muscle tremors

    References: p. 1022

    Descriptors:

1. 39	2. 06	3. Application
4. IV-1	5. Nursing Process	6. Moderate

    Rationale: Sleep apnea has been associated with cardiac arrhythmias.

24. The nurse is caring for a patient who experiences frequent somnambulism while sleeping in a second floor bedroom. A priority nursing diagnosis for this patient is
    a. Knowledge Deficit related to ways to control the somnambulism
    b. Risk for Injury related to somnambulism and environment*
    c. Anxiety related to fear of falling out of bed during the night
    d. Impaired Social Interaction related to fear of somnambulism

    Reference: p. 1026

    Descriptors:

1. 39	2. 07	3. Application
4. II-2	5. Teach/Learn	6. Moderate

    Rationale: The priority nursing diagnosis is Risk for Injury related to somnambulism and environment.

25. The nurse is caring for a 65-year-old patient who lives with her daughter and tells the nurse she doesn't sleep much at night. The nurse should suggest to the patient to obtain more specific data on the patient's sleep–wakefulness patterns, the patient should
    a. keep a sleep diary for 14 days*
    b. document what time she goes to sleep at night
    c. ask her daughter to keep a graph of her sleep
    d. record the type of medications she takes before sleep

    Reference: p. 1023

    Descriptors:

1. 39	2. 05	3. Application
4. IV-3	5. Nursing Process	6. Moderate

    Rationale: The patient should be instructed to keep a sleep diary for 14 days.

26. A hospitalized patient tells the nurse that he has been unable to sleep. To obtain more data related to the patient's sleep problem, the nurse should first say
    a. "How many hours of sleep do you need?"
    b. "Do you take naps during the day?"
    c. "Tell me about your sleep problem."*
    d. "Do you need a medication to help you sleep?"

    Reference: p. 1024

    Descriptors:

1. 39	2. 05	3. Application
4. IV-1	5. Teach/Learn	6. Moderate

    Rationale: The nurse should say "Tell me about your sleep problem" to obtain further data.

27. The nurse has instructed an adult patient about how to keep a sleep diary. The nurse determines that the patient understands the instructions when the patient says
    a "I should keep records of the time I fall asleep."
    b "It's important to record my mental and physical activities."*
    c. "It would be better if my husband kept the entire record for me."
    d. "It would be important to include any dreams I remember."

    Reference: p. 1023

    Descriptors:

1. 39	2. 05	3. Application
4. IV-1	5. Nursing Process	6. Moderate

    Rationale: A sleep diary should include the mental and physical activities prior to bedtime.

28. A 39-year-old patient is seen in the clinic because she has been sleeping 14 to 16 hours per day. The patient states that she is "depressed because my mother died from cancer 2 months ago." A priority nursing diagnosis for this patient is
    a. Risk for Spiritual Distress related to depression and grief response
    b. Depression related to loss of mother and excessive sleeping
    c. Sleep Pattern Alteration related to inability to resolve grief
    d. Sleep Pattern Disturbance related to grief process and loss of mother*

Reference: p. 1026

Descriptors:

1. 39	2. 07	3. Application
4. IV-1	5. Teach/Learn	6. Moderate

Rationale: The priority nursing diagnosis is Sleep Pattern Disturbance related to grief process and loss of mother.

29. Which of the following patients would be correctly diagnosed with Sleep Pattern Disturbance?
    a. a person with endogenous depression who complains of not having the energy to do almost anything but sleep
    b. a person on chemotherapy for cancer who is exhausted with completion of the activities of daily living
    c. a person who had difficulty falling asleep, wakes up at 3 AM, and is exhausted in the afternoon*
    d. a person with chronic obstructive pulmonary disease who becomes dyspneic with any activity

Reference: p. 1026

Descriptors:

1. 39	2. 07	3. Comprehensive
4. III-1	5. Nursing Process	6. Moderate

Rationale: The diagnosis of Sleep Pattern Disturbance consists of these symptoms.

30. The patient complains of difficulty falling asleep, awakening earlier than desired, and not feeling rested. She attributes these problems to leg pain that is secondary to her arthritis. What would be the appropriate nursing diagnosis for her?
    a. Sleep Pattern Disturbances related to arthritis
    b. Fatigue related to leg pain
    c. Knowledge Deficit regarding sleep hygiene measures
    d. Sleep Pattern Disturbance related to chronic leg pain*

Reference: p. 1029

Descriptors:

1. 39	2. 07	3. Comprehensive
4. IV-1	5. Nursing Process	6. Moderate

Rationale: The cause of the sleep pattern disturbance is the chronic leg pain.

31. While making a home visit to a 76-year-old patient, the patient tells the nurse that she often has trouble sleeping and then is "tired all day." The nurse should instruct the patient to
    a. watch television in bed before going to sleep
    b. take a short nap if she feels fatigued
    c. keep a routine of waking and sleeping*
    d. eat a light protein snack before bedtime

Reference: p. 1029

Descriptors:

1. 39	2. 08	3. Application
4. IV-1	5. Nursing Process	6. Moderate

Rationale: The patient should keep a routine of waking and sleeping and perhaps eat a light carbohydrate snack before bedtime.

32. The nurse is caring for a 3-year-old child hospitalized following an automobile injury. The nurse observes that the toddler awakens several times during the night. The nurse should
    a. administer an ordered pain medication
    b. ask the child why he keeps awakening
    c. ask the child's mother to stay with her
    d. provide comfort measures to the child*

Reference: p. 1029

Descriptors:

1. 39	2. 08	3. Application
4. IV-1	5. Teach/Learn	6. Moderate

Rationale: Providing comfort measures can help the child go back to sleep.

33. An adult patient is given a prescription for a sedative-hypnotic to aid in sleep. Following instructions about the medication, the nurse determines that the patient understands the instructions when he says
    a. "I can continue to take my Benadryl while on this medication."
    b. "This medication has no effect on REM sleep stages."
    c. "I should only take this medication temporarily."*
    d. "If the medication loses its effect, I can increase the dosage later."

Reference: p. 1029

Descriptors:

1. 39	2. 09	3. Application
4. II-1	5. Nursing Process	6. Moderate

Rationale: Sleeping medications are only for short-term use. Benadryl and a sleeping medication can seriously depress the central nervous system.

34. The nurse is caring for an adult patient who is being discharged from the hospital with a prescription for a sedative-hypnotic drug. The nurse plans to instruct the patient to
   a. take the medication every evening whether it is needed or not
   b. drink a glass of milk while taking the medication
   c. avoid alcoholic beverages while on the medication*
   d. contact the physician if the drug is no longer effective

Reference: pp. 1029–1031

Descriptors:

1. 39	2. 09	3. Application
4. IV-2	5. Teach/Learn	6. Moderate

Rationale: The patient should avoid drinking alcoholic beverages while taking the sleeping medication.

35. The nurse is caring for a patient who had a restless night due to postoperative pain. When the nurse enters the room at 7:30 AM for morning vital signs, the patient is sound asleep. The nurse should
   a. document that the patient was asleep at 7:30 AM and leave the room
   b. assess the patient's vital signs while trying not to disturb him
   c. ask the night shift nurse what the patient's vital signs were at 4 AM
   d. allow the patient to rest and assess the vital signs later in the morning*

Reference: p. 1029

Descriptors:

1. 39	2. 08	3. Application
4. IV-2	5. Teach/Learn	6. Moderate

Rationale: The nurse should avoid disturbing the patient until later in the morning if the procedure is routine and not lifesaving.

36. The nurse is planning care for the patient with a diagnosis of Sleep Pattern Disturbance related to environmental disturbances and sleep habit interruption. Which intervention would be appropriate?
   a. Turn off all lights in the patient's room to keep the patient comfortable.
   b. Synchronize schedules for medications and treatments to minimize interruptions.*
   c. Encourage exercise immediately before bedtime to decrease stress.
   d. Discuss with patient the advantages of long-term benzodiazepine use.

Reference: p. 1029

Descriptors:

1. 39	2. 09	3. Comprehensive
4. IV-1	5. Caring	6. Moderate

Rationale: To avoid numerous interruptions to the patient's sleep cycle, synchronize all necessary care.

37. A patient has been having difficulty falling asleep at night. Which of the following data would indicate progress toward the goal of alleviating a diagnosis of Sleep Pattern Disturbance?
   a. The person has had a drink of warm milk for the last three nights.
   b. The person reports falling asleep within 30 minutes of going to bed.*
   c. The person refuses a hypnotic as a sleep aid.
   d. The person changes the time of the evening meal from 5:00 to 6:00 PM.

Reference: p. 1031

Descriptors:

1. 39	2. 07	3. Comprehensive
4. IV-1	5. Nusing Process	6. Moderate

Rationale: In the evaluation step of the nursing process the goal is evaluated for whether the outcome was met. Falling asleep indicates goal achievement.

CHAPTER 40

Comfort

1. A patient has suffered a paper cut while writing a letter. The nurse should explain to the patient that this type of cut results in pain termed
   a. somatic
   b. referred
   c. cutaneous*
   d. deep
   Reference: p. 1039
   Descriptors:

1. 40	2. 01	3. Application
4. IV-1	5. Teach/Learn	6. Moderate

   Rationale: This type of pain is termed cutaneous.

2. While caring for patients with pain, the nurse should recognize that pain is a/an
   a. symptom of a severe disease or illness
   b. subjective experience*
   c. objective experience
   d. acute symptom of short duration
   Reference: p. 1039
   Descriptors:

1. 40	2. 02	3. Comprehensive
4. IV-1	5. Teach/Learn	6. Easy

   Rationale: Pain is a subjective experience and whatever the patient says it is.

3. Following abdominal surgery, an adult patient requests pain medication for incisional pain. The nurse determines that the patient is most likely experiencing pain termed
   a. visceral*
   b. referred
   c. somatic
   d. endogenous
   Reference: p. 1039
   Descriptors:

1. 40	2. 01	3. Application
4. IV-1	5. Nursing Process	6. Moderate

   Rationale: This type of pain is termed visceral.

4. The nurse is caring for a patient with terminal cancer and the patient reports that no matter what she does, the pain is never relieved. The nurse determines that the patient is experiencing pain termed
   a. intractable*
   b. intolerable
   c. diffuse
   d. acute
   Reference: p. 1039
   Descriptors:

1. 40	2. 03	3. Application
4. IV-1	5. Nursing Process	6. Moderate

   Rationale: Unrelieved pain is termed intractable.

5. An adult patient visits the emergency room complaining of pain that radiates down his right arm. The nurse determines that the patient is most likely experiencing pain termed
   a. psychogenic
   b. referred*
   c. transmitted
   d. cutaneous
   Reference: p. 1039
   Descriptors:

1. 40	2. 01	3. Application
4. IV-1	5. Nursing Process	6. Moderate

   Rationale: This type of pain is termed referred pain.

6. An injury to human tissue causes the release of histamine and pain receptors are then stimulated by
   a. substance K
   b. bradykinin*
   c. endorphins
   d. enkephalins

Reference: p. 1040

Descriptors:

1. 40	2. 01	3. Knowledge
4. None	5. None	6. Moderate

Rationale: The release of histamine and pain receptors are then stimulated by bradykinin.

7. Following an above-the-knee amputation as a result of diabetic complications, the 78-year-old patient continues to complain of pain in his amputated leg. The nurse determines that the patient is experiencing pain termed
   a. psychosomatic
   b. chronic
   c. myofascial
   d. phantom limb*

Reference: p. 1040

Descriptors:

1. 40	2. 03	3. Application
4. IV-1	5. Nursing Process	6. Moderate

Rationale: This type of pain is termed phantom limb pain.

8. Using the gate control theory of pain, an important nursing measure for a patient in pain is for the nurse to
   a. position the patient with several large pillows
   b. assist the patient with relaxation techniques
   c. provide pain medications as ordered
   d. give the patient a gentle backrub*

Reference: p. 1043

Descriptors:

1. 40	2. 04	3. Application
4. IV-1	5. Caring	6. Moderate

Rationale: To stop the pain at the "gate" the nurse should provide the patient with a backrub.

9. The nurse plans to instruct an adult patient about relaxation techniques to help relieve postoperative pain. Which of the following should be included in the teaching plan?
   a. Relaxation techniques can help close the pain gate.
   b. Meditation reduces the pain threshold.
   c. Endorphins are released during relaxation.*
   d. Exhaustion can be minimized with neuromuscular relaxation.

Reference: p. 1044

Descriptors:

1. 40	2. 07	3. Application
4. III-1	5. Nursing Process	6. Moderate

Rationale: Endorphins are released during relaxation.

10. The hospice nurse is planning a presentation on the topic of pain to a group of nursing students caring for terminally ill patients. Which of the following should be included in the nurse's teaching plan?
    a. Infants have little perception of pain until they are older.
    b. Pain in older adults is viewed as a normal part of the aging process.
    c. Individuals who have experienced more pain in their life have increased sensitivity.*
    d. Rested and relaxed individuals may experience pain in an acute manner.

Reference: p. 1047

Descriptors:

1. 40	2. 04	3. Application
4. IV-1	5. Teach/Learn	6. Moderate

Rationale: Individuals who have experienced more pain in their life have increased sensitivity. Past experiences can influence the patient's perception of pain.

11. The nurse has instructed a postoperative patient about pain and pain relief methods. The nurse determines that the patient needs further instructions when the patient says
    a. "If I am feeling pain, I should ask for my ordered pain medication."
    b. "All pain is real, regardless of its cause and there is a physical and mental component."
    c. "If I ask for something for pain, I may become addicted to the medication."*
    d. "Lack of pain expression does not necessarily mean lack of pain."

Reference: p. 1047

Descriptors:

1. 40	2. 04	3. Application
4. IV-1	5. Teach/Learn	6. Moderate

Rationale: The patient needs further instructions when he says "If I ask for something for pain, I may become addicted to the medication."

12. A family member tells the nurse that no matter what interventions are provided for a patient with cancer of the stomach, the patient continues to complain of pain. The best response by the nurse is to instruct the family member that
    a. "Individuals with prolonged pain have an increasingly low pain tolerance."*
    b. "Lying about the pain, or malingering, is common among adults."
    c. "People in pain should be given as much narcotics as they need to reduce the pain."
    d. "Pain is usually the result of an emotional or psychological problem."

Reference: p. 1047

Descriptors:

1. 40   2. 02   3. Application
4. IV-1   5. Teach/Learn 6. Moderate

Rationale: The best response by the nurse is to instruct the family member that "Individuals with prolonged pain have an increasingly low pain tolerance."

13. Two hours after receiving a pain medication, a postoperative patient tells the nurse that he is still having pain. To obtain more data, an appropriate response by the nurse is
    a. "Do you need your pain medication now?"
    b. "Tell me more about your pain."*
    c. "When did you last receive your pain medication?"
    d. "Tell me where the pain is located."

Reference: p. 1048

Descriptors:

1. 40   2. 05   3. Application
4. IV-2   5. Communication 6. Moderate

Rationale: To obtain additional data, the nurse should say to to the patient, "Tell me more about your pain."

14. The nurse is caring for a 4-year-old hospitalized child after cardiac surgery. To assess the child's pain level the nurse should
    a. assess the patient's vital signs and other symptoms of pain
    b. ask the child to compare his pain to a series of faces ranging from a broad smile to a grimace*
    c. ask the family members what symptoms in the child indicate he is having pain
    d. ask the child's mother to record the pain in a pain diary

Reference: p. 1054

Descriptors:

1. 40   2. 05   3. Application
4. IV-1   5. Nursing Process 6. Moderate

Rationale: The nurse can assess the child's pain level by asking the child to compare his pain to a series of faces ranging from a broad smile to a grimace.

15. The nurse has presented the topic of pain to a group of adults aged 65 years and older. The nurse determines that one of the participants needs further instruction when he says
    a. "People over 65 years of age have decreased pain sensitivity and tolerance."*
    b. "Boredom and loneliness can affect a person's perception of pain."
    c. "Having pain is not an expected outcome of the aging process."
    d. "The expression of pain varies based on a person's culture or ethnic background."

Reference: p. 1054

Descriptors:

1. 40   2. 05   3. Application
4. II-1   5. Teach/Learn   6. Moderate

Rationale: The participant needs further instructions when the patient says "People over 65 years of age have decreased pain sensitivity and tolerance."

16. The nurse is caring for an adult patient on the first postoperative day following thoracic surgery. The patient is reluctant to ask for pain medication yet appears to be in obvious pain. The priority nursing diagnosis for this patient is
    a. Ineffective Individual Coping related to past pain experience
    b. Pain: Postoperative related to fear of taking prescribed analgesics*
    c. Pain related to decreased blood supply to the thoracic cavity
    d. Knowledge Deficit related to appropriate pain management techniques

Reference: p. 1055

Descriptors:

1. 40   2. 06   3. Application
4. IV-1   5. Nursing Process 6. Moderate

Rationale: The priority nursing diagnosis for this patient is Pain: Postoperative related to fear of taking prescribed analgesics.

17. The nurse is caring for a hospitalized patient who is a quadriplegic and has had surgery on his right arm. The priority nursing diagnosis for this patient is
    a. Chronic Pain related to quadriplegia and surgery
    b. Risk for Social Isolation related to paralysis
    c. Risk for Injury related to decreased pain sensation*
    d. Anxiety related to heightened pain anticipation

    Reference: p. 1055

    Descriptors:

    1. 40   2. 06   3. Application
    4. IV-1   5. Nursing Process   6. Moderate

    Rationale: Because the patient is a quadriplegic and has no feeling in his arms, the priority diagnosis is Risk for Injury related to decreased pain sensation.

18. A patient with terminal cancer tells the nurse she has a great deal of pain and the medication is not working. She asks the nurse "I always tried to be a good person. Why is God punishing me like this?" A priority nursing diagnosis for the patient is
    a. Acute Pain related to ineffective analgesia
    b. Impaired Physical Mobility related to acute pain episode
    c. Risk of Self-Directed Violence related to loss of will to live
    d. Spiritual Distress related to belief that God is causing pain as punishment*

    Reference: p. 1055

    Descriptors:

    1. 40   2. 06   3. Application
    4. III-1   5. Nursing Process   6. Moderate

    Rationale: A priority nursing diagnosis for the patient is Spiritual Distress related to belief that God is causing pain as punishment.

19. The nurse has instructed a family member about caring for her father who is experiencing chronic pain and immobility from osteoarthritis. The nurse determines that the caregiver needs further instructions when the caregiver says
    a. "I should leave the room darkened with little stimuli."*
    b. "It's important to prevent him from becoming constipated."
    c. "I should encourage him to change positions frequently."
    d. "It's important that he be kept well hydrated throughout the day."

Reference: p. 1057

Descriptors:

1. 40   2. 07   3. Application
4. IV-1   5. Teach/Learn   6. Moderate

Rationale: The caregiver needs further instructions when the caregiver says "I should leave the room darkened with little stimuli." The patient needs some diversional activities.

20. The nurse is planning to instruct a patient with chronic pain from arthritis about the use of imagery to decrease pain sensation. The nurse should *first*
    a. ask the patient to take a cleansing deep breath
    b. identify the problem or goal*
    c. encourage images of the desired state of well-being
    d. inform the patient about therapeutic touch

    Reference: p. 1059

    Descriptors:

    1. 40   2. 07   3. Application
    4. IV-1   5. Nursing Process   6. Moderate

    Rationale: Before beginning imagery to decrease pain, the nurse should first identify the problem or goal with the patient.

21. The nurse is planning a presentation about relaxation techniques to a group of older adults. Which of the following would be important for the nurse to include in the teaching plan?
    a. Relaxation therapies do not provide distraction from pain.
    b. Acute pain benefits more from relaxation therapies than chronic pain.
    c. Relaxation is most effective when combined with slow, deep breathing.*
    d. Massage during relaxation techniques improves the effectiveness.

    Reference: p. 1059

    Descriptors:

    1. 40   2. 07   3. Application
    4. II-2   5. Teach/Learn   6. Moderate

    Rationale: Relaxation is most effective when combined with slow, deep-breathing techniques.

22. Which of the following is true among pain management practices among physicians and nurses?
    a. Physicians frequently prescribe higher analgesic doses than necessary.
    b. Nurses frequently overestimate the patient's need for pain medication.
    c. Nurses frequently give low priority to a patient's pain management.*
    d. Physicians frequently underestimate the duration of analgesics.

Reference: p. 1062

Descriptors:

1. 40	2. 09	3. Application
4. I-1	5. Caring	6. Moderate

Rationale: Nurses and physicians frequently give low priority to a patient's pain management.

23. The nurse is planning to instruct a patient about the use of nonsteroidal anti-inflammatory analgesics for arthritis pain. Which of the following should be included in the teaching plan?
    a. Patients with gastric ulcers can take these medications safely.
    b. Respiratory depression is a common side effect of these medications.
    c. Constipation can result from overuse of these medications.
    d. These medications can cause gastric irritation.*

Reference: p. 1062

Descriptors:

1. 40	2. 05	3. Application
4. IV-2	5. Teach/Learn	6. Moderate

Rationale: Nonsteroidal anti-inflammatory medications can cause bleeding and gastric irritation.

24. The nurse assesses a patient 3 hours after the patient received morphine for pain. The nurse determines that the patient's sedation level is 3. The nurse should
    a. contact the physician for an order for naloxone
    b. withhold the next dose of medication until the patient is less sedated*
    c. assess the patient's pulse rate for a full minute
    d. stimulate the patient and ask him to breathe deeply

Reference: p. 1062

Descriptors:

1. 40	2. 08	3. Application
4. IV-2	5. Nursing Process	6. Moderate

Rationale: For a patient with a level 3 sedation, the nurse should withhold the next dose of medication until the patient is less sedated.

25. A patient with terminal bone cancer has been taking a prescribed opioid medication for pain relief for 2 months. The nurse should assess the patient for
    a. constipation*
    b. respiratory depression
    c. addiction
    d. hypertension

Reference: p. 1062

Descriptors:

1. 40	2. 08	3. Application
4. IV-2	5. Nursing Process	6. Moderate

Rationale: Opioid medications can cause constipation.

26. Prior to giving a hospitalized 75-year-old patient an injection of morphine for pain, the nurse must assess the patient's
    a. heart rate
    b. respiratory rate*
    c. presence of pain
    d. temperature

Reference: p. 1062

Descriptors:

1. 40	2. 08	3. Application
4. IV-2	5. Nursing Process	6. Moderate

Rationale: Morphine can suppress a patient's respirations.

27. An Asian American patient appears in obvious pain following abdominal surgery; however, he rarely asks for pain medication. The nurse should instruct the patient that for the analgesic to be the most effective, the patient should
    a. ask for the medication only when the pain is severe
    b. take the medication every 4 hours as ordered
    c. request pain medication before the pain gets severe*
    d. take the pain medication only if other measures are ineffective

Reference: p. 1063

Descriptors:

1. 40	2. 04	3. Application
4. IV-2	5. Teach/Learn	6. Moderate

Rationale: For the medication to have its greatest effect, the patient should request pain medication before the pain gets severe.

28. A patient is transferred from the operating room to the nursing unit following abdominal surgery. The patient has a continuous epidural infusion in place for analgesia. The nurse should assess the patient for
    a. urine retention*
    b. hallucinations
    c. hypertension
    d. tremors

Reference: p. 1069

Descriptors:

1. 40	2. 08	3. Application
4. IV-2	5. Nursing Process	6. Moderate

Rationale: The bladder can be full and the patient would not feel any sensation, so the nurse should assess for urinary retention.

29. A patient with terminal cancer is being treated with continuous morphine epidural anesthesia. The nurse should tell the caregiver that an appropriate drug to have on hand in case of respiratory depression is
    a. thorazine
    b. naproxen
    c. meperidine
    d. naloxone*

Reference: p. 1062

Descriptors:

1. 40	2. 10	3. Application
4. IV-2	5. Teach/Learn	6. Moderate

Rationale: Respiratory depression due to morphine can be treated with naloxone (Narcan).

30. A patient has an intravenous patient-controlled analgesia pump (PCA) with morphine following thoracic surgery. The nurse should instruct the patient that one of the primary advantages of PCA is that
    a. the patient can administer the medication whenever the patient desires
    b. a family member can help with administration of the medication
    c. the nurse can more accurately assess the effectiveness of the analgesia
    d. consistent analgesic blood levels of the drug are maintained*

Reference: p. 1066

Descriptors:

1. 40	2. 10	3. Application
4. IV-2	5. Teach/Learn	6. Moderate

Rationale: One of the primary advantages of PCA is that consistent analgesic blood levels of the drug are maintained.

CHAPTER 41

Nutrition

1. The study of nutrients and how they are handled by the body is termed
   a. science
   b. nutrition*
   c. energy
   d. carbohydrates
   Reference: p. 1080
   Descriptors:

1. 41	2. 01	3. Knowledge
4. None	5. None	6. Easy

   Rationale: The science of nutrition encompasses the study of nutrients and how they are handled by the body, as well as the impact of human behavior and environment on the process of nourishment.

2. Biochemical substances used by the body for growth and development include
   a. carbohydrates
   b. vitamins
   c. minerals
   d. nutrients*
   Reference: p. 1080
   Descriptors:

1. 41	2. 01	3. Knowledge
4. None	5. None	6. Easy

   Rationale: Nutrients are specific biochemical substances used by the body for growth, development, activity, reproduction, lactation, health maintenance, and recovery from illness or injury.

3. Vitamins and minerals required in small amounts to regulate and control body processes are termed
   a. carbohydrates
   b. vitamins
   c. micronutrients*
   d. macronutrients

   Reference: p. 1080
   Descriptors:

1. 41	2. 01	3. Knowledge
4. None	5. None	6. Easy

   Rationale: Micronutrients, such as vitamins and minerals, are required in much smaller amounts to regulate and control body processes.

4. A patient consumes a diet with 55 grams of fat, 200 grams of carbohydrate, and 50 grams of protein. How many calories has the patient consumed from fat?
   a. 110 calories
   b. 495 calories*
   c. 220 calories
   d. 385 calories
   Reference: p. 1081
   Descriptors:

1. 41	2. 06	3. Comprehensive
4. II-2	5. Nursing Process	6. Moderate

   Rationale: The number of calories per gram of fat is 9. This assessment is important to determine if the patient is at risk for cardiovascular disease.

5. A person experiencing stress will have
   a. an increased basal metabolic rate*
   b. a decreased basal metabolic rate
   c. to use food to cope with the stress
   d. an increased amount of calories
   Reference: p. 1081
   Descriptors:

1. 41	2. 06	3. Application
4. III-1	5. Nursing Process	6. Moderate

   Rationale: The patient's basal metabolic rate will increase during stress.

6. A major difficulty with height and weight measurement charts is that they do not represent the
   a. male population
   b. female population
   c. minority population*
   d. young population

   Reference: p. 1081

   Descriptors:

1. 41	2. 05	3. Knowledge
4. None	5. None	6. Moderate

   Rationale: The standard height and weight measurement charts do not represent the minority population in the United States.

7. A 42-year-old female patient has a cholesterol of 200 and body mass index (BMI) of 31. The patient should be educated to
   a. stop gaining weight
   b. consume diary products
   c. lose 10% of body weight*
   d. have a stress test performed

   Reference: p. 1081

   Descriptors:

1. 41	2. 04	3. Application
4. IV-3	5.Teach/Learn	6. Moderate

   Rationale: A patient with a BMI above 29 with risk factors such as high blood pressure or elevated cholesterol should lose 10% of body weight.

8. An obese 50-year-old male patient would like to lose 2 pounds per week for the next 10 weeks. What is the most important diet aspect the nurse should teach? The patient should
   a. eat 1500 calories per day
   b. maintain current exercise schedule
   c. drink dietary supplements from herbs
   d. consume 1000 calories less per day*

   Reference: p. 1082

   Descriptors:

1. 41	2. 05	3. Application
4. II-2	5. Teach/Learn	6. Moderate

   Rationale: To lose 2 pounds per week the patient should reduce food intake by 1000 calories per day.

9. The most abundant source of calories in the diet is in the form of
   a. vitamins
   b. carbohydrates*
   c. protein
   d. fat

   Reference: p. 1082

   Descriptors:

1. 41	2. 03	3. Knowledge
4. None	5. None	6. Easy

   Rationale: Calories from carbohydrates may contribute to as much as 90% of total calories.

10. A patient is trying to reduce her weight by 6 pounds over the next 3 weeks. Her normal caloric intake is 1800 calories per day. The nurse should help the patient plan a diet with a caloric intake of
    a. 900 calories
    b. 1100 calories
    c. 1200 calories
    d. 1300 calories*

    Reference: p. 1082

    Descriptors:

1. 41	2. 01	3. Application
4. II-2	5. Nursing Process	6. Moderate

    Rationale: To lose 6 pounds in 3 weeks the patient should reduce her 1800-calorie diet to a diet containing 1300 calories.

11. A diabetic patient with hypoglycemia needs an immediate source of sugar to raise his blood sugar level. The nurse should offer the patient a
    a. polysaccharide
    b. triglyceride
    c. monosaccharide*
    d. disaccharide

    Reference: p. 1082

    Descriptors:

1. 41	2. 02	3. Application
4. IV-3	5. Nursing Process	6. Moderate

    Rationale: Monosaccharides are digested quickly and will raise the patient's blood sugar level.

12. In human beings, the hormones responsible for keeping serum glucose levels fairly constant during both feasting and fasting are insulin and
    a. adrenaline
    b. glucagon*
    c. thyroxine
    d. creatinine

Reference: p. 1082

Descriptors:

1. 41	2. 01	3. Application
4. None	5. None	6. Moderate

Rationale: The hormones responsible for keeping blood glucose steady are insulin and glucagon.

13. A patient following a vegetarian diet asks the nurse what he can do to get more protein with a meal that consists of a corn tortilla and refried beans. The nurse should suggest complementary protein such as
    a. lettuce and tomato salad
    b. cooked spinach
    c. lentil rice soup*
    d. granola bar

Reference: p. 1083

Descriptors:

1. 41	2. 02	3. Application
4. IV-3	5. Teach/Learn	6. Moderate

Rationale: Legumes or lentil soup is a complimentary protein.

14. In the body, carbohydrates are converted to
    a. glucose*
    b. fat
    c. sodium
    d. nitrogen

Reference: pp. 1082–1083

Descriptors:

1. 41	2. 01	3. Knowledge
4. None	5. None	6. Easy

Rationale: Carbohydrates are converted to glucose so they can be transported and used for energy.

15. The amount of carbohydrates needed to prevent ketosis is
    a. 25 to 50 grams
    b. 50 to 100 grams*
    c. 75 to 100 grams
    d. 100 to 125 grams

Reference: p. 1083

Descriptors:

1. 41	2. 02	3. Knowledge
4. None	5. None	6. Moderate

Rationale: At least 50 to 100 grams of carbohydrates is needed to prevent ketosis.

16. Recommendations for the average daily amounts that healthy population groups should consume over time are the
    a. recommended dietary allowances*
    b. Food Guide Pyramid
    c. essential vitamins and minerals
    d. American dietetic allowances

Reference: p. 1083

Descriptors:

1. 41	2. 01	3. Knowledge
4. None	5. None	6. Moderate

Rationale: The recommended dietary allowance of essential nutrients refers to recommendations for average daily amounts that healthy population groups should consume over time.

17. A patient with a draining decubitus ulcer requires a diet with an increased amount of
    a. vitamins
    b. carbohydrates
    c. fats
    d. proteins*

Reference: p. 1085

Descriptors:

1. 41	2. 08	3. Application
4. IV-3	5. Nursing Process	6. Difficult

Rationale: Proteins are essential for the formation of all body structures, including genes, enzymes, muscle, bone matrix, and hemoglobin.

18. Of the following foods, which is a complete protein?
    a. eggs*
    b. carrots
    c. squash
    d. cereal

Reference: pp. 1083–1084

Descriptors:

1. 41	2. 03	3. Application
4. None	5. None	6. Moderate

Rationale: Complete dietary proteins contain sufficient amounts and proportions of all the essential amino acids to support growth. Generally, animal proteins (eggs, dairy products, and meats) are complete.

19. One month following major abdominal surgery, an 80-year-old patient tells the nurse that she has lost 20 pounds. The nurse should assess the patient for
    a. positive nitrogen balance
    b. negative nitrogen balance*
    c. anabolism
    d. catabolism

    Reference: p. 1085

    Descriptors:

1. 41	2. 02	3. Application
4. IV-3	5. Nursing Process	6. Moderate

    Rationale: Because of the patient's recent weight loss, the nurse should assess the patient for a negative nitrogen balance.

20. The nurse is planning a presentation to a group of adult patients on the topic of healthy diets. Which of the following would be important for the nurse to include in the teaching plan?
    a. Heart disease and obesity have been correlated with high-fat diets.*
    b. Protein deficiency is a widespread problem in the United States.
    c. Dietary experts recommend eating more animal protein and less vegetable protein.
    d. Carbohydrate intake should comprise only 30% of the daily diet.

    Reference: p. 1085

    Descriptors:

1. 41	2. 02	3. Application
4. II-1	5. Teach/Learn	6. Moderate

    Rationale: Heart disease and obesity have been correlated with high-fat diets.

21. The nurse is caring for a 4-year-old child who has had frequent infections during the last year. The nurse should instruct the patient's mother that to help ward off infections, the mother should offer the child foods that are high in
    a. carbohydrates
    b. calories
    c. protein*
    d. water-soluble fiber

    Reference: p. 1085

    Descriptors:

1. 41	2. 02	3. Application
4. II-2	5. Teach/Learn	6. Moderate

    Rationale: Foods that are high in protein will boost the child's immune system and prevent anemia.

22. A negative nitrogen balance is noted in which of the following situations?
    a. lactation
    b. growth
    c. edema
    d. trauma*

    Reference: p. 1085

    Descriptors:

1. 41	2. 06	3. Application
4. IV-4	5. Nursing Process	6. Moderate

    Rationale: A negative nitrogen balance, an undesirable state that occurs in situations such as starvation and the catabolism that immediately follows surgery, illness, trauma, and stress, indicates that more nitrogen is being excreted than consumed.

23. In developing countries, the leading cause of infant death is
    a. infection
    b. kwashiorkor*
    c. nystagmus
    d. pneumocystis

    Reference: p. 1085

    Descriptors:

1. 41	2. 04	3. Knowledge
4. None	5. None	6. Moderate

    Rationale: In developing countries, protein deficiency alone (kwashiokor) or combined (marasmus) is a leading cause of infant death.

24. Of the following foods, which contains cholesterol?
    a. olive oil
    b. eggs*
    c. corn
    d. fish

    Reference: p. 1086

    Descriptors:

1. 41	2. 01	3. Application
4. None	5. None	6. Moderate

    Rationale: Cholesterol is a fatlike substance found only in animal products.

25. Fat in the diet increases
    a. metabolism
    b. vitamins
    c. minerals
    d. palatability*

Reference: p. 1086

Descriptors:

1. 41	2. 03	3. Knowledge
4. None	5. None	6. Easy

Rationale: Fat increases the palatability of the diet.

26. An adult patient tells the nurse that he needs to increase his intake of water-soluble vitamins. The nurse assesses the patient to determine if he likes
    a. oatmeal
    b. wheat germ
    c. sunflower oil
    d. orange juice*

Reference: p. 1087

Descriptors:

1. 41	2. 03	3. Application
4. II-2	5. Teach/Learn	6. Moderate

Rationale: Orange juice is an excellent sourse of water soluble vitamins, especially vitamin C.

27. The nurse is caring for a patient who has been instructed about fat-soluble vitamins. The nurse determines that the patient understands the instructions when she says she should eat foods such as
    a. grapefruit juice
    b. seafood
    c. fortified milk*
    d. strawberries

Reference: p. 1087

Descriptors:

1. 41	2. 03	3. Application
4. II-2	5. Teach/Learn	6. Moderate

Rationale: Fortified milk contains vitamin D, which is a fat-soluble vitamin.

28. An adult patient has been diagnosed with biliary disease. An important nutritional assessment for the nurse to make for this patient is his intake of vitamin
    a. C
    b. B_{12}
    c. folate
    d. A*

Reference: p. 1086

Descriptors:

1. 41	2. 04	3. Application
4. IV-3	5. Nursing Process	6. Moderate

Rationale: Biliary disease can result in a deficiency of vitamin A.

29. Which of the following vitamins in the patient's diet is not stored?
    a. vitamin C*
    b. vitamin D
    c. vitamin E
    d. vitamin K

Reference: p. 1086

Descriptors:

1. 41	2. 03	3. Knowledge
4. None	5. None	6. Moderate

Rationale: Water-soluble vitamins include vitamin C and the B-complex vitamins. Because water-soluble vitamins are not stored, amounts consumed in excess of need are excreted in the urine.

30. When instructing a patient in food preparation, the nurse should
    a. discourage excess amounts of vitamin B complex in the diet
    b. discourage the soaking of foods due to mineral loss*
    c. have the patient always count the number of calories
    d. encourage a diet with large amounts of animal products

Reference: p. 1086

Descriptors:

1. 41	2. 04	3. Comprehensive
4. II-2	5. Teach/Learn	6. Difficult

Rationale: Excessive soaking and cooking in water can cause loss of minerals from food.

31. A patient with fatigue and pallor has been instructed by the nurse to consume foods that are high in folate. The nurse determines that the patient understands the instructions when the nurse observes the patient eating
    a. scrambled eggs
    b. spinach salad*
    c. whole grapefruit
    d. broccoli

Reference: p. 1087

Descriptors:

1. 41	2. 02	3. Application
4. II-2	5. Teach/Learn	6. Moderate

Rationale: Spinach is a food with a high folate content.

32. The nurse is caring for a patient who is on a fluid-restricted diet. The nurse should instruct the patient that
    a. large amounts of water are stored in the body
    b. most people have above average fluid intake
    c. water intake averages about 2000 mL daily
    d. solid foods may have a high water content*

    Reference: p. 1088

    Descriptors:

1. 41	2. 04	3. Application
4. IV-3	5. Teach/Learn	6. Moderate

    Rationale: Individuals on a fluid-restricted diet need to be aware that solid foods may have a high water content, for example, watermelon.

33. The major dietary problem noted in the United States is
    a. poverty
    b. malnutrition
    c. overnutrition*
    d. lifestyle

    Reference: p. 1088

    Descriptors:

1. 41	2. 04	3. Comprehensive
4. None	5. None	6. Moderate

    Rationale: Nutritional concerns in the United States focus on overnutrition.

34. The Food Guide Pyramid places the cereal and grain group
    a. near the peak
    b. with the vegetables
    c. at the base*
    d. with the fats

    Reference: p. 1090

    Descriptors:

1. 41	2. 03	3. Knowledge
4. None	5. None	6. Easy

    Rationale: The Food Guide Pyramid places the grain and cereal group at the base of the pyramid followed by the fruit and vegetable group.

35. The nurse is caring for a patient who complains of being thirsty and appears thin and dehydrated. The nurse explains to the patient that water loss can occur through urine, feces, expired air, and
    a. pancreatic secretions
    b. circulation
    c. perspiration*
    d. metabolism

    Reference: p. 1088

    Descriptors:

1. 41	2. 04	3. Application
4. IV-3	5. Teach/Learn	6. Moderate

    Rationale: Water loss can occur from perspiration.

36. A patient tells the nurse that she takes "lots of vitamins every day but seems to be losing her hair." The nurse should assess the patient's daily intake of vitamin
    a. A*
    b. folate
    c. B_{12}
    d. C

    Reference: p. 1087

    Descriptors:

1. 41	2. 02	3. Application
4. II-2	5. Nursing Process	6. Moderate

    Rationale: Hair loss can result from a deficiency in vitamin A.

37. A patient visits the Urgent Care Center and tells the nurse he has had chills, fever, nausea, and vomiting for 3 days and thinks he has the flu. The nurse should assess the patient for symptoms of
    a. adequate fiber intake
    b. chronic fatigue
    c. vitamin C deficiency
    d. dehydration*

    Reference: p. 1088

    Descriptors:

1. 41	2. 04	3. Application
4. IV-3	5. Nursing Process	6. Moderate

    Rationale: A patient who has had nausea and vomiting for 3 days should be assessed for dehydration.

38. A patient tells the nurse he needs to increase his intake of potassium. The nurse should instruct the patient that a good source of potassium is
    a. pork chops
    b. squash
    c. bananas*
    d. nuts

    Reference: p. 1089

    Descriptors:

1. 41	2. 02	3. Application
4. II-2	5. Teach/Learn	6. Moderate

    Rationale: A good source of potassium is a banana.

39. A patient tells the nurse that he needs more copper in his diet. The nurse should assess whether the patient likes
a. whole-grain bread
b. shellfish*
c. broccoli
d. carrots

Reference: p. 1089

Descriptors:

| 1. 41 | 2. 04 | 3. Application |
| 4. IV-3 | 5. Nursing Process | 6. Moderate |

Rationale: A good source of copper is shellfish such as shrimp and crabmeat.

40. An adult patient from Turkey is diagnosed with goiter. The nurse determines that the patient's diet was most likely deficient in
a. potassium
b. iron
c. iodine*
d. magnesium

Reference: p. 1089

Descriptors:

| 1. 41 | 2. 04 | 3. Application |
| 4. IV-3 | 5. Nursing Process | 6. Moderate |

Rationale: Goiter can result from a deficiency in iodine.

41. An adult female patient tells the nurse that her fingernails are brittle and she is experiencing fatigue although she gets 9 to 10 hours of sleep per night. The nurse should assess the patient's dietary intake of
a. selenium*
b. chromium
c. potassium
d. sodium

Reference: p. 1090

Descriptors:

| 1. 41 | 2. 04 | 3. Application |
| 4. II-1 | 5. Nursing Process | 6. Moderate |

Rationale: Brittle fingernails and toenails and fatigue are associated with selenium deficiency.

42. The nurse has instructed a group of high school students about the Food Guide Pyramid. Following the instructions, the nurse determines that one of the students needs further instructions when she says
a. "I should eat the minimum number of servings from the lower five groups."
b. "A serving size of meat equals 2½ to 3 ounces of cooked meat."
c. "Foods at the top of the pyramid should be eaten the most."*
d. "One serving of bread is equal to one slice of bread."

Reference: p. 1090

Descriptors:

| 1. 41 | 2. 03 | 3. Application |
| 4. II-1 | 5. Teach/Learn | 6. Moderate |

Rationale: Foods at the top of the pyramid (eg, fats) should be eaten the least.

43. A 65-year-old male patient who lives alone tells the nurse that he needs to decrease his sodium intake but doesn't know how to tell how much sodium is actually in the food he purchases. The nurse should instruct the patient to
a. buy a nutrition book
b. read the product labels*
c. check the RDA chart
d. follow the Food Guide Pyramid

Reference: pp. 1091–1092

Descriptors:

| 1. 41 | 2. 02 | 3. Application |
| 4. IV-3 | 5. Teach/Learn | 6. Moderate |

Rationale: The nurse should instruct the patient to read the food labels for the amount of sodium content.

44. An infant weighing 6 pounds 10 ounces at birth should weigh
a. 9 pounds at 6 months
b. 10 pounds at 6 months
c. 13 pounds at 6 months*
d. 16 pounds at 6 months

Reference: p. 1093

Descriptors:

| 1. 41 | 2. 05 | 3. Application |
| 4. II-1 | 5. Nursing Process | 6. Moderate |

Rationale: Birth weight doubles in 4 to 6 months and triples by 1 year of age.

45. At menarche, girls experience
   a. weight loss
   b. fat deposition*
   c. muscle mass
   d. weight loss

Reference: p. 1093

Descriptors:

1. 41	2. 05	3. Application
4. II-1	5. Nursing Process	6. Moderate

Rationale: At menarche, girls begin menstruation and experience fat deposition.

46. A mother brings her 15-year-old daughter to the clinic. She has lost 15 pounds in 3 weeks, complains of increased stress, and describes low self-esteem. The nurse practitioner suspects that this adolescent is suffering from
   a. overnutrition
   b. leukemia
   c. anorexia nervosa*
   d. bulimia

Reference: p. 1093

Descriptors:

1. 41	2. 04	3. Application
4. II-1	5. Nursing Process	6. Difficult

Rationale: Anorexia nervosa is characterized by extreme muscle wasting, weight loss, bizarre eating habits, and low self-esteem.

47. Of the following, which patient is at most nutritional risk?
   a. pregnant teenager*
   b. middle-aged adult
   c. adolescent
   d. pregnant woman

Reference: p. 1093

Descriptors:

1. 41	2. 04	3. Application
4. II-1	5. Nursing Process	6. Easy

Rationale: In teenage pregnancy, both mother and fetus are at increased nutritional risk.

48. A 58-year-old construction worker visits the occupational health nurse with the complaint of constipation. This symptom is related to
   a. increased fat intake
   b. decreased basal metabolic rate
   c. decreased peristalsis*
   d. increased alcohol intake

Reference: p. 1094

Descriptors:

1. 41	2. 05	3. Application
4. II-1	5. Nursing Process	6. Difficult

Rationale: Aging causes a decrease in peristalsis resulting in constipation.

49. An 85-year-old female patient complains of light-headedness and has a blood pressure of 88/50. It is important to assess
   a. fat intake
   b. carbohydrate intake
   c. vitamin intake
   d. fluid intake*

Reference: p. 1094

Descriptors:

1. 41	2. 06	3. Application
4. IV-3	5. Nursing Process	6. Difficult

Rationale: Elderly people are prone to dehydration and decreased interest in food.

50. The nurse plans to discuss nutritional needs with a group of adult patients. Which of the following would be important to include in the teaching plan?
   a. Adult women should have an intake of 200 mg of calcium daily.
   b. Adult men have higher iron requirements than women.
   c. Adult women require a greater number of calories than men.
   d. Adult men require higher protein and vitamin B intake than women.*

Reference: p. 1095

Descriptors:

1. 41	2. 05	3. Application
4. II-1	5. Teach/Learn	6. Moderate

Rationale: Adult men require higher protein and vitamin B complex intake than women. Women need fewer calories and more iron in their diets.

51. An adult patient with moderate obesity is taking prescription medications for hypertension and he tells the nurse he suffers from constipation. The nurse should suggest to the patient that he
   a. chew his food thoroughly
   b. avoid spicy foods
   c. eat foods that are soft
   d. increase his fluid intake*

Reference: p. 1095

Descriptors:

| 1. 41 | 2. 05 | 3. Application |
| 4. IV-3 | 5. Teach/Learn | 6. Moderate |

Rationale: Increased fluid, fiber, and exercise can help to minimize constipation.

52. The nurse is caring for a patient who has been diagnosed with hypoglycemia. The nurse should instruct the patient to
a. decrease protein intake
b. eat 3 large meals daily with no snacks
c. avoid sugar-rich foods*
d. take a multivitamin supplement

Reference: p. 1105

Descriptors:

| 1. 41 | 2. 09 | 3. Application |
| 4. IV-3 | 5. Teach/Learn | 6. Moderate |

Rationale: A patient who is diagnosed with hypoglycemia should avoid sugar-rich foods and eat 6 to 8 smaller meals per day.

53. A patient tells the nurse that her 15-month-old child has developed erratic eating patterns and frequently goes on a food jag requesting only "tater tots and chicken nuggets." The nurse should instruct the patient that the child
a. is exhibiting normal behavior for this age group*
b. needs to be assessed for iron-deficiency anemia
c. may not be receiving adequate protein
d. will develop poor nutritional habits later in life

Reference: p. 1093

Descriptors:

| 1. 41 | 2. 05 | 3. Application |
| 4. II-1 | 5. Teach/Learn | 6. Moderate |

Rationale: Toddlers frequently develop food jags and eat only one specific food for a period of time. This is normal and the child typically outgrows the behavior.

54. The nurse is planning to conduct a nutrition class for a group of parents with third- and fourth-grade children. Which of the following would be important to include in the teaching plan?
a. Children of this age group have a dramatic decrease in their appetites.
b. Fluoride, vitamins A and D, and calcium are important for dental health.*
c. Nutrient needs decrease toward the end of the school-age period.
d. Food attitudes develop later on in the child's life.

Reference: pp. 1089–1090

Descriptors:

| 1. 41 | 2. 05 | 3. Application |
| 4. II-1 | 5. Teach/Learn | 6. Moderate |

Rationale: Fluoride, vitamins A and D, and calcium are important for dental health for this age group. Nutrient needs increase as the child grows older.

55. The nurse is caring for a patient who has just learned that she is about 10 weeks pregnant. Which of the following would be important for the nurse to include when counseling the patient about nutritional needs during pregnancy? During pregnancy,
a. a weight gain of 6 to 8 pounds during the first trimester is recommended
b. iron supplements are usually necessary to prevent iron-deficiency anemia*
c. the amount of weight gained is more important than the pattern of weight gain
d. key nutrients include carbohydrates and fats for the developing fetus

Reference: p. 1093

Descriptors:

| 1. 41 | 2. 05 | 3. Application |
| 4. II-1 | 5. Teach/Learn | 6. Moderate |

Rationale: Iron supplements, and sometimes folic acid supplements, are prescribed to prevent deficiencies. The pattern of weight gain is more important than the total amount, although pregnant women should gain 25 to 35 pounds.

56. The nurse is caring for an alert 79-year-old patient who appears to have a decreased appetite and refuses to eat any meat. The nurse should assess the patient for symptoms of
a. gastrointestinal distress
b. diarrhea or loose stools
c. metabolic disorders
d. periodontal or jaw disease*

Reference: p. 1087

Descriptors:

1. 41	2. 05	3. Application
4. II-1	5. Nursing Process	6. Moderate

Rationale: In older people, periodontal, jaw disease, or poorly fitting dentures can cause them to lose their appetite or not eat meat because they cannot chew properly.

57. The nurse makes a home visit to an 86-year-old patient who is being cared for by her daughter. The daughter tells the nurse that she is concerned because her mother uses a large amount of salt on all of her food. The nurse should explain to the daughter that
    a. as people age, the taste threshold for sugar and salt increases*
    b. the patient may develop gallstones if salt intake is not decreased
    c. salt should be removed from the patient's dietary intake
    d. excessive salt intake may lead to urinary frequency

Reference: p. 1094

Descriptors:

1. 41	2. 05	3. Application
4. II-1	5. Teach/Learn	6. Moderate

Rationale: As people age, the taste threshold for sugar and salt increases.

58. The nurse is caring for an adult patient who practices Orthodox Judaism and adheres to a Kosher diet. To increase the patient's protein intake, the nurse should recommend that the patient consume
    a. a ham sandwich
    b. crabcakes on rice
    c. shrimp cocktail
    d. roast beef*

Reference: p. 1095

Descriptors:

1. 41	2. 08	3. Application
4. IV-1	5. Cultural	6. Moderate

Rationale: Orthodox Jewish people avoid shellfish and pork products. Roast beef is the best choice.

59. Alcohol consumption requires the increased need for
    a. vitamin A
    b. vitamin C
    c. vitamin B complex*
    d. vitamin E

Reference: p. 1095

Descriptors:

1. 41	2. 07	3. Application
4. IV-3	5. Nursing Process	6. Difficult

Rationale: The need for vitamin B increases because it is used to metabolize alcohol.

60. A 16-year-old girl visits the clinic with her mother because the patient has developed bizarre eating patterns, such as binge eating and then vomiting. The nurse determines that the patient is most likely experiencing
    a. bulimia*
    b. yo-yo dieting
    c. anorexia nervosa
    d. normal adolescent rebellion

Reference: p. 1096

Descriptors:

1. 41	2. 05	3. Application
4. II-1	5. Nursing Process	6. Moderate

Rationale: Bulimia is associated with starvation, binge eating, and purging or vomiting in an effort to be thin.

61. The nurse is caring for a patient who has recently moved to the United States from Italy. The nurse should assess the patient for a dietary deficiency of
    a. calcium*
    b. protein
    c. vitamin C
    d. carbohydrates

Reference: p. 1096

Descriptors:

1. 41	2. 07	3. Application
4. II-1	5. Cultural	6. Moderate

Rationale: Milk and milk products may not have been readily available in the patient's home country of Italy, so an assessment of the patient's calcium intake is warranted.

62. The nurse is caring for a hospitalized postoperative patient from Greece who has just been ordered a regular diet. While assisting the patient to complete his diet menu, the nurse should suggest that the patient choose
    a. bacon and tomato sandwich
    b. broiled lamb chops*
    c. spaghetti with meat sauce
    d. ham and cheese sandwich

Reference: p. 1096

Descriptors:

1. 41	2. 08	3. Application
4. IV-1	5. Cultural	6. Moderate

Rationale: Lamb and veal are plentiful in Greece and this would provide the patient with added protein, necessary for healing.

63. An obese patient visits the clinic and expresses a desire to be placed on a weight loss program. To begin collecting dietary data on the patient, the nurse should
   a. determine if the patient is really motivated to diet
   b. ask the patient about food likes and dislikes
   c. determine if the patient takes vitamin and mineral supplements
   d. ask about foods eaten in the last 24 hours*

Reference: p. 1098

Descriptors:

1. 41	2. 08	3. Application
4. IV-3	5. Nursing Process	6. Moderate

Rationale: Most individuals can provide a 24-hour dietary recall, but keeping a food diary for 3 to 7 days can provide the best data for dietary assessment.

64. A thorough assessment of the patient's dietary habits is best accomplished with
   a. asking the family what the patient ate
   b. a 3- to 7-day food diary*
   c. verbal recall by the patient
   d. determining who does the cooking

Reference: p. 1098

Descriptors:

1. 41	2. 06	3. Application
4. IV-1	5. Nursing Process	6. Easy

Rationale: Food frequency or food diaries may provide a better overall picture of nutrient intake because the patient records all food and beverage consumed in a specified period, usually 3 to 7 days.

65. Height and weight are examples of
   a. caloric restrictions
   b. laboratory values
   c. anthropometric measures*
   d. nutritional assessments

Reference: p. 1099

Descriptors:

1. 41	2. 06	3. Comprehensive
4. None	5. None	6. Easy

Rationale: Anthropometric measurements are used to determine body dimensions.

66. The product of the breakdown of amino acids is
   a. urea*
   b. creatinine
   c. lipoproteins
   d. hemoglobin

Reference: p. 1100

Descriptors:

1. 41	2. 06	3. Knowledge
4. None	5. None	6. Easy

Rationale: Urea is the breakdown product of amino acids, which can be measured in the urine and blood.

67. The nurse makes a home visit to a 67-year-old postoperative patient who tells the nurse that she has "lost a lot of weight since the surgery." To obtain anthropometric data from the patient, the nurse should
   a. measure skin folds from several body sites*
   b. ask the patient to recall foods consumed over the last 24 hours
   c. determine the patient's current weight
   d. gather information about medication usage

Reference: p. 1101

Descriptors:

1. 41	2. 06	3. Application
4. IV-3	5. Nursing Process	6. Moderate

Rationale: Anthropometric data are obtained by measuring the patient's skin folds from various sites on the body.

68. An obese female patient diagnosed with hypertension has been placed on a 1200-calorie low-fat diet and prescribed medications. The patient asks the nurse to tell her about what kinds of foods she should cook. A priority nursing diagnosis for this patient is
   a. Alteration in Nutrition: More than Body Requirements related to poor metabolism
   b. Altered Health Maintenance related to hypertension and medications
   c. Knowledge Deficit related to lack of information about low-fat foods*
   d. Obesity related to inappropriate eating patterns and decreased activity

Reference: p. 1101

Descriptors:

1. 41	2. 07	3. Application
4. II-2	5. Nursing Process	6. Moderate

Rationale: The priority nursing diagnosis is Knowledge Deficit related to lack of information about low-fat foods because the patient is requesting such information.

69. A 48-year-old patient visits the clinic 4 weeks after being placed on a weight reduction and exercise program. The patient has gained 2 pounds since the last visit. She tells the nurse that she enjoys eating and frequently goes out with her friends for lunch and exercises infrequently. A priority nursing diagnosis for this patient is
   a. Noncompliance with Low-Calorie Diet and Exercise Program related to lack of motivation*
   b. Knowledge Deficit related to lack of interest in appropriate nutrition and need for exercise
   c. Altered Nutrition: More than Body Requirements related to inability to maintain proper weight
   d. Altered Nutrition related to overeating and lack of exercise in daily activities

Reference: p. 1101

Descriptors:

1. 41	2. 07	3. Application
4. II-2	5. Nursing Process	6. Moderate

Rationale: The priority nursing diagnosis is Noncompliance with Low-Calorie Diet and Exercise Program related to lack of motivation.

70. A 20-year-old patient tells the nurse that she has been on a 1200-calorie diet for the last month and lately has become very fatigued when walking from the parking lot to her office. A laboratory value that the nurse should assess is the patient's
   a. blood urea nitrogen
   b. serum albumin
   c. hemoglobin*
   d. total lymphocyte count

Reference: p. 1100

Descriptors:

1. 41	2. 09	3. Application
4. IV-3	5. Nursing Process	6. Moderate

Rationale: Fatigue is associated with anemia and the patient should have her hemoglobin and hematocrit assessed.

71. A 22-year-old patient visits the clinic and tells the nurse that although she has been on a 1200-calorie diet for the last month, she continues to gain weight. The patient also complains of fatigue, dry skin, and amenorrhea. The nurse suspects the patient may be experiencing a deficiency of
   a. albumin
   b. thyroxine*
   c. glucose
   d. lipase

Reference: p. 1103

Descriptors:

1. 41	2. 04	3. Comprehensive
4. IV-3	5. Nursing Process	6. Moderate

Rationale: The patient's symptoms are associated with hypothyroidism or a deficiency of thyroxine.

72. The nurse is caring for a postoperative patient following bowel surgery when the patient tells the nurse that she has had several frothy stools and has lost 10 pounds since the surgery. The patient appears fatigued and malnourished. An important laboratory value for the nurse to assess is the patient's
   a. basal metabolic rate
   b. serum thyroxine
   c. serum magnesium
   d. serum albumin*

Reference: p. 1103

Descriptors:

1. 41	2. 04	3. Application
4. IV-3	5. Nursing Process	6. Moderate

Rationale: The patient's symptoms are associated with low serum albumin (protein) levels.

73. After instructing a patient and his wife about low-fat, low-calorie foods, the nurse determines that the patient has understood the instructions when he says
   a. "I should avoid drinking all beverages with caffeine."
   b. "I shouldn't eat sandwiches made with bologna."*
   c. "A granola bar once a day is acceptable for a snack."
   d. "I should eat cheese at least twice a day."

Reference: pp. 1089, 1091

Descriptors:

1. 41   2. 06   3. Application

4. IV-3   5. Teach/Learn   6. Moderate

Rationale: Processed meats, such as ham and bologna are high in fat and calories. Granola bars and some cheeses are high in fat and calories.

74. The nurse visits an 84-year-old patient whose husband is caring for the patient following abdominal surgery. The husband tells the nurse that his wife has a poor appetite and seems to be losing weight. After giving suggestions for stimulating the patient's appetite, the nurse determines that the husband needs further instructions when he says

a. "It doesn't matter what the food looks like, as long as it tastes good."*

b. "It's important to offer alternatives if she doesn't like what I've served her."

c. "I should avoid giving her medications just prior to giving her a meal."

d. "Small, frequent meals and snacks may be better than three large meals."

Reference: p. 1104

Descriptors:

1. 41   2. 09   3. Application

4. II-1   5. Teach/Learn   6. Moderate

Rationale: Eating a meal begins with one's eyes and nose. If the food doesn't look or smell appealing, the patient will not want to eat it.

75. An adult patient hospitalized following cardiac surgery has been instructed about a clear liquid diet. The nurse determines that the patient understands the instructions when the patient when he says he can have

a. milk shakes

b. pineapple juice

c. lime gelatin*

d. frozen yogurt

Reference: p. 1106

Descriptors:

1. 41   2. 09   3. Application

4. IV-3   5. Teach/Learn   6. Moderate

Rationale: A clear liquid diet includes broths, gelatin, and water.

76. The nurse visits a patient at home who will be on a full liquid diet for 4 days after abdominal surgery. The nurse should suggest to the patient that he increase his intake of

a. pureed squash

b. chicken broth

c. melted cheese sandwiches

d. protein supplements*

Reference: p. 1106

Descriptors:

1. 41   2. 07   3. Application

4. IV-3   5. Teach/Learn   6. Moderate

Rationale: A full liquid diet includes protein supplements so the patient doesn't develop anemia. Other foods that can be included are milk shakes, ice cream, and frozen yogurt products.

77. A patient tells the nurse that she is a vegetarian and asks whether additional vitamins are necessary. The nurse should instruct the patient that she may need to supplement the vegetarian diet with

a. iron*

b. magnesium

c. calcium

d. vitamin C

Reference: p. 1106

Descriptors:

1. 41   2. 08   3. Application

4. II-2   5. Teach/Learn   6. Moderate

Rationale: Because vegetarian diets do not include meat products, the diet may be deficient in protein and iron.

78. The nurse has instructed a patient and family members about the nasal intestinal tube feedings the patient will need after surgery. The nurse determines that the patient understands the instructions when the patient says

a. "This type of feeding is appropriate if I don't have any appetite."

b. "Nasal intestinal tube feedings often can result in aspiration."

c. "Dumping syndrome may occur with this type of feeding."*

d. "I may develop hypercalcemia with this type of feeding."

Reference: p. 1106

Descriptors:

| 1. 41 | 2. 09 | 3. Application |
| 4. IV-1 | 5. Teach/Learn | 6. Moderate |

Rationale: Dumping syndrome is common in patients receiving nasal tube feedings. Aspiration is a risk, but it is not common.

79. The nurse is caring for a patient who has a nasogastric tube for intermittent feedings. Before beginning the next feeding the nurse plans to
a. prepare the patient for an x-ray examination
b. measure the pH of the stomach aspirate*
c. remove air from the tubing
d. flush the tube with sterile water

Reference: p. 1109

Descriptors:

| 1. 41 | 2. 08 | 3. Application |
| 4. IV-1 | 5. Nursing Process | 6. Moderate |

Rationale: Before beginning the next feeding, the nurse should measure the pH of the contents to be certain that the tube is still in the patient's stomach and not the lungs.

80. The nurse is preparing to insert a rubber nasogastric tube into an adult patient. Before beginning the insertion the nurse should first
a. position the patient in a side-lying position
b. measure the distance from the patient's nostril to the xiphoid process
c. don sterile gloves after opening the tube package
d. place the tube in a basin with ice for 5 to 10 minutes*

Reference: p. 1107

Descriptors:

| 1. 41 | 2. 08 | 3. Application |
| 4. IV-1 | 5. Nursing Process | 6. Moderate |

Rationale: The nurse should first place the tubing in ice, which will make insertion of the tubing easier.

81. While inserting a nasogastric tube into an adult patient, the patient begins to gag. The nurse should
a. instruct the patient to take deep breaths for several minutes
b. check the tube position with a tongue blade and flashlight*
c. discontinue the procedure and remove the tubing
d. ask the patient to hold his neck in a hyperextended position

Reference: p. 1108

Descriptors:

| 1. 41 | 2. 08 | 3. Application |
| 4. IV-1 | 5. Nursing Process | 6. Moderate |

Rationale: If the patient begins to gag, the nurse should check the tube position with a tongue blade and flashlight to be certain the tube is in the esophagus.

82. The nurse is caring for a patient with nasogastric tube feedings. After several attempts to aspirate gastrointestinal fluid from the tube with a syringe, the nurse has been unsuccessful in obtaining fluid. The nurse should
a. remove the tube and reinsert a new nasogastric tube
b. flush the tube with 100 mL of water
c. change the patient's position and raise the head of the bed*
d. instill air and leave the large syringe in place for 2 hours

Reference: p. 1112

Descriptors:

| 1. 41 | 2. 08 | 3. Application |
| 4. IV-1 | 5. Nursing Process | 6. Moderate |

Rationale: To try to obtain fluid from the tube, the nurse should change the patient's position and raise the head of the bed.

83. The nurse is caring for a patient who is receiving intermittent feedings through a nasogastric tube. The nurse has aspirated the gastric contents and measured 120 mL of residual fluid. The nurse should
a. report these findings to the patient's physician*
b. inform the oncoming nurse during the shift report
c. dispose of the gastric contents in the patient's commode
d. flush the tube with 110 mL of sterile water

Reference: p. 1113

Descriptors:

1. 41	2. 08	3. Application
4. IV-1	5. Nursing Process	6. Moderate

Rationale: A residual of 100 mL or more should be reported to the physician immediately because the feeding is not being digested.

84. The nurse is caring for a patient who is receiving continuous feedings through a nasogastric tube. While caring for this patient the nurse plans to
   a. hang the feeding solution 20 inches above the patient's stomach
   b. check the tubing for residual every 4 to 8 hours*
   c. ask the patient to remain in a supine position for 1 hour after the feeding
   d. assess for bowel sounds every hour

Reference: p. 1114

Descriptors:

1. 41	2. 09	3. Application
4. IV-1	5. Nursing Process	6. Moderate

Rationale: The tubing should be flushed every 4 hours and the residual should be checked every 4 to 8 hours.

85. The nurse has instructed a caregiver of a patient how to administer tube feedings through a jejunostomy tube. The nurse determines that the caregiver needs further instructions when the caregiver says
   a. "I should refrigerate the formula and discard it after 24 hours."
   b. "If the skin around the area becomes reddened, I should cleanse the area."*
   c. "I should change the delivery set every 24 hours using aseptic technique."
   d. "I should flush the tube with water before and after feeding."

Reference: p. 1116

Descriptors:

1. 41	2. 09	3. Application
4. IV-1	5. Teach/Learn	6. Moderate

Rationale: Reddened skin may indicate an infectious process and should be reported to the physician.

86. When the nurse prepares to remove a nasogastric feeding tube from an adult patient, the nurse should
   a. instruct the patient to take a deep breath and hold it*
   b. don sterile gloves before beginning the procedure
   c. inject 50 mL of sterile water to clear the tube
   d. remove the tube slowly while the patient exhales deeply

Reference: p. 1118

Descriptors:

1. 41	2. 09	3. Application
4. IV-1	5. Teach/Learn	6. Moderate

Rationale: The nurse who is discontinuing a tube feeding should instruct the patient to take a deep breath and hold it while the nurse removes the tube. The nurse should wear clean gloves.

87. The nurse is caring for a hospitalized patient who has a Salem sump tube in place for decompression following surgery. The nurse plans to
   a. flush the tube with 30 mL of sterile water every 4 hours
   b. remove 60 mL of air from the air vent on the tube
   c. irrigate the tube with 30 mL of normal saline every 4 hours*
   d. position the patient in a side-lying position

Reference: p. 1119

Descriptors:

1. 41	2. 08	3. Application
4. IV-1	5. Nursing Process	6. Moderate

Rationale: The nurse should irrigate the Salem pump with 30 mL of normal saline every 4 hours to keep the tubing clear.

88. The nurse is caring for a patient who will be receiving parenteral nutrition through a central vein for several weeks. The nurse plans to
   a. weigh the patient once per shift
   b. monitor serum protein levels q. 8 hours
   c. assess blood glucose levels q. 6 hours*
   d. assess the patient for symptoms of hypercalcemia

Reference: p. 1120

Descriptors:

1. 41	2. 10	3. Application
4. IV-1	5. Nursing Process	6. Moderate

Rationale: Because of the high glucose content of the feeding solutions, the nurse should monitor the patient's blood glucose levels every 6 hours.

89. The nurse has instructed a moderately obese patient about a weight loss program. The patient will be receiving a 1200-calorie daily diet. The nurse determines that the patient needs further instructions when she says
    a. "I should keep low-calorie foods toward the front of the refrigerator."
    b. "It's important to try to lose at least 4 to 5 pounds per week."*
    c. "I shouldn't weigh myself too often during the week."
    d. "I should wait 10 minutes after feeling the urge to eat."

    Reference: p. 1082

    Descriptors:

1. 41	2. 09	3. Application
4. IV-1	5. Teach/Learn	6. Moderate

    Rationale: The patient needs further instructions when she says she should try to lose 4 to 5 pounds per week.

90. A patient who has been diagnosed with iron-deficiency anemia asks the nurse how to improve her hemoglobin levels. The nurse should instruct the patient to
    a. eat a source of heme iron at least once per day
    b. include a rich source of magnesium with every meal
    c. drink a cup of hot milk chocolate with every meal
    d. eat citrus fruits or cantaloupe with every meal*

    Reference: p. 1087

    Descriptors:

1. 41	2. 08	3. Application
4. II-2	5. Teach/Learn	6. Moderate

    Rationale: Citrus juices and fruits help absorb iron. The patient should get a minimum of 3 to 4 servings of foods high in iron daily.

91. A young mother tells the nurse that her 3½-year-old son consumes 1 to 2 quarts of milk daily and is a "picky eater." The nurse should assess the toddler for
    a. malabsorption syndrome
    b. failure to thrive syndrome
    c. malnutrition
    d. iron-deficiency anemia*

    Reference: p. 1093

    Descriptors:

1. 41	2. 04	3. Application
4. II-1	5. Nursing Process	6. Moderate

    Rationale: A child who consumes large quantities of milk and is a picky eater may not be getting enough protein and iron in the diet. Iron-deficiency anemia may result.

92. Hypothyroidism can lead to the establishment of which of the following nursing diagnoses?
    a. Altered Nutrition: Less than Body Requirements
    b. Altered Nutrition: More than Body Requirements*
    c. Altered Endocrine Status
    d. Altered Skin Integrity

    Reference: p. 1100

    Descriptors:

1. 41	2. 07	3. Application
4. IV-1	5. Nursing Process	6. Difficult

    Rationale: The diagnosis is Altered Nutrition: More than Body Requirements related to overeating manifested by the decreased basal metabolic rate associated with hypothyroidism.

93. Following an episode of vomiting, it is important to provide the patient with a
    a. clear liquid diet*
    b. full liquid diet
    c. soft diet
    d. regular diet

    Reference: p. 1088

    Descriptors:

1. 41	2. 07	3. Application
4. IV-1	5. Nursing Process	6. Moderate

    Rationale: A clear liquid diet after an episode of vomiting will help prevent dehydration and will often decrease the vomiting episodes.

94. The nurse is caring for a 3-year-old child with diarrhea. Which of the following foods should not be administered?
    a. applesauce
    b. bananas
    c. toast
    d. oranges*

Reference: p. 1106

Descriptors:

1. 41   2. 07 3   . Application

4. II-1   5. Nursing Process   6. Moderate

Rationale: A patient experiencing diarrhea should be advanced from liquids to the BRAT diet. The BRAT diet consists of bananas, rice, applesauce, and toast.

95. The administration of formula through a tube to provide nutrition is called
    a. oral feeding
    b. intravenous feeding
    c. enteral feeding*
    d. endogenous feeding

Reference: p. 1106

Descriptors:

1. 41   2. 07   3. Application

4. IV-1   5. Nursing Process   6. Moderate

Rationale: Enteral nutrition involves passing a tube into the gastrointestinal tract to administer a formula containing nutrients.

CHAPTER 42

Urinary Elimination

1. The most significant function of this organ of elimination is to maintain the composition and volume of body fluids. This organ is the
   a. kidney*
   b. bladder
   c. urethra
   d. ureters
   Reference: p. 1132
   Descriptors:

1. 42	2. 02	3. Knowledge
4. None	5. None	6. Easy

   Rationale: One of the more significant functions of the kidneys is to help maintain the composition and volume of body fluids.

2. The unit of the kidney that removes the end products of metabolism such as urea, creatinine, and uric acid is the
   a. glomerulus
   b. nephron*
   c. tubule
   d. bladder
   Reference: p. 1132
   Descriptors:

1. 42	2. 02	3. Knowledge
4. None	5. None	6. Easy

   Rationale: The nephron is the basic structural and functional unit of the kidney. Nephrons remove the end products of metabolism such as urea, creatinine, and uric acid.

3. The three layers of the bladder are called the
   a. abdominal muscle
   b. peritoneal muscle
   c. detrusor muscle*
   d. pelvic muscle
   Reference: p.1132
   Descriptors:

1. 42	2. 02	3. Knowledge
4. None	5. None	6. Easy

   Rationale: There are three layers of muscle tissue in the bladder: the inner longitudinal layer, the middle circular layer, and the outer longitudinal layer. These three layers are known as the detrusor muscle.

4. In human beings, as urine collects in the bladder, the desire to void is experienced due to stimulation of the
   a. sympathetic nervous system
   b. urinary meatus
   c. stretch receptors*
   d. external sphincter
   Reference: p. 1133
   Descriptors:

1. 42	2. 02	3. Knowledge
4. None	5. None	6. Moderate

   Rationale: In human beings, as urine collects in the bladder, the desire to void is experienced due to stimulation of the stretch receptors in the bladder.

5. An older adult patient tells the nurse that she is "very embarrassed and just not able to obtain a requested urine sample." The nurse determines that the patient's inability to obtain the sample is due to
   a. urinary retention related to the aging process
   b. small bladder capacity related to aging process
   c. inability to relax the restraining muscles of the bladder*
   d. loss of muscle tone in the bladder walls
   Reference: p. 1134
   Descriptors:

1.42	2. 03	3. Application
4. II-1	5. Nursing Process	6. Moderate

   Rationale: An inability to relax the restraining muscles of the walls of the bladder can prevent a patient from voiding.

6. The process of emptying the bladder is called voiding, urination, or
   a. evacuation
   b. expectoration
   c. micturition*
   d. evacuation
   Reference: p. 1133
   Descriptors:
   1. 42   2. 02   3. Knowledge
   4. None   5. None   6. Easy
   Rationale: The process of emptying the bladder is known as micturition, voiding, or urination.

7. A 30-year-old pregnant woman states to the nurse, "I don't know what is wrong with me. Every time I cough I urinate." The nurse's best response is
   a. "What you are describing is called urinary incontinence. That often happens due to the pressure of the fetus on the bladder."*
   b. "Urination when you cough is a normal occurrence with older women who are pregnant. However, not at your age."
   c. "I will need to notify your physician of the urinary incontinence you are experiencing because you will need a urologist."
   d. "This is symptom is called urinary incontinence. I will need to assess you and determine if you have an infection."
   Reference: p. 1135
   Descriptors:
   1. 42   2. 03   3. Application
   4. II-1   5. Nursing Process   6. Difficult
   Rationale: An involuntary loss of urine that causes a problem is referred to as urinary incontinence. The pressure of the fetus on the bladder can cause urinary incontinence.

8. An 18-year-old woman is paralyzed from the chest down as the result of a motor vehicle accident. She is unable to control her bladder function following the accident. This is referred to as
   a. mixed incontinence
   b. urinary retention
   c. autonomic bladder*
   d. stress incontinence
   Reference: p. 1134
   Descriptors:
   1. 42   2. 03   3. Application
   4. IV-1   5. Nursing Process   6. Moderate
   Rationale: People whose bladders are no longer controlled by the brain because of injury or disease void by reflex only. This is called autonomic bladder.

9. An adult patient tells the nurse that she voids frequently in small amounts and has done this most of her life. The nurse determines that the patient is most likely experiencing
   a. stress incontinence
   b. a normal pattern of voiding*
   c. decreased bladder sensation
   d. urinary retention
   Reference: p. 1134
   Descriptors:
   1. 42   2. 03   3. Application
   4. II-1   5. Nursing Process   6. Moderate
   Rationale: Some patients void frequently in small amounts and this is a normal pattern of voiding for them.

10. Individuals who are able to go 8 to 12 hours without voiding are
    a. children
    b. adolescents
    c. young adults
    d. older adults*
    Reference: p. 1135
    Descriptors:
    1. 42   2. 03   3. Application
    4. II-1   5. Nursing Process   6. Moderate
    Rationale: Some individuals may go 8 to 12 waking hours or longer without urinating. A habitual low fluid intake or decrease in the sensation of thirst associated with aging may be the reason.

11. Toilet training for a toddler should not begin until the child can
    a. hold urine for 4 hours
    b. sit on the toilet unassisted
    c. communicate voiding needs*
    d. drink easily from a cup

Reference: p. 1134
Descriptors:

| 1. 42 | 2. 03 | 3. Application |
| 4. II-1 | 5. Nursing Process | 6. Easy |

Rationale: Toilet training should not begin until the child is able to (1) hold urine for 1 to 2 hours, (2) recognize the feeling bladder fullness, and (3) communicate the need to void and control urination while seated on the toilet.

12. A new mother tells the nurse that she is concerned because her 14-month-old child still uses diapers and refuses to use the potty chair to void. The nurse should instruct the mother that
a. most children begin to control urination voluntarily at 18 to 24 months*
b. she should keep trying by placing the child on the potty chair at frequent intervals
c. the child may need further evaluation by a urologist to determine the problem
d. some children are just more stubborn than others and she should offer treats

Reference: p. 1134
Descriptors:

| 1. 42 | 2. 02 | 3. Application |
| 4. II-1 | 5. Nursing Process | 6. Moderate |

Rationale: Most children begin to control urination voluntarily at 18 to 24 months when they are developmentally ready.

13. The nurse has instructed a caregiver of a 79-year-old patient with occasional urinary incontinence about the effects of aging on urination patterns. The nurse determines that the caregiver needs further instructions when the caregiver says
a. "Decreased bladder muscle tone may result in increased frequency."
b. "Neuromuscular problems and weakness may interfere with voluntary control."
c. "Decreased ability of the kidneys to concentrate urine may result in nocturia."
d. "Increased bladder capacity may lead to urinary incontinence."*

Reference: p. 1134–1135
Descriptors:

| 1. 42 | 2. 03 | 3. Application |
| 4. II-1 | 5. Teach/Learn | 6. Moderate |

Rationale: The caregiver needs further instructions when she says "Increased bladder capacity may lead to urinary incontinence." Decreased bladder capacity can contribute to incontinence.

14. The mother of a 6-year-old boy states to the pediatric nurse, "My son still has accidents at night." The nurse's best response is
a. "When a child urinates past the age of toilet training at night it is called enuresis."*
b. "Enuresis is seen in male children not female children and requires surgery."
c. "I'm sure enuresis is nothing to be concerned about; other children experience it."
d. "Be sure your child drinks only water and no carbonated beverages. Soda causes it."

Reference: p. 1134
Descriptors:

| 1. 42 | 2. 03 | 3. Application |
| 4. II-1 | 5. Teach/Learn | 6. Difficult |

Rationale: Involuntary urination that occurs after an age when continence should be present is termed enuresis.

15. An elderly woman complains of stress incontinence. As the nurse caring for the patient it is important to educate her that she should avoid
a. potato chips
b. milk
c. lemonade
d. caffeine*

Reference: p. 1135
Descriptors:

| 1. 42 | 2. 03 | 3. Application |
| 4. IV-3 | 5. Teach/Learn | 6. Moderate |

Rationale: Caffeine-containing beverages have a diuretic effect and increase urine production.

16. A child is admitted to the pediatric unit with dehydration after several episodes of vomiting. The nurse should expect
a. increased blood pressure
b. decreased temperature
c. decreased urination*
d. increased sweating

Reference: p. 1135
Descriptors:

| 1. 42 | 2. 04 | 3. Application |
| 4. IV-1 | 5. Nursing Process | 6. Moderate |

Rationale: Vomiting will cause the kidneys to conserve body fluids.

CHAPTER 42 ■ **Urinary Elimination** **419**

17. The nurse is planning to obtain a urine specimen from a dehydrated hospitalized patient with a temperature of 101.4°F. The nurse anticipates that the urine will be
   a. reddish colored
   b. diluted
   c. frothy
   d. concentrated*

Reference: p. 1139

Descriptors:

1. 42	2. 03	3. Application
4. IV-1	5. Nursing Process	6. Moderate

Rationale: A dehydrated patient typically has very concentrated urine.

18. A patient tells the nurse that he voids frequently throughout the day and must get out of bed at night to void. The nurse should assess the patient's intake prior to bedtime, especially the use of
   a. orange juice
   b. cranapple juice
   c. beer*
   d. hot milk

Reference: p. 1135; 1138

Descriptors:

1. 42	2. 03	3. Application
4. IV-1	5. Nursing Process	6. Moderate

Rationale: Caffeinated products such as cola, coffee, and alcohol can contribute to nighttime voiding.

19. The nurse makes a home visit to a 86-year-old patient who is moderately immobile due to arthritis. While assessing the patient's urinary elimination patterns the nurse should pay particular attention to symptoms of
   a. straw-colored urine
   b. urinary stasis*
   c. bladder spasms
   d. kidney disorders

Reference: p. 1135

Descriptors:

1. 42	2. 04	3. Application
4. II-1	5. Nursing Process	6. Moderate

Rationale: The nurse should pay particular attention to symptoms of urinary stasis, which can occur in the elderly when fluid intake is decreased and the patient ignores the urge to void.

20. An adult patient has been given a prescription for oral Pyridium as a urinary tract analgesic. The nurse should instruct the patient that the medication may cause
   a. hematuria
   b. greenish colored urine
   c. urinary retention
   d. orange-colored urine*

Reference: p. 1136

Descriptors:

1. 42	2. 03	3. Application
4. IV-2	5. Teach/Learn	6. Moderate

Rationale: Pyridium can cause the urine to become orange in color.

21. An adult female patient visits the clinic and tells the nurse that the color of her urine is blue. The nurse should assess the patient for
   a. intake of B-complex vitamins*
   b. use of opioid medications
   c. intake of vitamin E
   d. frequency of douching

Reference: p. 1136

Descriptors:

1. 42	2. 03	3. Application
4. IV-3	5. Nursing Process	6. Moderate

Rationale: Excessive intake of vitamin B complex vitamins can turn the urine a bluish color.

22. A patient taking anticoagulants should report which of the following symptoms immediately to her primary health provider?
   a. lethargy
   b. dysphagia
   c. afebrile
   d. hematuria*

Reference: p. 1136

Descriptors:

1. 42	2. 04	3. Application
4. IV-2	5. Teach/Learn	6. Difficult

Rationale: Anticoagulants may cause hematuria.

23. The right kidney can be assessed by
   a. palpating at the 12th rib on inspiration*
   b. palpating at the 12th rib on expiration
   c. palpating at the 11th rib on inspiration
   d. palpating at the 11th rib on expiration

Copyright © 2001 Lippincott Williams & Wilkins. **Instructor's Manual and Testbank to Accompany** Taylor, Lillis, LeMone: Fundamentals of Nursing: The Art and Science of Nursing Care, 4th ed.

Reference: p. 1137

Descriptors:

1. 42	2. 05	3. Knowledge
4. IV-1	5. Nursing Process	6. Easy

Rationale: The right kidney is at the level of the 12th rib, lower than the left kidney. The right kidney can be palpated if it is pushed down by the diaphragm when the patient inhales.

24. While performing a physical examination of an adult patient, the nurse should assess the patient's kidneys by
    a. gently tapping the flank area with the palm of the hand
    b. deeply palpating while under supervision*
    c. moderately palpating the costovertebral angle
    d. using the dominant hand to palpate the spinal area

Reference: p. 1137

Descriptors:

1. 42	2. 05	3. Application
4. IV-1	5. Nursing Process	6. Moderate

Rationale: To assess the patient's kidneys, the nurse should palpate deeply while under supervision because this can cause discomfort and injury to the patient.

25. While percussing an adult patient's bladder above the symphysis pubis, the nurse hears a dull sound. The nurse determines that the patient is most likely experiencing a/an
    a. full bladder*
    b. empty bladder
    c. bladder tumor
    d. urinary infection

Reference: p. 1137

Descriptors:

1. 42	2. 05	3. Application
4. IV-1	5. Nursing Process	6. Moderate

Rationale: A full bladder will produce a dull sound on percussion.

26. After an adult patient has voided, the nurse assesses the patient's bladder and would normally find that the bladder is
    a. above the symphysis pubis
    b. barely palpable
    c. unable to be palpated*
    d. tender to touch

Reference: p. 1137

Descriptors:

1. 42	2. 05	3. Application
4. IV-1	5. Nursing Process	6. Moderate

Rationale: After the patient has voided, the bladder should be unable to be palpated.

27. To obtain a urine sample for a routine urinalysis from an adult patient who has voided into a bedpan, the nurse should
    a. wear clean gloves*
    b. take the specimen to the laboratory
    c. measure the amount in the specimen container
    d. test the sample for glucose and protein

Reference: p. 1141

Descriptors:

1. 42	2. 05	3. Application
4. IV-1	5. Nursing Process	6. Easy

Rationale: To obtain the sample of urine, the nurse should wear clean gloves for blood and bodily fluid precautions.

28. A postoperative adult patient with an indwelling catheter needs to have his urine output measured hourly. After measuring the amount of urine produced during the last hour, the nurse should
    a. empty the urine into the patient's toilet while wearing gloves
    b. notify the physician if the amount of urine is less than 100 mL
    c. encourage the patient to keep track of his fluid intake
    d. tilt the measuring chamber and allow the urine to enter the collection bag*

Reference: p. 1142

Descriptors:

1. 42	2. 05	3. Application
4. IV-1	5. Nursing Process	6. Moderate

Rationale: After measuring the amount of urine, the nurse should tilt the measuring chamber and allow the urine to enter the collection bag.

29. A hospitalized adult patient tells the nurse that during the last two voidings he has experienced pain and burning. The nurse should notify the physician of the patient's
    a. dysuria*
    b. polyuria
    c. pyuria
    d. oliguria

Reference: p. 1138

Descriptors:

| 1. 42 | 2. 04 | 3. Application |
| 4. II-2 | 5. Communication | 6. Easy |

Rationale: Pain and burning with urination is termed dysuria.

30. The nurse is caring for an adult patient whose urine output was 500 mL during the last 24 hours. The nurse documents the patient's
    a. urinary retention
    b. dysuria
    c. pyuria
    d. oliguria*

Reference: p. 1138

Descriptors:

| 1. 42 | 2. 01 | 3. Application |
| 4. IV-1 | 5. Document | 6. Moderate |

Rationale: A urine output of 500 mL in 24 hours is considered oliguria.

31. The nurse obtains a straw-colored, clear urine sample from an adult patient and determines that the urine pH is 6.0 with a specific gravity of 1.020. The nurse determines that the patient's urine most likely indicates
    a. overhydration
    b. underhydration
    c. effects of medications
    d. normal findings*

Reference: p. 1139

Descriptors:

| 1. 42 | 2. 04 | 3. Application |
| 4. IV-1 | 5. Nursing Process | 6. Moderate |

Rationale: A pH of 6.0 and specific gravity of 1.020 are considered normal findings.

32. An adult patient who is very athletic and eats a high-protein diet daily provides a urine sample. The nurse anticipates that because of the high-protein intake, the patient's urine will likely be
    a. frothy
    b. acidic*
    c. alkaline
    d. concentrated

Reference: p. 1139

Descriptors:

| 1. 42 | 2. 04 | 3. Application |
| 4. II-1 | 5. Nursing Process | 6. Moderate |

Rationale: Because of the high-protein diet, the nurse can anticipate that the patient's urine will be acidic.

33. The nurse requests an adult male patient to obtain an ordered clean-catch urine specimen. The nurse should instruct the patient to
    a. collect the urine in a sterile container*
    b. void first, then collect the specimen 1 hour later
    c. use a clean container to collect 50 mL of urine
    d. cleanse the meatus with an alcohol wipe before voiding

Reference: p. 1141

Descriptors:

| 1. 42 | 2. 05 | 3. Application |
| 4. IV-1 | 5. Nursing Process | 6. Moderate |

Rationale: The patient should be instructed to void a small amount, then collect the specimen into a sterile container.

34. The nurse is planning to collect a clean-catch specimen from a female patient on bed rest when the patient says "I don't think I can void with you in the room." The nurse plans to ask the patient to
    a. perform self-catheterization to obtain a sterile specimen
    b. use a sterile bedpan to collect the specimen for transfer to a container*
    c. discard the first 100 mL of urine and collect the remainder
    d. collect all urine into a clean bedpan, then measure 30 mL for a specimen

Reference: p. 1141–1142

Descriptors:

| 1. 42 | 2. 03; 05 | 3. Application |
| 4. IV-1 | 5. Nursing Process | 6. Moderate |

Rationale: The nurse should offer the patient a sterile bedpan to collect the specimen and then the nurse can transfer the specimen to a container. The nurse should offer the patient privacy by leaving the room until the patient has voided.

35. When collecting a specimen from an indwelling catheter the nurse should
    a. insert an irrigation syringe in the catheter
    b. insert a sterile syringe in the catheter port*
    c. disconnect the catheter and collect urine
    d. insert an new catheter and collect urine

Reference: p. 1142

Descriptors:

1. 42	2. 05	3. Comprehensive
4. IV-1	5. Nursing Process	6. Easy

Rationale: Collection of a sterile urine specimen is obtained from the port with a sterile syringe.

36. The physician has ordered a 24-hour urine collection for an adult patient. The nurse begins the collection procedure at 7 AM by
    a. starting a new intake and output flow sheet
    b. asking the patient to void and discard the specimen*
    c. putting a sign on the patient's entry door
    d. placing the collection container in the patient's bathroom

Reference: p. 1143

Descriptors:

1. 42	2. 05	3. Application
4. IV-1	5. Nursing Process	6. Moderate

Rationale: The nurse should first ask the patient to void and discard the specimen. All urine collected after this for the next 24 hours should be saved.

37. A patient is being discharged to home care and is to have his urine tested for protein using plastic testing strips with a special coating. The nurse should instruct the patient that when the color of the strip changes after contact with the urine, this is due to the strip's
    a. preservative
    b. alkalinity
    c. reagent*
    d. reactivity

Reference: p. 1143

Descriptors:

1. 42	2. 05	3. Application
4. IV-1	5. Teach/Learn	6. Moderate

Rationale: The color changes are due to the strip's reagent.

38. When using a hydrometer to assess the specific gravity of a patient's urine, the nurse should
    a. read the measurement at eye level at the bottom of the meniscus*
    b. shake the hydrometer briefly before taking the measurement
    c. hold the hydrometer above eye level and read above the meniscus
    d. allow 15 minutes before taking the measurement to allow time for settling

Reference: p. 1144

Descriptors:

1. 42	2. 05	3. Application
4. IV-1	5. Nursing Process	6. Moderate

Rationale: The nurse should read the measurement at eye level at the bottom of the meniscus.

39. Urine specific gravity indicates the urine
    a. amount
    b. dilution*
    c. color
    d. content

Reference: p. 1143

Descriptors:

1. 42	2. 05	3. Comprehensive
4. None	5. None	6. Easy

Rationale: The density or dilution of the urine floats the hydrometer. If the urine is concentrated, the urinometer is buoyed up. If the urine is diluted, the hydrometer will float lower in the urine with a low specific gravity.

40. The nurse plans to collect a urine specimen for a routine urinalysis from an alert, adult male patient who has been ambulating. To collect the specimen, the nurse plans to use a
    a. clean urinal*
    b. sterile container
    c. clean bedpan
    d. clean catheter

Reference: p. 1141

Descriptors:

1. 42	2. 05	3. Application
4. IV-1	5. Nursing Process	6. Moderate

Rationale: To obtain a routine urinalysis from an alert, mobile adult patient, the nurse should obtain a clean container.

41. The nurse is caring for an 86-year-old patient at home when the patient tells the nurse that she "is afraid to go anywhere because I often lose my urine." A priority nursing diagnosis for this patient is
    a. Risk for Skin Breakdown related to urinary incontinence
    b. Potential for Sleep Pattern Disturbance related to urge incontinence
    c. Risk for Toileting Self-Care Deficit related to urinary frequency
    d. Self-Esteem Disturbance related to urinary incontinence*

    Reference: p.1144

    Descriptors:

1. 42	2. 06	3. Application
4. II-1	5. Nursing Process	6. Moderate

    Rationale: The priority nursing diagnosis is Self-Esteem Disturbance related to urinary incontinence because the patient is afraid to go anywhere owing to her incontinence.

42. An adult patient who is active in sports activities tells the nurse that she often dribbles her urine when she least expects it. The nurse should instruct the patient to
    a. ask the physician for a medication to stop the dribbling
    b. limit fluid intake while active in sports
    c. practice Kegel exercises at least 30 or more times per day*
    d. decrease the number of sports activities

    Reference: p. 1148

    Descriptors:

1. 42	2. 07	3. Application
4. IV-1	5. Nursing Process	6. Moderate

    Rationale: The nurse should instruct the patient that to strengthen the muscles she should practice Kegel exercises at least 30 to 80 times per day for at least 6 weeks.

43. An adult patient has been instructed about how to perform Kegel exercises. The nurse determines that the patient understands the instructions when she says
    a. "I should contract the pelvic floor muscles for 10 seconds."*
    b. "It's important that I do the exercises daily for at least a week."
    c. "I need to do these exercises for the rest of my life."
    d. "I should contract and then relax the muscles for at least 20 to 30 seconds."

    Reference: p. 1148

    Descriptors:

1. 42	2. 07	3. Application
4. IV-3	5. Teach/Learn	6. Moderate

    Rationale: The nurse should instruct the woman to perform the exercises by contracting the pelvic floor muscles for 10 seconds, then relaxing them for 10 seconds. These exercises should be done 30 to 80 times per day for 6 weeks.

44. A female patient tells the nurse that she sometimes experiences hesitancy when trying to void. After instructing the patient about various methods to resolve this problem, the nurse determines that the patient needs further instructions when the patient says she should
    a. use Credé's maneuvers to stimulate a urine stream*
    b. run warm water over her fingers while trying to void
    c. void when the urge to void is first experienced
    d. use warm water over the perineal area to stimulate voiding

    Reference: p. 1148

    Descriptors:

1. 42	2. 07	3. Application
4. IV-1	5. Nursing Process	6. Moderate

    Rationale: The patient needs further instructions when the patient says she should use Credé's maneuvers to stimulate a urine stream because this is not necessary for this patient.

45. The nurse is assisting a female patient on bed rest with perineal care following urination on a bedpan. Following instructions about the proper technique, the nurse determines that the patient understands the instructions when the nurse observes the patient clean the perineal area
    a. in a circular motion around the meatus
    b. once a day with mild soap and water
    c. from front to back toward the rectum*
    d. from the back toward the front

    Reference: p. 1151

    Descriptors:

1. 42	2. 07	3. Application
4. IV-3	5. Teach/Learn	6. Moderate

    Rationale: Female patients should always be instructed to clean the perineum from front to back.

46. An adult patient is scheduled for a cystoscopy in the morning. The nurse should instruct the patient that she will
    a. remain NPO after midnight the day of the procedure
    b. have a Foley catheter in place after the procedure
    c. need to sign an informed consent statement before the procedure*
    d. be given pain medication after the procedure is completed

    Reference: p. 1145
    Descriptors:
    1. 42   2. 05   3. Application
    4. IV-1   5. Teach/Learn   6. Moderate

    Rationale: The patient will need to sign an informed consent before the procedure. Liquids are allowed and sedation will be given before the procedure.

47. The nurse has instructed an alert adult patient about intravenous pyelography, which is scheduled the next day. The nurse determines that the patient understands the instructions when the patient says
    a. "I will need to void before the examination." *
    b. "No preparation is needed for this procedure."
    c. "I can maintain my normal eating patterns before the procedure."
    d. "There are no side effects from this procedure."

    Reference: p. 1145
    Descriptors:
    1. 42   2. 05   3. Application
    4. IV-1   5. Nursing Process   6. Moderate

    Rationale: Intravenous pyelography requires an injection of dye, so preparation is involved. The patient should void before the procedure.

48. An adult patient hospitalized after a serious fall from a ladder is scheduled for a retrograde pyelography examination in the morning. The nurse should plan to
    a. provide the patient with a clear liquid breakfast in the morning
    b. ask the patient to refrain from voiding on the morning of the examination
    c. give the patient an ordered laxative the evening before the examination*
    d. administer an ordered analgesic the evening before the examination

    Reference: p. 1145
    Descriptors:
    1. 42   2. 05   3. Application
    4. IV-1   5. Nursing Process   6. Moderate

    Rationale: The nurse should plan to give the patient an ordered laxative the evening before the examination.

49. An adult patient is scheduled for an ultrasound of her kidneys on the following day. Following instructions about the procedure, the nurse determines that the patient needs further instruction when the patient says
    a. "It is OK for me to chew gum before the procedure."*
    b. "This procedure is painless but I may get uncomfortable."
    c. "I will need to sign a consent form before the procedure."
    d. "The results of the test are usually ready 1 to 2 days after the procedure."

    Reference: p. 1145
    Descriptors:
    1. 42   2. 05   3. Application
    4. IV-1   5. Teach/Learn   6. Moderate

    Rationale: The patient needs further instruction when she says she can chew gum before the procedure because this may cause air to be swallowed.

50. An adult patient is scheduled for a computed tomography scan of his bladder and a contrast dye is to be used. The nurse should
    a. keep the patient NPO for 12 hours before the test
    b. withhold any prescribed medications usually taken
    c. tape the patient's wedding rings in place
    d. assess the patient for history of an allergic reaction to shellfish*

    Reference: p. 1146
    Descriptors:
    1. 42   2. 05   3. Application
    4. IV-3   5. Nursing Process   6. Moderate

    Rationale: The dye contains iodine, which is found in shellfish. Some patients are allergic to iodine and shellfish.

51. An obese patient with three children tells the nurse that when she laughs suddenly, she dribbles urine down the side of her leg. The nurse suspects that the patient is experiencing
    a. urge incontinence
    b. urinary frequency
    c. stress incontinence*
    d. reflex relaxation

    Reference: p. 1147

    Descriptors:

    1. 42   2. 01   3. Comprehensive
    4. IV-3   5. Nursing Process 6. Moderate

    Rationale: When urine dribbles after exercise or laughing, this is termed stress incontinence because stress is placed on the bladder and muscles.

52. The nurse makes a home visit to an 80-year-old patient who tells the nurse that she "has trouble making it to the bathroom on time and urinates before she gets there." The nurse determines that the patient is experiencing
    a. nocturnal frequency
    b. polyuria
    c. urge incontinence*
    d. reflex incontinence

    Reference: p. 1147

    Descriptors:

    1. 42   2. 01   3. Comprehensive
    4. II-1   5. Nursing Process 6. Moderate

    Rationale: The patient is experiencing urge incontinence when she has trouble getting to the bathroom on time and urinates before she gets there.

53. A caregiver of a 90-year-old patient tells the nurse that her mother frequently experiences nocturia and is sometimes incontinent. Following instructions about strategies to resolve the elimination problems, the nurse determines that the caregiver understands the instructions when she says
    a. "I should keep her in adult-sized diapers continuously until this stops."
    b. "I should be sure that my mother drinks at least 2500 mL of fluid before 5 PM."
    c. "Beverages with caffeine and Nutrasweet should be avoided before bedtime."*
    d. "My mother may need to have an indwelling catheter in place."

    Reference: p. 1148

    Descriptors:

    1. 42   2. 08   3. Application
    4. II-1   5. Teach/Learn   6. Moderate

    Rationale: Long-term use of adult diapers is not recommended. Beverages with caffeine and Nutrasweet may irritate the bladder and result in incontinence.

54. The nurse is preparing to assist a patient on complete bed rest to use the bedpan for voiding. The nurse should *first*
    a. don clean gloves before offering the bedpan*
    b. place the bed in the lowest position
    c. offer the patient some soft tissues
    d. be certain the call light is available

    Reference: p. 1150

    Descriptors:

    1. 42   2. 05   3. Application
    4. IV-1   5. Nursing Process 6. Moderate

    Rationale: The nurse should first don clean gloves before the procedure.

55. After a patient has voided, the nurse measures the patient's postvoid residual as 5 mL. The nurse determines that that the patient is most likely experiencing
    a. normal bladder function*
    b. stress incontinence
    c. urinary retention
    d. functional incontinence

    Reference: p. 1152

    Descriptors:

    1. 42   2. 04   3. Application
    4. IV-1   5. Nursing Process 6. Moderate

    Rationale: A postvoid residual of 5 mL indicates normal bladder function.

56. The nurse is caring for a postoperative patient who has had frequent urinary incontinence since the surgery. The patient's husband says "Why don't the doctors just order a catheter for her?" The best response by the nurse is to instruct the patient's husband that urinary catheters
    a. can affect the patient's future voiding patterns
    b. require constant monitoring for output
    c. affect the patient's mobility patterns
    d. are the most prominent cause of nosocomial infections*

Reference: p. 1154

Descriptors:

1. 42	2. 08	3. Application
4. IV-1	5. Teach/Learn	6. Moderate

Rationale: Urinary catheters are the most prominent cause of nosocomial infections.

57. The nurse makes a home visit to an adult patient who has had a urologic stent inserted 2 days ago. While assessing the stent, the nurse observes that the urine from the stent is bright red in color. The nurse should
   a. continue to monitor the output daily
   b. notify the patient's physician immediately*
   c. irrigate the stent with normal saline
   d. offer the patient an acidic juice drink

Reference: p. 1155

Descriptors:

1. 42	2. 04	3. Application
4. IV-3	5. Communication	6. Moderate

Rationale: Bloody drainage from the stent requires immediate notification of the physician.

58. The nurse is preparing to catheterize an 80-year-old patient with rheumatoid arthritis and a left hip joint replacement. The nurse plans to position the patient in which of the following positions?
   a. Sims'*
   b. dorsal recumbent
   c. lithotomy
   d. prone

Reference: p. 1157

Descriptors:

1. 42	2. 05	3. Application
4. IV-1	5. Nursing Process	6. Moderate

Rationale: The Sims' position is most appropriate for a patient with rheumatoid arthritis.

59. The nurse is planning to insert an indwelling catheter in an adult male patient. The nurse plans to
   a. ask the patient to void into the urinal if he can
   b. use an 8 French catheter for the procedure
   c. insert the catheter ½ to 1 inch beyond the point where urine flows
   d. insert the catheter to the bifurcation of the catheter tubing*

Reference: p. 1164

Descriptors:

1. 42	2. 05	3. Application
4. IV-1	5. Nursing Process	6. Moderate

Rationale: The nurse should plan to insert the catheter to the bifurcation of the catheter tubing.

60. The nurse is preparing to insert an indwelling catheter into an adult female patient. Before inserting the catheter, the nurse should *first*
   a. spread the labia with the dominant hand to begin the procedure
   b. test the catheter balloon with a syringe and sterile water for patency*
   c. wear clean gloves to pour the antiseptic solution into the container
   d. clean the meatus by moving the moistened cotton ball toward the rectum

Reference: p. 1159

Descriptors:

1. 42	2. 05	3. Application
4. IV-1	5. Nursing Process	6. Moderate

Rationale: The nurse should first test the catheter balloon with a syringe and sterile water for patency.

61. A patient has not voided for 9 hours and a straight catheterization is ordered. After removing 750 mL of urine through the catheter, the nurse stops the procedure to prevent the patient from experiencing
   a. a potential risk for a nosocomial infection
   b. engorgement of pelvic floor muscles and hypotension*
   c. further relaxation of the urethral sphincter
   d. irritability of the bladder muscle, which may cause discomfort

Reference: p. 1160

Descriptors:

1. 42	2. 05	3. Application
4. IV-1	5. Nursing Process	6. Moderate

Rationale: The nurse stops the procedure to prevent the patient from experiencing engorgement of pelvic floor muscles and possible hypotension.

62. While performing a catheterization on an adult female patient, there is not an immediate flow of urine from the catheter. The nurse should
   a. obtain a larger sized catheter for another catheterization
   b. remove the catheter and reinsert another catheter
   c. rotate the catheter slightly while leaving it in place*
   d. ask the patient to turn to the side slightly

Reference: p. 1160

Descriptors:

1. 42	2. 05	3. Application
4. IV-1	5. Nursing Process	6. Moderate

Rationale: The nurse should rotate the catheter slightly while leaving it in place to obtain the urine.

63. The nurse is preparing to give a continuous bladder irrigation to an adult male patient. The nurse plans to
   a. hang the solution bag on a pole 2½ to 3 feet above the patient's bladder*
   b. allow air from the solution bag tubing to flow slowly into the catheter
   c. use aseptic technique to attach the solution bag tubing to the catheter
   d. clamp the tubing of the solution bag periodically to prevent bladder distention

Reference: p. 1167

Descriptors:

1. 42	2. 05	3. Application
4. IV-1	5. Nursing Process	6. Moderate

Rationale: The nurse plans to hang the solution bag on a pole 2½ to 3 feet above the patient's bladder. Sterile technique should be used.

64. The nurse has instructed a caregiver of an adult patient about care of the patient with an indwelling catheter. The nurse determines that the caregiver understands the instructions when the nurse observes the caregiver
   a. use mild hand lotion around the labia to moisten the tissues
   b. wash the perineal area with mild soap and water at least twice daily*
   c. apply baby powder to the perineal area and thighs after cleansing
   d. open the closed drainage system to measure the amount of urine

Reference: p. 1169

Descriptors:

1. 42	2. 05	3. Application
4. IV-1	5. Teach/Learn	6. Moderate

Rationale: The nurse determines that the caregiver is following the instructions when the nurse observes the caregiver wash the perineal area of the patient with mild soap and water twice daily.

65. The nurse is caring for an adult female patient with an indwelling catheter. To help keep the urine acidic, the nurse suggests to the patient that she drink
   a. buttermilk
   b. fruit punch
   c. grape juice
   d. cranberry juice*

Reference: p. 1166

Descriptors:

1. 42	2. 09	3. Application
4. IV-3	5. Teach/Learn	6. Moderate

Rationale: Cranberry juice is helpful for preventing bacteria from adhering to the bladder wall.

66. The nurse is planning to remove an indwelling catheter from an adult male patient. During the procedure, the nurse plans to
   a. cleanse the perineal area before removing the catheter
   b. measure the amount of urine in the catheter tubing
   c. aspirate the fluid in the inflated balloon*
   d. use sterile scissors to cut the tubing and drain the balloon

Reference: p. 1168

Descriptors:

1. 42	2. 05	3. Application
4. IV-1	5. Nursing Process	6. Moderate

Rationale: The nurse should plan to aspirate the fluid from the inflated balloon before removing the catheter.

67. The nurse has instructed the patient about care following the removal of an indwelling catheter. The nurse determines that the patient needs further instruction when the patient says
    a. "I need to keep track of my intake for the next 2 days."*
    b. "I should continue to drink plenty of fluids during the day."
    c. "The first time or two that I void I might have a slight burning sensation."
    d. "I should tell the nurse if I see any blood in my urine when I void."

Reference: p. 1168

Descriptors:

1. 42	2. 10	3. Application
4. IV-1	5. Teach/Learn	6. Moderate

Rationale: The patient needs further instruction when he says "I need to keep track of my intake for the next 2 days." While fluid intake is important, the patient needs to monitor his output for the next few days.

68. The nurse has instructed a home care patient about self-catheterization. The nurse determines that the patient understands the instruction when she says
    a. "I should plan to catheterize myself at least every hour."
    b. "I should drink at least 1½ to 2 quarts of fluid daily."*
    c. "The catheter should be washed with a bleach solution after use."
    d. "When the catheter is in place, I should press down on the meatus to fully empty the bladder."

Reference: p. 1162

Descriptors:

1. 42	2. 10	3. Application
4. IV-3	5. Teach/Learn	6. Moderate

Rationale: The patient understands the instructions when she says she should drink at least 1½ to 2 quarts of water daily.

69. An ambulatory patient is being discharged with an indwelling catheter and drainage bag. The nurse should instruct the patient to clean the leg bag with water and
    a. vinegar
    b. mild detergent
    c. alcohol
    d. chlorine bleach*

Reference: p. 1169

Descriptors:

1. 42	2. 10	3. Application
4. IV-3	5. Teach/Learn	6. Easy

Rationale: The leg bag can be disinfected with a solution of 5 ounces of water and 2 ounces of chlorine bleach.

70. The nurse is preparing to change a male patient's condom catheter. The nurse plans to
    a. don sterile gloves before removing the previous condom catheter
    b. keep the tip of the tubing 2½ to 5 inches beyond the tip of the penis
    c. wash and dry the penis thoroughly after removing the condom catheter*
    d. position the tubing of the new condom catheter close to the penis

Reference: p. 1169

Descriptors:

1. 42	2. 07	3. Application
4. IV-1	5. Nursing Process	6. Moderate

Rationale: Clean gloves should be worn. To change the condom catheter, the nurse should wash the penis and dry thoroughly before replacing the catheter.

71. The nurse is caring for a patient who has an ileal conduit following surgery. The nurse should instruct the patient that
    a. fluid restriction is necessary because a limited amount of urine will be produced
    b. the appliance to collect urine should be emptied frequently throughout the day*
    c. the patient will need assistance in ambulating at least every 4 hours
    d. no tub baths will be allowed, but the patient can shower daily

Reference: p. 1169–1171

Descriptors:

1. 42	2. 07	3. Application
4. IV-3	5. Teach/Learn	6. Moderate

Rationale: The nurse should instruct the patient that the appliance to collect urine should be emptied frequently throughout the day.

72. A 75-year-old male patient tells the nurse that he has had a great deal of difficulty voiding during the past week. The nurse determines that the most likely reason for the patient's urinary retention is a/an
a. enlarged prostate gland*
b. sexually transmitted disease
c. diminished bladder capacity
d. neurologic injury

Reference: p. 1147

Descriptors:

1. 42   2. 09   3. Application
4. II-2   5. Nursing Process   6. Moderate

Rationale: The 75-year-old male patient is most likely experiencing symptoms of an enlarged prostate gland.

73. The nurse is caring for a patient with an indwelling catheter when the nurse observes that the patient's urine culture shows 100,000 bacterial colonies per milliliter. The nurse should
a. notify the patient's physician*
b. provide fluids often to the patient
c. continue to monitor the patient's output
d. flush the catheter with normal saline

Reference: p. 1139; 1149

Descriptors:

1. 42   2. 09   3. Application
4. IV-1   5. Communication   6. Moderate

Rationale: The patient has a urinary tract infection and the physician should be notified.

CHAPTER 43

Bowel Elimination

1. The amount of chyme processed daily by the large intestine is about
   a. 500 mL
   b. 1000 mL
   c. 1500 mL*
   d. 2000 mL

   Reference: p. 1182

   Descriptors:

1. 43	2. 02	3. Knowledge
4. None	5. None	6. Easy

   Rationale: The amount of chyme processed by the body is 1500 mL daily.

2. Functions of the human body's large intestine include finishing absorption, formation and explusion of feces, and
   a. fat storage
   b. manufacturing of vitamins*
   c. digestion of lactose
   d. initiation of peristalsis

   Reference: p. 1182

   Descriptors:

1. 43	2. 02	3. Knowledge
4. None	5. None	6. Easy

   Rationale: The large intestine also manufactures vitamins in the body.

3. The nurse is caring for a first-time mother who is breastfeeding her neonate. The nurse plans to instruct the patient that stools of breastfed infants
   a. are firm and yellow to brown in color
   b. are soft and dark brown in color
   c. usually average from 2 to 4 per day*
   d. usually average from 6 to 8 per day

   Reference: p. 1185

   Descriptors:

1. 43	2. 03	3. Application
4. II-1	5. Teach/Learn	6. Moderate

   Rationale: Stools of breastfed infants are yellow, soft, and average 2 to 4 per day.

4. A young mother visits the clinic with her 16-month-old son. The mother tells the nurse that no matter what she does, the child just isn't interested in using the potty chair for a bowel movement. The nurse should instruct the mother that
   a. she should wait until the child seems interested in potty training
   b. she should schedule an appointment for a comprehensive evaluation
   c. it is possible that the father of the child would have greater success
   d. children usually attain bowel control by the age of 30 months*

   Reference: p. 1185

   Descriptors:

1. 43	2. 03	3. Application
4. II-1	5. Teach/Learn	6. Moderate

   Rationale: Children usually begin toilet training at around 18 to 24 months and usually attain bowel control by 30 months.

5. A patient with chronic constipation tells the nurse that he would like to improve his diet. Besides encouraging high-fiber foods, the nurse should instruct the patient to
   a. drink 2000 to 3000 mL of fluid daily*
   b. refrain from eating spicy foods
   c. eat more soft cheese daily
   d. avoid dairy products

   Reference: p. 1185

   Descriptors:

1. 43	2. 03; 07	3. Application
4. IV-3	5. Teach/Learn	6. Moderate

   Rationale: Increasing fluid intake to 2000 to 3000 mL daily will ease constipation.

6. The nurse has instructed a patient with chronic
constipation about high-fiber foods. The nurse
determines that the patient understands the
instructions when he says high fiber in the diet
a. decreases gas formation before the stool is
passed
b. increases the water reabsorption process
c. serves as a stimulus for peristalsis*
d. moves the stool more slowly through the
intestine
Reference: p. 1185
Descriptors:

1. 43 2. 03; 07 3. Application
4. IV-1 5. Teach/Learn 6. Moderate

Rationale: High fiber removes cholesterol and
serves as a stimulus for peristalsis.

7. A patient tells the nurse that he has been eating a
high-fiber diet for 2 months. The nurse should
explain to the patient that when the transit time
for feces through the colon is decreased, the
amount of toxins absorbed is reduced, which can
decrease the chance of developing
a. stomach cancer
b. colon cancer*
c. diarrhea
d. hemorrhoids
Reference: p. 1185
Descriptors:

1. 43 2. 03; 07 3. Application
4. IV-3 5. Teach/Learn 6. Moderate

Rationale: High-fiber foods have been shown to
decrease the incidence of colon cancer.

8. An adult patient tells the nurse that she gets
diarrhea and feels bloated when she eats ice cream
and other dairy products. The nurse determines
that the patient is most likely experiencing
a. lactose intolerance*
b. diverticulitis
c. colon polyps
d. gallbladder disease
Reference: p. 1186
Descriptors:

1. 43 2. 03 3. Application
4. IV-1 5. Nursing Process 6. Moderate

Rationale: Lactose intolerance can result in
bloating after eating dairy products.

9. A hospitalized adult patient on a regular diet tells
the nurse that she had two episodes of diarrhea
yesterday. In helping the patient to select items
from the hospital's menu, the nurse should instruct
the patient to choose
a. coleslaw
b. lean meat*
c. cauliflower
d. chocolate brownie
Reference: p. 1186
Descriptors:

1. 43 2. 03, 07 3. Application
4. IV-1 5. Teach/Learn 6. Moderate

Rationale: Lean meat is advised for a patient who
has experienced diarrhea. High-fiber foods and
chocolate should be temporarily avoided.

10. An adult patient tells the nurse that she has been
experiencing a great amount of flatulence in recent
weeks and constantly feels "bloated." The nurse
should instruct the patient to avoid foods such as
a. tomatoes
b. oranges
c. cabbage*
d. potatoes
Reference: p. 1186
Descriptors:

1. 43 2. 07 3. Application
4. IV-1 5. Teach/Learn 6. Moderate

Rationale: Foods such as cabbage and brussels
sprouts can cause flatulence and bloating.

11. A patient who has been receiving intravenous
antibiotics for 2 days for a wound infection tells
the nurse that she is now experiencing diarrhea
and asks the nurse to have the doctor order an
antidiarrheal medication. The nurse should
a. instruct the patient to restrict her fluid intake to
800 mL
b. contact the physician for an order for oral
Prilosec
c. further assess the patient because the antibiotics
may be the cause*
d. contact the physician to see if the antibiotic can
be discontinued

Reference: p. 1188
Descriptors:

| 1. 43 | 2. 09 | 3. Application |
| 4. IV-3 | 5. Nursing Process | 6. Moderate |

Rationale: The nurse should further assess the patient because the antibiotics may be the cause of the diarrhea. The physician should be notified of the patient's recent diarrhea.

12. A patient visits the clinic with her 8-month-old child and tells the nurse that the child has had bulky stools that appear greasy and foul smelling. The nurse should instruct the mother that the child should be evaluated for
a. cystic fibrosis*
b. biliary disease
c. meconium ileus
d. liver disease

Reference: p. 1187
Descriptors:

| 1. 43 | 2. 03 | 3. Comprehensive |
| 4. II-2 | 5. Nursing Process | 6. Moderate |

Rationale: Foul-smelling, greasy stools in a child are associated with cystic fibrosis.

13. A patient tells the nurse that he frequently takes an antacid with aluminum for heartburn. The nurse should assess the patient for
a. increased bowel sounds
b. abdominal distention
c. diarrhea
d. constipation*

Reference: p. 1188
Descriptors:

| 1. 43 | 2. 03 | 3. Application |
| 4. IV-3 | 5. Nursing Process | 6. Moderate |

Rationale: Antacids with aluminum can lead to constipation.

14. A patient has been given a prescription for antibiotics for 10 days. The nurse should instruct the patient that his stool may appear
a. tarry black
b. greenish gray*
c. pinkish red
d. whitish gray

Reference: p. 1188
Descriptors:

| 1. 43 | 2. 03 | 3. Application |
| 4. IV-2 | 5. Teach/Learn | 6. Moderate |

Rationale: Some antibiotics may make the stool appear greenish gray in color.

15. A pregnant patient has been taking iron supplements and tells the nurse that her bowel movements produce dark black-colored stools. The nurse determines that the patient is most likely experiencing
a. hemorrhoids
b. colon polyps
c. biliary blockage
d. normal results from iron salts*

Reference: p. 1188
Descriptors:

| 1. 43 | 2. 03 | 3. Comprehensive |
| 4. IV-2 | 5. Nursing Process | 6. Moderate |

Rationale: Iron salts can contribute to dark black-colored stools.

16. The nurse is preparing to perform a physical assessment of an adult patient's abdomen. The nurse should *first*
a. palpate the abdomen for nodules
b. place the patient in Sims' position
c. auscultate for bowel sounds*
d. use percussion in all four quadrants

Reference: p. 1188
Descriptors:

| 1. 43 | 2. 04 | 3. Application |
| 4. IV-1 | 5. Nursing Process | 6. Moderate |

Rationale: Auscultation of bowel sounds should precede palpation and percussion because palpation and percussion can influence the sounds.

17. While auscultating an adult patient's abdomen, the nurse hears abnormally intense and frequent bowel sounds. The nurse determines that the patient is experiencing
a. borborygmus*
b. gastric ulcers
c. hyperresonance
d. diarrhea

Reference: p. 1188

Descriptors:

| 1. 43 | 2. 04 | 3. Application |
| 4. IV-1 | 5. Nursing Process | 6. Moderate |

Rationale: Borborygmus is associated with abnormally intense and frequent bowel sounds.

18. To determine if a patient is experiencing no bowel sounds after surgery, the nurse plans to auscultate for
    a. 3 minutes
    b. 4 minutes
    c. 5 minutes*
    d. 6 minutes

Reference: p. 1188

Descriptors:

| 1. 43 | 2. 02 | 3. Application |
| 4. IV-1 | 5. Nursing Process | 6. Easy |

Rationale: A full 5 minutes to auscultate bowel sounds in each quadrant is necessary to determine if bowel sounds are present.

19. While auscultating a 2-day postoperative patient's abdomen following chest surgery, the nurse determines that no bowel sounds are present. The nurse suspects that the patient may be experiencing
    a. tympany
    b. paralytic ileus*
    c. increased acid production
    d. malabsorption syndrome

Reference: p. 1188

Descriptors:

| 1. 43 | 2. 04 | 3. Application |
| 4. IV-1 | 5. Nursing Process | 6. Moderate |

Rationale: A patient who is 2 days postoperative with no bowel sounds present may be experiencing paralytic ileus. The physician should be notified.

20. The nurse has instructed an adult patient how to obtain a stool specimen. The nurse determines that the patient understands the directions when she says
    a. "I should wait to void until after I obtain the stool specimen."
    b. "It's acceptable to place toilet tissue into the container as it is easily removed."
    c. "I should have my regular bowel movement in the bedpan, then place a specimen in the container."
    d. "I should void first to avoid contaminating the stool specimen."*

Reference: p. 1191

Descriptors:

| 1. 43 | 2. 05 | 3. Application |
| 4. IV-3 | 5. Teach/Learn | 6. Moderate |

Rationale: The patient should be instructed to void first, because sometimes the act of defecation causes voiding to occur.

21. A patient is diagnosed with a bile obstruction and will need surgical intervention. The nurse should instruct the patient that bile obstruction can result in the stool to be the color
    a. white*
    b. yellow
    c. red
    d. black

Reference: p. 1190

Descriptors:

| 1. 43 | 2. 04 | 3. Application |
| 4. IV-1 | 5. Teach/Learn | 6. Moderate |

Rationale: A patient with a bile obstruction will most likely have a stool that is white in color because there is no bile in the stool.

22. The physician asks the nurse to determine if a 4-year-old hospitalized patient has pinworms. To observe for pinworms, the nurse plans to obtain
    a. a sterile specimen container
    b. two tongue blades
    c. silver foil
    d. clear cellophane tape*

Reference: p. 1192

Descriptors:

| 1. 43 | 2. 05 | 3. Application |
| 4. IV-1 | 5. Nursing Process | 6. Moderate |

Rationale: Clear cellophane tape should be used to collect the stool and check for pinworms.

23. The nurse has instructed an adult patient how to obtain a stool sample at home to test for fecal occult blood. The nurse determines that the patient needs further instructions when the patient says
    a. "If the color on the slide changes to black, I should report this immediately."*
    b. "Multiple specimens are usually collected to validate the results."
    c. "The hemoccult slide test requires 2 drops of developer solution."
    d. "If the color on the slide changes to blue, I should report this immediately."

Reference: p. 1192

Descriptors:

1. 43	2. 05	3. Application
4. IV-1	5. Teach/Learn	6. Moderate

Rationale: The patient needs further instruction when he says "If the color on the slide changes to black, I should report this immediately." A blue discoloration should be reported to the physician.

24. A patient is scheduled for a biopsy while having a sigmoidoscopy. The nurse should instruct the patient that he will have a procedure that uses
    a. a radiopaque dye
    b. a barium solution
    c. a flexible fiberoptic instrument
    d. two rigid instruments*

    Reference: p. 1193

    Descriptors:

1. 43	2. 05	3. Application
4. IV-1	5. Teach/Learn	6. Moderate

    Rationale: Two rigid instruments are used during a sigmoidoscopy.

25. An adult patient is scheduled to have a series of diagnostic tests for a bowel disorder. Which of the following should the nurse schedule *first*?
    a. Upper GI series with barium
    b. Lower GI series with barium
    c. Endoscopy
    d. Fecal occult blood test*

    Reference: p. 1193

    Descriptors:

1. 43	2. 05	3. Application
4. IV-1	5. Nursing Process	6. Moderate

    Rationale: The fecal occult blood test should be done first before the administration of barium.

26. The nurse has explained the esophagogastroduodenoscopy procedure to an adult patient. The nurse determines that the patient needs further instructions about the procedure when the patient says
    a. "I should empty my bladder before going for this procedure."
    b. "I can leave my dentures in place during the procedure."*
    c. "Before the test, I need to sign a consent form."
    d. "A bitter tasting local anesthetic may be sprayed in my mouth."

Reference: pp. 1192, 1194

Descriptors:

1. 43	2. 05	3. Application
4. IV-1	5. Teach/Learn	6. Moderate

Rationale: The patient needs further instructions about the procedure when the patient says "I can leave my dentures in place during the procedure." The patient should remove the dentures to prevent damage to the dentures during the procedure.

27. A 65-year-old patient visits the clinic with symptoms of the flu, which include nausea, vomiting, and diarrhea. The patient tells the nurse she has been unable to tolerate food or fluids for 3 days. A priority nursing diagnosis for the patient is
    a. Self-Care Deficit related to weakness and flu
    b. Body Image Disturbance related to diarrhea
    c. Risk for Self-Esteem Disturbance related to nausea and vomiting
    d. Fluid Volume Deficit related to prolonged vomiting and diarrhea*

    Reference: p. 1193

    Descriptors:

1. 43	2. 06	3. Application
4. IV-1	5. Nursing Process	6. Moderate

    Rationale: The patient who has been vomiting and had nausea and diarrhea is at risk for Fluid Volume Deficit and dehydration.

28. The nurse is caring for a patient who has had diarrhea for the past 3 days. After instructing the patient about how to cope with diarrhea, the nurse determines that the patient understands the instructions when he says
    a. "I should avoid hot foods because this can aggravate the problem."
    b. "Cold and spicy foods should be avoided."*
    c. "It's important to use wet wipes around the anus."
    d. "I should continue to take my Metamucil or mineral oil daily."

    Reference: p. 1195

    Descriptors:

1. 43	2. 09	3. Application
4. IV-3	5. Teach/Learn	6. Moderate

    Rationale: The patient understands the instructions when he says that cold and spicy foods should be avoided because this can aggravate the problem.

29. After 3 days of diarrhea, the nurse determines that the patient's diarrhea has subsided when the patient has a regularly formed stool. To aid in restoring the patient's normal bowel flora, the nurse should encourage the patient to consume
   a. yogurt*
   b. whole-grain breads
   c. green leafy vegetables
   d. skim milk

   Reference: p. 1198

   Descriptors:

1. 43	2. 09	3. Application
4. IV-1	5. Teach/Learn	6. Moderate

   Rationale: Yogurt will help to restore the normal flora.

30. The nurse visits an adult patient who had a permanent colostomy 6 weeks ago. He tells the nurse that he hasn't felt like having sexual intercourse with his wife since his surgery because he has to wear the ostomy bag. A priority nursing diagnosis for this patient is
   a. Self-Care Deficit related to lack of information
   b. Risk for Spiritual Distress related to body image changes
   c. Sexual Dysfunction related to perceived change in body image*
   d. Altered Elimination Pattern related to colostomy

   Reference: p. 1193

   Descriptors:

1. 43	2. 06	3. Application
4. III-1	5. Nursing Process	6. Moderate

   Rationale: The priority nursing diagnosis is Sexual Dysfunction related to perceived change in body image.

31. The nurse has instructed an adult patient with a colostomy about nutrition. The nurse determines that the patient needs further instruction when he says
   a. "I should avoid low-fiber foods such as ice cream."*
   b. "Brussels sprouts may lead to flatulence."
   c. "I shouldn't eat peanuts or popcorn."
   d. "If I eat an apple, I should remove the skin first."

   Reference: p. 1213

   Descriptors:

1. 43	2. 08	3. Application
4. IV-1	5. Teach/Learn	6. Moderate

   Rationale: The patient needs further instructions when he says he should avoid low-fiber foods, because this is not necessary.

32. The nurse is caring for a 74-year-old patient on the first postoperative day following abdominal surgery. To aid the patient's bowel elimination, the nurse plans to
   a. encourage high-fiber food intake
   b. ambulate the patient as soon as possible*
   c. obtain an elevated commode
   d. turn the patient every 4 to 6 hours

   Reference: p. 1196

   Descriptors:

1. 43	2. 09	3. Application
4. IV-3	5. Nursing Process	6. Moderate

   Rationale: To aid in the patient's circulation and bowel elimination, the nurse should plan to ambulate the patient as soon as possible.

33. An adult patient has been given a prescription for Paragoric to control acute diarrhea. The nurse plans to advise the patient to
   a. take the medication for 2 weeks to stop the diarrhea
   b. avoid operating heavy equipment while taking the medication*
   c. take the medication with Kaopectate for the greatest effectiveness
   d. limit fluid intake to a maximum of 500 mL while taking the medication

   Reference: p. 1199

   Descriptors:

1. 43	2. 09	3. Application
4. IV-2	5. Teach/Learn	6. Moderate

   Rationale: Paragoric can make an individual sleepy so the patient should avoid operating heavy equipment while taking the medication.

34. The nurse is caring for an adult patient who is taking Colace to assist with bowel elimination. The nurse should instruct the patient to
   a. increase the intake of foods high in fat-soluble vitamins*
   b. decrease the intake of high-fiber foods
   c. drink three glasses of Gatorade daily
   d. increase the intake of foods high in vitamin C

Reference: p. 1188

Descriptors:

| 1. 43 | 2. 09 | 3. Application |
| 4. IV-2 | 5. Teach/Learn | 6. Moderate |

Rationale: Colace can result in excess fat soluble vitamin excretion.

35. The nurse has instructed a 60-year-old patient with frequent constipation about bulk-forming products, such as Metamucil. The nurse determines that the patient needs further instructions when she says
   a. "I shouldn't use Metamucil if I have hard, formed stools."*
   b. "It takes about 24 hours for this to work for most people."
   c. "This product works by absorbing water and stimulating peristalsis."
   d. "I need to eat more high-iron foods, such as meat."

Reference: p. 1197

Descriptors:

| 1. 43 | 2. 09 | 3. Application |
| 4. IV-2 | 5. Teach/Learn | 6. Moderate |

Rationale: The patient needs further instructions when she says she shouldn't take Metamucil if she has hard, formed stools. The product stimulates peristalsis, but may interfere with metabolism of iron and calcium.

36. An 74-year-old patient visits the clinic and tells the nurse she has had acute diarrhea for the past 3 days. The nurse should assess the patient for
   a. dehydration*
   b. fluid retention
   c. distention
   d. hemorrhoids

Reference: p. 1199

Descriptors:

| 1. 43 | 2. 04; 09 | 3. Application |
| 4. IV-1 | 5. Nursing Process | 6. Moderate |

Rationale: The patient who is 74 and who has had diarrhea for 3 days may be becoming dehydrated.

37. The nurse has instructed an adult patient about rectal suppositories that have been ordered for the patient. The nurse determines that the patient needs further instructions when the patient says
   a. "I should leave the suppository in place for at least 5 minutes."*
   b. "After insertion of the suppository, I should ambulate in the room."
   c. "The suppository will be inserted about 4 inches into my rectum."
   d. "The suppository will be lubricated prior to insertion."

Reference: p. 1205

Descriptors:

| 1. 43 | 2. 07 | 3. Application |
| 4. IV-2 | 5. Teach/Learn | 6. Moderate |

Rationale: The suppository should be left in place for 30 to 45 minutes for maximum effectiveness.

38. The nurse is caring for an adult patient on the second postoperative day following chest surgery. The patient tells the nurse he is "bloated and has a lot of gas." The nurse should encourage the patient to
   a. ambulate in the room and hallway as much as possible*
   b. lie in a prone position before and after meals
   c. perform abdominal strengthening exercises daily
   d. ask the physician if an oil retention enema is needed

Reference: p. 1199

Descriptors:

| 1. 43 | 2. 07; 09 | 3. Application |
| 4. IV-1 | 5. Nursing Process | 6. Moderate |

Rationale: The nurse should encourage the patient to ambulate in the room and hallway as much as possible. This will help the patient to pass the flatus.

39. The physician has ordered a rectal tube for an adult patient. The nurse caring for the patient plans to
   a. obtain a size 12 French tube
   b. leave the tube in place for 45 minutes
   c. ask the patient to lie in a supine position after insertion of the tube
   d. use the tube intermittently every 2 to 3 hours*

Reference: p. 1199

Descriptors:

1. 43	2. 09	3. Application
4. IV-1	5. Nursing Process	6. Moderate

Rationale: A size 22 French tube should be used and left in place for 20 minutes. The tube should be used intermittently every 2 to 3 hours.

40. The nurse has instructed an adult patient about the physician's order for a hypertonic solution enema. The nurse determines that the patient understands the instructions when the patient says
    a. "I'll feel full because there will be 700 mL of solution administered."
    b. "This type of enema may result in water intoxication."
    c. "I will receive about 100 ml of solution during the procedure."*
    d. "This type of enema may result in calcium retention."

Reference: p. 1200

Descriptors:

1. 43	2. 09	3. Application
4. IV-1	5. Teach/Learn	6. Moderate

Rationale: The patient has understood the instructions when the patient says that she will receive about 100 mL of the solution during the procedure.

41. The nurse is caring for a patient in the home who tells the nurse that her stools "look like rock-hard marbles." The nurse should contact the patient's physician for an order for an enema termed
    a. oil retention*
    b. carminative
    c. hypertonic
    d. normal saline

Reference: p. 1200

Descriptors:

1. 43	2. 09	3. Application
4. IV-1	5. Communication	6. Moderate

Rationale: Oil retention enemas are used for hard, formed stools to soften the stool.

42. The nurse is planning to administer an enema to a 75-year-old patient with chronic obstructive pulmonary disease (COPD) and rheumatoid arthritis. The nurse plans to place the patient in which of the following positions?
    a. Fowler's position
    b. knee–chest with head of bed lowered
    c. side-lying while flat in bed
    d. side-lying with head of bed elevated*

Reference: p. 1201

Descriptors:

1. 43	2. 09	3. Application
4. IV-1	5. Nursing Process	6. Moderate

Rationale: The nurse should position the patient in the side-lying position with the head of the bed elevated because of the patient's respiratory problems.

43. The nurse is preparing to administer an oil retention enema. Following instructions about the procedure, the nurse determines that the patient understands the procedure when he says
    a. "I need to hold the enema for at least 30 minutes if possible."*
    b. "This enema is being given to help me with my flatus."
    c. "The solution will feel cold when the procedure starts."
    d. "I shouldn't use this type of enema if I have hemorrhoids."

Reference: p. 1201

Descriptors:

1. 43	2. 09	3. Application
4. IV-1	5. Teach/Learn	6. Moderate

Rationale: The nurse determines that the patient understands the procedure when he says "I need to hold the enema for at least 30 minutes if possible."

44. The nurse prepares to give an adult patient a solution of Colyte the night before the patient's surgery. The nurse should instruct the patient that he will
    a. have a full liquid diet the evening before surgery
    b. begin having a bowel movement within 30 minutes after consuming the solution
    c. tolerate the solution more readily if it is warmed to room temperature
    d. have a clear liquid diet 24 hours before the administration of the Colyte solution*

Reference: p. 1204

Descriptors:

1. 43	2. 07	3. Application
4. IV-2	5. Teach/Learn	6. Moderate

Rationale: Before administration of the Colyte solution, the patient will have a clear liquid diet for 24 hours.

45. The nurse is caring for an 85-year-old patient who tells the nurse that she has not had a bowel movement for 3 days and is having stool seepage on her bed sheets. The nurse suspects the patient is most likely experiencing
    a. fecal impaction*
    b. hemorrhoids
    c. constipation
    d. rectal polyps

Reference: p. 1204

Descriptors:

1. 43	2. 07	3. Application
4. IV-1	5. Nursing Process	6. Moderate

Rationale: Seepage of stool and no bowel movement for 3 days is most likely due to a fecal impaction.

46. The nurse is preparing to administer a cleansing enema to an adult patient. After donning disposable gloves, the nurse should
    a. elevate the solution to 8 to 10 inches above the patient's anus
    b. give the solution slowly over a period of 5 to 10 minutes*
    c. position the patient on his right side in the Sims' position
    d. ask the patient to hold his breath if cramping occurs

Reference: p. 1203

Descriptors:

1. 43	2. 07	3. Application
4. IV-1	5. Nursing Process	6. Moderate

Rationale: The nurse should administer the solution slowly over a period of 5 to 10 minutes.

47. The physician has ordered "enemas until clear" for an ambulatory 60-year-old patient prior to a barium enema. The nurse should instruct the patient that
    a. 200 mL of solution will be administered
    b. the patient will be placed on a bedpan
    c. no more than three enemas will be administered*
    d. the last enema given should be retained for 20 minutes

Reference: p. 1204

Descriptors:

1. 43	2. 07	3. Application
4. IV-1	5. Teach/Learn	6. Moderate

Rationale: No more than three enemas should be administered before the barium enema procedure.

48. The nurse is caring for a patient with a temporary colostomy on the second postoperative day. While assessing the patient's stoma, the nurse should notify the physician if the stoma color is
    a. pink
    b. red
    c. pale
    d. blue*

Reference: p. 1208

Descriptors:

1. 43	2. 08	3. Application
4. IV-3	5. Communication	6. Moderate

Rationale: The nurse should notify the physician if the stoma is bluish or purple in color because this indicates cyanosis.

49. The nurse has instructed a patient about care of his colostomy. The nurse determines that the patient understands the instructions when he says
    a. "I should plan to drain the pouch when it is completely full."
    b. "I should take only liquid medications if I need them."
    c. "It's important to cleanse around the stoma with alcohol."
    d. "If I need to go on a trip, I should pack extra pouches and equipment."*

Reference: p. 1213

Descriptors:

1. 43	2. 08	3. Application
4. IV-1	5. Teach/Learn	6. Moderate

Rationale: The pouch should be emptied when only partially full and time-release medications should be avoided. Alcohol is drying to the skin. The patient understands the instructions when he says "If I need to go on a trip, I should pack extra pouches and equipment."

50. The enterostomy nurse has instructed an adult patient with a permanent colostomy about control of odors. The nurse determines that the patient needs further instructions when she says she should
    a. avoid milk and dairy products*
    b. use bismuth subgallate with meals
    c. eat dark green leafy vegetables daily
    d. avoid foods such as cauliflower

Reference: p. 1213

Descriptors:

1. 43	2. 08	3. Application
4. IV-1	5. Teach/Learn	6. Moderate

Rationale: The patient does not need to avoid milk or dairy products to decrease the odors; however, gas-producing foods such as cauliflower should be avoided.

CHAPTER 44

Oxygenation

1. In the human body, lungs will become stiff and alveoli will collapse when there is a reduction in
   a. cilia
   b. mucus
   c. surfactant*
   d. pleurae

   Reference: p. 1223

   Descriptors:

1. 44	2. 01	3. Knowledge
4. None	5. None	6. Easy

   Rationale: Lungs will become stiff and alveoli will collapse when the amount of surfactant is reduced.

2. Oxygen and carbon dioxide are exchanged in the
   a. pleural space
   b. tracheobronchial tree
   c. alveoli*
   d. visceral pleurae

   Reference: p. 1223

   Descriptors:

1. 44	2. 01	3. Knowledge
4. None	5. None	6. Easy

   Rationale: Oxygen and carbon dioxide are exchanged in the alveoli.

3. In the human body, the stimulus for respiration is
   a. positive pressure in the pleural spaces
   b. decreased air pressure in the terminal alveoli
   c. increased blood carbon dioxide levels*
   d. movement of the intercostal muscles

   Reference: p. 1225

   Descriptors:

1. 44	2. 02	3. Knowledge
4. None	5. None	6. Easy

   Rationale: The stimulus for respiration is increased blood carbon dioxide levels.

4. A patient diagnosed with atelectasis will have decreased
   a. diffusion*
   b. infusion
   c. inhalation
   d. friction

   Reference: p. 1224

   Descriptors:

1. 44	2. 02	3. Knowledge
4. IV-3	5. None	6. Easy

   Rationale: Atelectasis results in decreased lung diffusion.

5. While assessing a newborn infant, the nurse observes that the infant has an irregular abdominal breathing pattern with a respiratory rate of 40 per minute. The nurse should
   a. continue to monitor the infant*
   b. notify the pediatrician as soon as possible
   c. turn the infant to a side-lying position
   d. elevate the head of the crib

   Reference: p. 1226

   Descriptors:

1. 44	2. 03	3. Application
4. II-1	5. Nursing Process	6. Moderate

   Rationale: A respiratory rate of 40 per minute and irregular abdominal breathing in a newborn is normal.

6. While assessing a 65-year-old patient, the nurse observes that the patient appears to be leaning forward while sitting upright in a chair. The nurse determines that this is most likely due to
   a. kyphosis*
   b. senile emphysema
   c. rheumatoid arthritis
   d. scoliosis

   Reference: p. 1226

   Descriptors:

1. 44	2. 03	3. Application
4. II-1	5. Nursing Process	6. Moderate

Rationale: Kyphosis is typically the reason that a patient appears to be leaning forward while sitting upright in the chair.

7. The nurse is performing a physical assessment on a 12-year-old child. The nurse anticipates that normal findings for the patient's breath sounds will be
   a. swooshing with harsh crackles at end of deep inspiration
   b. a harsh expiration longer than inspiration
   c. clear inspiration longer than expiration*
   d. clear inspiration equal to expiration
   Reference: p. 1226
   Descriptors:
   1. 44   2. 03   3. Application
   4. II-1   5. Nursing Process   6. Moderate
   Rationale: In children, the clear inspiration is longer than expiration.

8. While assessing breath sounds of a moderately obese patient, the nurse would anticipate that the patient frequently experiences
   a. asthmatic attacks
   b. pleural friction rubs
   c. hypoxic episodes
   d. chronic bronchitis*
   Reference: p. 1227
   Descriptors:
   1. 44   2. 04   3. Application
   4. IV-3   5. Nursing Process   6. Moderate
   Rationale: Chronic bronchitis is frequently experienced by obese individuals.

9. Before administering morphine intramuscularly to an adult postoperative patient, the nurse should assess the patient's
   a. pain tolerance
   b. pulse
   c. blood pressure
   d. respirations*
   Reference: p. 1227
   Descriptors:
   1. 44   2. 04   3. Application
   4. IV-2   5. Nursing Process   6. Moderate
   Rationale: Morphine can depress the patient's respirations, so the respiratory rate should be documented before administering morphine.

10. When assessing a patient with severe kyphosis, the nurse would expect a decreased
    a. diffusion of gases
    b. diaphragm movement
    c. vital capacity*
    d. hypoxic receptor
    Reference: p. 1226
    Descriptors:
    1. 44   2. 04   3. Comprehensive
    4. IV-1   5. Nursing Process   6. Moderate
    Rationale: Kyphosis is a curvature of the spine leading to decreased ability of the lungs to expand and contract.

11. While caring for a patient with bronchial asthma, the nurse should instruct the patient that asthmatic attacks have been associated with
    a. morbid obesity
    b. generalized anxiety*
    c. decreased fluid intake
    d. food allergies
    Reference: p. 1227
    Descriptors:
    1. 44   2. 04   3. Application
    4. IV-3   5. Teach/Learn   6. Moderate
    Rationale: Anxiety can increase the number of asthmatic episodes.

12. While assessing an adult patient, the nurse detects a loud, low, booming sound in both lungs. The nurse determines that the patient needs further evaluation because this finding most likely indicates
    a. pneumonia
    b. emphysema*
    c. tuberculosis
    d. bronchitis
    Reference: p. 1230
    Descriptors:
    1. 44   2. 05   3. Application
    4. IV-1   5. Nursing Process   6. Moderate
    Rationale: A loud booming sound in both lungs is associated with emphysema.

13. The nurse is assessing a patient's respiratory system when the nurse detects high-pitched sounds at the end of inspiration at the base of the lungs. The nurse should document these sounds as
    a. fine crackles*
    b. coarse crackles
    c. wheezes
    d. rhonchi

Reference: p. 1230

Descriptors:

1. 44	2. 05	3. Application
4. IV-1	5. Documentation	6. Moderate

Rationale: High-pitched sounds at the end of inspiration are termed fine crackles.

14. While performing a respiratory assessment of an adolescent patient, the nurse detects high-pitched, squeaky sounds on both inspiration and expiration. The nurse determines that the patient is most likely experiencing
    a. pneumonia
    b. bronchitis
    c. pleural effusion
    d. asthma*

Reference: p. 1230

Descriptors:

1. 44	2. 05	3. Application
4. IV-3	5. Nursing Process	6. Moderate

Rationale: High-pitched, squeaky sounds on both inspiration and expiration are associated with asthma.

15. While assessing an adult patient's respiratory system, the nurse detects a dry, grating sound while auscultating the lungs. The sound appears on inspiration and is unaffected by the patient's coughing. The nurse determines that the patient is most likely experiencing
    a. asthma
    b. chronic bronchitis
    c. emphysema
    d. pleural friction rub*

Reference: p. 1230

Descriptors:

1. 44	2. 05	3. Application
4. IV-1	5. Nursing Process	6. Moderate

Rationale: A dry, grating sound heard while auscultating the lungs, which appears on inspiration and is unaffected by the patient's coughing, is associated with a pleural friction rub.

16. The nurse has instructed a patient about thoracentesis. The nurse determines that the patient understands the instructions when she says
    a. "Fluid will be removed from the pleural cavity using a large syringe."*
    b. "I will probably need to have a general anesthetic."
    c. "I'll be transferred to the operating room for the procedure."
    d. "This will be done while I am lying supine in bed."

Reference: p. 1232

Descriptors:

1. 44	2. 08	3. Application
4. IV-1	5. Teach/Learn	6. Moderate

Rationale: The patient understands the instructions when she says that fluid will be removed from the pleural cavity using a large syringe.

17. Following a thoracentesis, the nurse should prepare the patient for
    a. excessive sputum output
    b. intravenous therapy
    c. frequent blood pressure checks*
    d. computed tomography scan

Reference: p. 1232

Descriptors:

1. 44	2. 08	3. Application
4. IV-1	5. Nursing Process	6. Moderate

Rationale: A large amount of fluid can result in vasodilation, hypovolemia, and syncope; therefore, the nurse should take the patient's blood pressure immediately after the procedure and every 15 minutes until stable.

18. The nurse has instructed a preoperative adult patient about spirometry testing after surgery. The nurse determines that the patient needs further instructions when the patient says
    a. "I should wear the nose clip while breathing through the mouthpiece."
    b. "If I take bronchodilator drugs, I should not take them before the test."
    c. "I should wear a tight belt during the procedure."*
    d. "I may feel very fatigued after I do the procedure."

Reference: p. 1238

Descriptors:

1. 44   2. 08   3. Application
4. IV-3   5. Teach/Learn   6. Moderate

Rationale: The nurse determines that the patient needs further instructions when the patient says. "I should wear a tight belt during the procedure." Loose clothing or a hospital gown should be worn.

19. The nurse is preparing an adult patient who is to have an arterial blood gas drawn. The nurse should instruct the patient that the
    a. preferred site is the femoral artery for adult patients
    b. procedure is less uncomfortable than having an intravenous solution
    c. normal pH of the blood is between 7.46 and 7.56
    d. procedure requires a pressure dressing for 3 minutes after the blood is drawn*

Reference: p. 1231

Descriptors:

1. 44   2. 08   3. Application
4. IV-1   5. Teach/Learn   6. Moderate

Rationale: Following an arterial blood gas draw, the procedure requires a pressure dressing for 3 minutes.

20. An adult patient is ordered to have a cytologic study performed on his sputum. The nurse plans to
    a. collect the specimen in the morning before breakfast*
    b. collect the specimen in the evening before bedtime
    c. use the patient's saliva if sputum cannot be obtained
    d. offer the patient a mouthwash after the specimen is collected

Reference: p. 1231

Descriptors:

1. 44   2. 08   3. Application
4. IV-1   5. Nursing Process   6. Moderate

Rationale: The nurse should plan to collect the specimen in the morning before breakfast because this is when the sputum is most abundant.

21. Which of the following is an appropriate nursing strategy to maintain the respiratory system of an immobilized patient?
    a. Encourage the use of incentive spirometry.*
    b. Maintain maximum fluid intake of 1500 mL daily.
    c. Apply an abdominal binder continuously while in bed.
    d. Turn the patient every 4 hours.

Reference: p. 1238

Descriptors:

1. 44   2. 08   3. Application
4. IV-3   5. Nursing Process   6. Moderate

Rationale: Incentive spirometry is used to maximize lung expansion in an immobilized patient.

22. An adult patient is scheduled for an endoscopy. The nurse should instruct the patient that he will most likely have
    a. clear liquids the evening before the procedure
    b. no food or fluids for 8 hours after the procedure
    c. cold salt-water gargles after the procedure
    d. a sedative about 30 minutes before the procedure*

Reference: p. 1231

Descriptors:

1. 44   2. 08   3. Application
4. IV-1   5. Teach/Learn   6. Moderate

Rationale: The patient will most likely receive a sedative about 30 minutes before the test.

23. A patient has just returned to his hospital room following endoscopy where a biopsy was obtained. The nurse plans to observe the patient for
    a. hypoxia
    b. nausea
    c. syncope
    d. hemoptysis*

Reference: p. 1231

Descriptors:

1. 44   2. 08   3. Application
4. IV-1   5. Nursing Process   6. Moderate

Rationale: The nurse should assess the patient for return of the gag reflex, edema, hemoptysis or bleeding, and dyspnea after the procedure.

24. The nurse has instructed a patient about a ventilation detection scan. The nurse determines that the patient needs further instructions when she says
    a. "I will breathe radioactive gas by mask and then exhale it into room air."
    b. "A radiopaque dye will be injected and then my chest will be scanned."*
    c. "The radioactive isotope disintegrates in about 8 hours."
    d. "This procedure is usually done after the perfusion scan in the x-ray department."

    Reference: p. 1231

    Descriptors:

1. 44	2. 08	3. Application
4. IV-1	5. Teach/Learn	6. Moderate

    Rationale: The patient needs further instructions when the patient says "A radiopaque dye will be injected and then my chest will be scanned." The radioactive drug will be inhaled.

25. A moderately obese adult patient with emphysema tells the nurse that she becomes short of breath after walking one block. A priority nursing diagnosis for the patient is
    a. Ineffective Individual Coping related to inactivity
    b. Fatigue related to overeating and obesity
    c. Activity Intolerance related to shortness of breath*
    d. Fear related to disabling respiratory illness

    Reference: p. 1234

    Descriptors:

1. 44	2. 06	3. Application
4. IV-1	5. Nursing Process	6. Moderate

    Rationale: The priority nursing diagnosis is Activity Intolerance related to shortness of breath.

26. An adult patient is receiving morphine every 3 hours for terminal lung cancer and is semiconscious. A priority nursing diagnosis for this patient is
    a. Impaired Verbal Communication related to comatose state
    b. Activity Intolerance related to pain and medication
    c. Altered Oral Mucous Membranes related to morphine therapy

    d. Risk for Aspiration related to reduced level of consciousness*

    Reference: p. 1234

    Descriptors:

1. 44	2. 06	3. Application
4. IV-2	5. Nursing Process	6. Moderate

    Rationale: A priority nursing diagnosis for this patient is Risk for Aspiration related to reduced level of consciousness.

27. A hospitalized adult patient is ordered to have pulse oximetry with a spring tension sensor. The nurse plans to
    a. cleanse the site with antibacterial soap solution every hour
    b. assess the patient's pulse at a site farthest from the oximetry sensor
    c. remove the sensor every 2 hours and assess skin irritation*
    d. allow the sensor to remain in place continuously

    Reference: pp. 1233–1234

    Descriptors:

1. 44	2. 08	3. Application
4. IV-1	5. Nursing Process	6. Moderate

    Rationale: The nurse should plan to remove the sensor every 2 hours and assess skin irritation. The site does not need to be cleansed every hour.

28. The nurse is caring for a patient on the first postoperative day after abdominal surgery. The physician has ordered incentive spirometry for the patient. The nurse should instruct the patient to
    a. complete the breathing exercises 10 times every hour*
    b. hold his breath and count to 10 before using the spirometer
    c. breathe through his nose while using the spirometer
    d. leave any dentures in place during the exercises

    Reference: p. 1238

    Descriptors:

1. 44	2. 08	3. Application
4. IV-1	5. Teach/Learn	6. Moderate

    Rationale: The nurse should instruct the patient to complete the breathing exercises 10 times every hour.

29. A patient returns to the hospital unit with a chest tube in place because of a pneumothorax. The nurse should explain to the patient that the purpose of the chest tube is to
    a. apply suction to the ribcage
    b. provide adequate oxygenation
    c. allow the compressed lung to re-expand*
    d. drain fluid from the thoracic space

    Reference: p. 1238

    Descriptors:

1. 44	2. 07	3. Application
4. IV-1	5. Teach/Learn	6. Moderate

    Rationale: The purpose of the chest tube is to allow the compressed lung to re-expand.

30. The nurse is caring for patient on the first postoperative day postoperative; the patient has been taught deep-breathing and coughing exercises. The nurse plans to
    a. frequently remind the patient to perform these exercises*
    b. instruct the patient to cough after eating a meal
    c. use endotracheal suctioning to stimulate the gag reflex
    d. encourage the patient to cough while in a side-lying position

    Reference: p. 1237

    Descriptors:

1. 44	2. 08	3. Application
4. IV-1	5. Nursing Process	6. Moderate

    Rationale: The nurse should frequently remind the patient to perform these exercises to improve lung expansion. The exercises should be performed before meals.

31. A patient is given a prescription for oral codeine as a cough suppressant. Following instructions, the nurse determines that the patient needs further instructions when he says that the medication
    a. can be addictive to humans
    b. may cause sleepiness
    c. is a very effective expectorant*
    d. prevents the release of histamine

    Reference: p. 1240

    Descriptors:

1. 44	2. 07	3. Application
4. IV-3	5. Teach/Learn	6. Moderate

    Rationale: Codeine is a narcotic that prevents the release of histamine and thus decreases the need to cough. It is addictive and causes sleepiness.

32. A patient with very thick, tenacious secretions is given a prescription for an expectorant. Following instructions about the medication, the nurse determines that the patient needs further instructions when she says
    a. "I should use a humidifier in my room at night."
    b. "I should drink an adequate amount of fluids."
    c. "It's acceptable to take an antihistamine with this medicine."*
    d. "Guaifenesin is widely used as an expectorant in cough medicines."

    Reference: p. 1240

    Descriptors:

1. 44	2. 07	3. Application
4. IV-3	5. Teach/Learn	6. Moderate

    Rationale: The patient needs further instructions when he says an antihistamine can be used with the expectorant. This can elevate the patient's blood pressure and the expectorant usually has an antihistamine in the medication.

33. The nurse is caring for an 86-year-old patient with unilateral lung disease on her left side. The nurse plans to
    a. alternate the patient's position from Fowler's to lying on the left side
    b. keep the patient in a supine position most of the day
    c. use oxygen at 8 liters per minute by nasal cannula as ordered.
    d. alternate the patient's position from semi-Fowler's to lying in the prone position.*

    Reference: p. 1241

    Descriptors:

1. 44	2. 07	3. Application
4. IV-1	5. Nursing Process	6. Moderate

    Rationale: The nurse should plan to alternate the patient's position from semi-Fowler's to lying in a prone position. This will assist the patient's breathing pattern.

34. An adult patient has been ordered percussion to loosen pulmonary secretions. The nurse should
    a. allow the patient to wear a nightgown or underwear during the procedure*
    b. percuss the area below the ribcage then move upward toward the ribs
    c. percuss the patient's lungs over bare skin to better hear the sounds
    d. continue the procedure even if the patient expresses pain

Reference: p. 1241

Descriptors:

1. 44   2. 08   3. Application
4. IV-1   5. Nursing Process   6. Moderate

Rationale: The nurse should allow the patient to wear a nightgown or underwear during the procedure. Percussion should be stopped if there is pain.

35. The nurse has instructed a caregiver how to perform postural drainage on her daughter. The nurse determines that the patient's caregiver needs further instructions when the caregiver says
    a. "I should perform the procedure 1 to 2 hours after meals."
    b. "I should perform the procedure at least once a day for 45 minutes."*
    c. "The Trendelenburg position helps drain the lower lobes of the lungs."
    d. "The procedure should be performed 2 to 4 times a day for 20 to 30 minutes."

Reference: p. 1242

Descriptors:

1. 44   2. 07   3. Application
4. IV-1   5. Teach/Learn   6. Moderate

Rationale: The patient's caregiver needs further instructions when the caregiver says, "I should perform the procedure at least once a day for 45 minutes." The procedure should be performed 2 to 4 times per day for 20 to 30 minutes.

36. A patient has been prescribed a bronchodilator that is to be administered using a metered-dose inhaler. The nurse should instruct the patient to
    a. agitate the container and then hold upside down before using it
    b. inhale the medication rapidly through the nose
    c. exhale after inhaling the medication
    d. inhale the medication through the mouth and not the nose*

Reference: p. 1243

Descriptors:

1. 44   2. 07   3. Application
4. IV-3   5. Teach/Learn   6. Moderate

Rationale: The patient should inhale the medication through the mouth and not the nose.

37. The physician has ordered epinephrine subcutaneously for a dyspneic patient. The nurse plans to
    a. position the patient in an upright position*
    b. instruct the patient to reduce calcium intake
    c. observe the patient for prolonged bleeding
    d. monitor the patient's blood glucose level

Reference: p. 1244

Descriptors:

1. 44   2. 08   3. Application
4. IV-3   5. Nursing Process   6. Moderate

Rationale: The nurse should plan to position the patient in an upright position to aid in lung expansion and help the patient to breathe.

38. A patient is to be discharged on home oxygen therapy at 2 L/min using a nasal cannula. The nurse plans to instruct the patient to
    a. humidify the oxygen with sterile water
    b. avoid open flames and smoking*
    c. humidify the oxygen with distilled water
    d. wear only synthetic fabric clothing

Reference: p. 1247

Descriptors:

1. 44   2. 07   3. Application
4. IV-3   5. Teach/Learn   6. Moderate

Rationale: The patient should be instructed to avoid open flames and smoking because oxygen is highly flammable.

39. A patient is to have oxygen therapy at home using a nasal cannula. The nurse should explain that one of the disadvantages of the nasal cannula is that it
    a. requires a tight seal around the nose
    b. is impractical for long-term therapy
    c. can easily become dislodged*
    d. makes it difficult to eat or talk

Reference: p. 1248

Descriptors:

1. 44   2. 07   3. Application
4. IV-3   5. Teach/Learn   6. Moderate

Rationale: Oxygen therapy via nasal cannula can easily become dislodged.

40. Nursing care for a patient receiving oxygen via nasal cannula should include an assessment of the patient's
    a. hydration status
    b. peripheral edema
    c. infection status
    d. mucosal irritation*

Reference: p. 1248

Descriptors:

1. 44	2. 07	3. Application
4. IV-1	5. Nursing Process	6. Moderate

Rationale: Oxygen can be very drying to the nasal mucosa and the nasal prongs can cause irritation.

41. Nursing care for a patient receiving oxygen therapy should include
    a. using mineral oil on the nasal mucosa
    b. encouraging milk products in the daily diet
    c. positioning the patient to ease respiratory efforts*
    d. suctioning per clean technique every hour

Reference: pp. 1249–1250

Descriptors:

1. 44	2. 07	3. Application
4. IV-1	5. Nursing Process	6. Moderate

Rationale: Positioning the patient in a high Fowler's position helps the lungs to expand and makes breathing easier.

42. The nurse is caring for a patient who is to have a very precise oxygen concentration delivered because of respiratory problems. The nurse plans to obtain a
    a. partial rebreather mask
    b. nonrebreather mask
    c. simple mask
    d. Venturi mask*

Reference: p. 1250

Descriptors:

1. 44	2. 08	3. Application
4. IV-1	5. Nursing Process	6. Moderate

Rationale: The Venturi mask should be used for patients requiring a very precise oxygen concentration to be delivered.

43. A hospitalized patient is ordered to have continuous oxygen by mask. The nurse plans to
    a. remove the mask every 2 to 3 hours*
    b. place baby oil around the mask for greater comfort
    c. place the mask loosely around the patient's nose and mouth
    d. use powder around the patient's ears and scalp

Reference: p. 1251

Descriptors:

1. 44	2. 08	3. Application
4. IV-1	5. Nursing Process	6. Moderate

Rationale: Powder and oils should not be used. The nurse should plan to remove the mask every 2 to 3 hours for assessment and comfort.

44. The nurse is caring for a 4-year-old patient who is receiving oxygen through an oxygen tent. The nurse plans to
    a. open the tent every hour to monitor the patient
    b. keep the tent secured under the patient's pillow
    c. check the oxygen concentration every 4 hours*
    d. fill the nebulizer with normal saline

Reference: p. 1252

Descriptors:

1. 44	2. 08	3. Application
4. IV-1	5. Nursing Process	6. Moderate

Rationale: The nurse should plan to check the oxygen concentration every 4 hours. The care should be synchronized so the tent is not opened often.

45. An adult patient is receiving humidified oxygen by mask. The nurse should explain to the patient that the purpose of humidifying the oxygen is to
    a. prevent oxygen toxicity
    b. prevent drying of the mucous membranes*
    c. decrease the potential for combustion
    d. provide a route for inhalation medication

Reference: p. 1247

Descriptors:

1. 44	2. 08	3. Application
4. IV-1	5. Teach/Learn	6. Moderate

Rationale: The purpose of humidifying the oxygen is to prevent drying of the mucous membranes. Oxygen can irritate the nasal mucosa.

46. The nurse is preparing to insert an oropharygeal airway into an adult patient. The nurse should
    a. rotate the airway 90 degrees as it passes the uvula in the patient's mouth
    b. position the patient in a prone position before beginning the procedure
    c. leave dentures in place unless they are chipped or broken
    d. insert the airway with the curved tip pointing upward toward roof of the mouth*

    Reference: p. 1253

    Descriptors:

1. 44	2. 08	3. Application
4. IV-1	5. Nursing Process	6. Moderate

    Rationale: The nurse should insert the airway with the curved tip pointing upward toward roof of the mouth. Dentures should always be removed to prevent damage.

47. The nurse has instructed a caregiver of an adult patient how to care for the patient's cuffed tracheostomy tube. The nurse determines that the caregiver needs further instructions when the caregiver says
    a. "The outer cannula can be removed for cleaning and replaced."*
    b. "The tube should be deflated before oral feeding."
    c. "The tracheostomy dressing should be kept dry."
    d. "I should avoid using cotton balls to clean around the opening."

    Reference: pp. 1253–1260

    Descriptors:

1. 44	2. 08	3. Application
4. IV-1	5. Teach/Learn	6. Moderate

    Rationale: The nurse determines that the caregiver needs further instructions when the caregiver says. "The outer cannula can be removed for cleaning and replaced." The inner cannula can be removed but not the outer cannula.

48. The nurse is preparing to perform tracheal suction of a postoperative patient who has an endotracheal tube. The nurse should
    a. remove the gloves to clean the inner cannula with normal saline
    b. use a suction catheter of the same size as the endotracheal tube
    c. wear sterile gown and gloves to perform the suctioning
    d. stop suctioning immediately if the patient becomes cyanotic*

    Reference: p. 1254

    Descriptors:

1. 44	2. 08	3. Application
4. IV-1	5. Nursing Process	6. Moderate

    Rationale: The nurse should stop suctioning immediately if the patient becomes cyanotic. A clean gown can be worn.

49. The nurse is preparing to suction an unconscious adult patient with an endotracheal tube. The nurse plans to
    a. use sterile technique for the procedure*
    b. place the patient in a supine position
    c. adjust the wall suction to 10 to 15 mm Hg
    d. apply suction while inserting the catheter

    Reference: p. 1255

    Descriptors:

1. 44	2. 08	3. Application
4. IV-1	5. Nursing Process	6. Moderate

    Rationale: The nurse should always use sterile technique for this procedure. Suctioning while inserting the catheter can damage mucosa.

50. Following oropharyngeal suctioning of a postoperative patient, it is important for the nurse to assess the patient's
    a. blood pressure
    b. apical pulse rate
    c. appetite
    d. breath sounds*

    Reference: p. 1257

    Descriptors:

1. 44	2. 08	3. Application
4. IV-1	5. Nursing Process	6. Moderate

    Rationale: After suctioning, it is important for the nurse to assess breath sounds to determine if the suctioning has been effective.

51. The nurse is preparing to suction an adult patient with a tracheostomy tube in place. The nurse should
    a. use aseptic technique
    b. hyperoxygenate the patient*
    c. place the patient in a supine position
    d. set the portable suction unit at 100 to 120 mm Hg

Reference: p. 1258

Descriptors:

1. 44   2. 08   3. Application
4. IV-1   5. Nursing Process 6. Moderate

Rationale: The nurse should hyperoxygenate the patient because the suctioning may cause the patient's oxygen level to decrease during the procedure. Sterile technique is used.

52. A nurse is caring for a patient when the patient begins to choke while eating. The patient becomes cyanotic and clutches his throat. The nurse should
   a. ask the patient if he needs assistance
   b. administer six thrusts to the patient's back
   c. instruct the patient to cough forcefully
   d. administer four abdominal thrusts to the patient*

Reference: p. 1261

Descriptors:

1. 44   2. 08   3. Application
4. IV-3   5. Nursing Process 6. Moderate

Rationale: The nurse should begin the Heimlich maneuver by administering four abdominal thrusts to the patient to dislodge the food caught in the throat.

53. The nurse is planning to clean the nondisposable inner cannula of a patient with a tracheostomy. The nurse should obtain
   a. hydrogen peroxide*
   b. Betadine solution
   c. sterile water
   d. mild soap and water

Reference: p. 1260

Descriptors:

1. 44   2. 08   3. Application
4. IV-1   5. Nursing Process 6. Moderate

Rationale: Hydrogen peroxide should be used to clean the inner cannula.

54. The nurse has instructed a group of nursing students how to perform cardiopulmonary resuscitation in a setting outside the hospital. The nurse determines that one of the students needs further instructions when the student says
   a. "I should stay with the person until paramedics arrive with the ambulance."
   b. "The automated external defibrillator can analyze a person's heart rhythm."
   c. "I should call for assistance before beginning to administer breaths."
   d. "I should administer four quick breaths, then call for help."*

Reference: p. 1261

Descriptors:

1. 44   2. 08   3. Application
4. IV-1   5. Teach/Learn   6. Moderate

Rationale: The student needs further instructions when the student says "I should administer four quick breaths, then call for help." The call for help or dialing 911 (emergency number) should be done first, then administer two quick breaths.

CHAPTER 45

Fluid, Electrolyte, and Acid–Base Balance

1. Plasma is a type of fluid termed
   a. intracellular
   b. interstitial
   c. intravascular*
   d. hypertonic

   Reference: p. 1273

   Descriptors:

1. 45	2. 02	3. Knowledge
4. None	5. None	6. Easy

   Rationale: Plasma is a type of fluid termed intravascular fluid.

2. Which of the following patients would be more prone to fluid volume deficits due to a greater amount of extracellular fluid? A/an
   a. obese 35-year-old man
   b. thin 50-year-old woman
   c. average weight 68-year-old woman
   d. 6-month-old female infant*

   Reference p. 1273

   Descriptors:

1. 45	2. 02	3. Knowledge
4. None	5. None	6. Easy

   Rationale: Infants are more prone to fluid volume deficits due to a greater amount of extracellular fluid.

3. Which of the following substances would be considered a nonelectrolyte?
   a. glucose*
   b. sodium
   c. potassium
   d. magnesium

   Reference: pp. 1274–1276

   Descriptors:

1. 45	2. 02	3. Knowledge
4. None	5. None	6. Easy

   Rationale: Urea and glucose are considered nonelectrolytes.

4. The chief electrolyte of extracellular fluid is
   a. potassium
   b. magnesium
   c. glucose
   d. sodium*

   Reference p. 1274

   Descriptors:

1. 45	2. 02	3. Knowledge
4. None	5. None	6. Easy

   Rationale: The chief electrolyte of extracellular fluid is sodium.

5. A patient tells the nurse that he needs to have greater amounts of potassium in his diet. The nurse should suggest that the patient eat
   a. nuts
   b. whole-grain breads
   c. peaches*
   d. spinach

   Reference: p. 1275

   Descriptors:

1. 45	2. 03	3. Application
4. IV-3	5. Teach/Learn	6. Moderate

   Rationale: Peaches, bananas, and kiwis are good sources of potassium.

6. A solution that has the same concentration of particles as plasma is considered to be
   a. hypertonic
   b. isotonic*
   c. hypotonic
   d. normotonic

   Reference p. 1276

   Descriptors:

1. 45	2. 03	3. Knowledge
4. None	5. None	6. Easy

   Rationale: An isotonic solution has the same concentration of particles as plasma.

7. The type of pressure whereby force is exerted by a fluid against the container wall is termed
   a. filtration
   b. continuous
   c. metabolic
   d. hydrostatic*

   Reference: p. 1277

   Descriptors:

1. 45	2. 04	3. Knowledge
4. None	5. None	6. Easy

   Rationale: The type of pressure whereby force is exerted by a fluid against the container wall is termed hydrostatic pressure.

8. The role of the adrenal glands in maintaining fluid homeostasis is to
   a. regulate the conservation of magnesium
   b. regulate the conservation of sodium*
   c. increase glomerular filtration
   d. inhibit the release of antidiuretic hormone

   Reference: p. 1279

   Descriptors:

1. 45	2. 05	3. Knowledge
4. None	5. None	6. Easy

   Rationale: The role of the adrenal glands in maintaining fluid homeostasis is to regulate the conservation of sodium.

9. In the body, the parathyroid glands regulate
   a. blood pressure
   b. cortisol
   c. calcium*
   d. extracellular fluid

   Reference: p. 1279

   Descriptors:

1. 45	2. 03	3. Knowledge
4. None	5. None	6. Easy

   Rationale: The parathyroid glands regulate calcium and phosphate through parathormone.

10. If a patient is experiencing alkalosis, the patient's kidneys will
    a. retain hydrogen ions*
    b. retain bicarbonate ions
    c. excrete sodium ions
    d. excrete potassium ions

    Reference: p. 1282

    Descriptors:

1. 45	2. 06	3. Knowledge
4. None	5. None	6. Easy

    Rationale: If a patient is experiencing alkalosis, the patient's kidneys will retain hydrogen ions.

11. In human beings, fluid intake is regulated primarily by the thirst mechanism. The thirst control center is located within the
    a. parathyroid
    b. parathyroid
    c. hypothalamus*
    d. pituitary

    Reference: p. 1277

    Descriptors:

1. 45	2. 05	3. Application
4. None	5. None	6. Easy

    Rationale: The thirst center is located in the hypothalamus.

12. The nurse is caring for a newly admitted patient who has experienced severe burns as a result of an automobile accident. The nurse plans to assess the patient for
    a. excessive thirst
    b. hypovolemia
    c. hypervolemia
    d. third-space shift*

    Reference p. 1282

    Descriptors:

1. 45	2. 07	3. Application
4. IV-3	5. Nursing Process	6. Moderate

    Rationale: For a patient with severe burns, the nurse should plan to assess the patient for third-space shift of fluid.

13. The nurse is caring for a patient who is in congestive heart failure. The nurse plans to assess the patient for
    a. edema*
    b. hyponatremia
    c. weight loss
    d. hunger

Reference: p. 1282

Descriptors:

1. 45	2. 07	3. Application
4. IV-3	5. Nursing Process	6. Moderate

Rationale: Edema and hypernatremia are associated with congestive heart failure. These patients are usually prescribed diuretics to alleviate the edema.

14. The nurse is caring for a hospitalized adult patient after thoracic surgery. The nurse observes that the patient has decreased skin turgor, dry mucous membranes, and a weak radial pulse rate of 100 beats/min. The nurse determines that the patient is most likely experiencing
    a. hypervolemia
    b. interstitial-to-plasma shift
    c. hypernatremia
    d. hypovolemia*

Reference: p. 1282

Descriptors:

1. 45	2. 07	3. Application
4. IV-3	5. Nursing Process	6. Moderate

Rationale: The patient's symptoms are associated with hypovolemia.

15. The nurse is caring for a patient with congestive heart failure who is taking diuretics. Following instructions about decreasing the edema, the nurse determines that the patient needs further instructions when she says
    a. "I should avoid eating bananas until the edema is decreased."*
    b. "I should lie down frequently to rest during the day."
    c. "I need to maintain a sodium-restricted diet."
    d. "I should avoid over-the-counter medications until checking with the physician."

Reference: p. 1282

Descriptors:

1. 45	2. 07	3. Application
4. IV-2	5. Teach/Learn	6. Moderate

Rationale: The patient needs further instructions when she says she should avoid eating bananas until the edema is decreased. Diuretics can deplete potassium and foods such as peaches and bananas are good sources of potassium.

16. The nurse is caring for a patient who is at risk for hyperkalemia because of kidney disease. The nurse should notify the patient's physician immediately if the nurse observes that the patient has
    a. brawny edema
    b. a 1-pound weight loss
    c. nausea and vomiting
    d. an irregular pulse rate*

Reference: pp. 1283, 1299

Descriptors:

1. 45	2. 07	3. Application
4. IV-3	5. Communication	6. Moderate

Rationale: An irregular pulse is associated with hyperkalemia.

17. The nurse is caring for a postoperative patient after thyroid surgery. The patient complains of tingling in her fingers and muscle cramps. The nurse notifies the patient's physician as the patient is most likely experiencing
    a. hypocalcemia*
    b. hypercalcemia
    c. hypermagnesemia
    d. hypokalemia

Reference: pp. 1284, 1299

Descriptors:

1. 45	2. 07	3. Application
4. IV-3	5. Communication	6. Moderate

Rationale: Tingling and muscle cramps are associated with hypocalcemia.

18. The nurse has instructed a caregiver of a homebound patient with breast cancer about the potential for hypercalcemia. The nurse determines that the caregiver needs further instructions when the caregiver says
    a. "I should reduce her fluid intake during the day."*
    b. "She shouldn't take any antacids for an upset stomach."
    c. "I should call the physician if she demonstrates confusion."
    d. "I should be sure she gets adequate fiber in her diet."

Reference: pp. 1284, 1299

Descriptors:

1. 45	2. 07	3. Application
4. IV-3	5. Teach/Learn	6. Moderate

Rationale: A patient with the potential for hypercalcemia should receive adequate fluid intake, not reduced fluid intake. Confusion may be an early sign of hypercalcemia.

19. The nurse is caring for a patient who has had diabetic ketoacidosis and has been taking calcium supplements. To determine if the patient is experiencing hypomagnesemia, the nurse should assess the patient for
    a. flushing of the skin
    b. hypotension
    c. decreased reflexes
    d. tachyarrhythmia*

    Reference: pp. 1284, 1299

    Descriptors:

1. 45	2. 07	3. Application
4. IV-3	5. Nursing Process	6. Moderate

    Rationale: Tachyarrhythmias are associated with hypomagnesemia.

20. While caring for a patient with compromised renal function, the nurse notes that the patient is scheduled to receive magnesium citrate in preparation for a lower GI diagnostic test. The nurse should
    a. administer the medication the evening before the test
    b. assess the patient's blood pressure
    c. reschedule the lower GI diagnostic test for another date
    d. withhold the medication and contact the patient's physician*

    Reference p. 1296

    Descriptors:

1. 45	2. 07	3. Application
4. IV-3	5. Communication	6. Moderate

    Rationale: Giving the patient magnesium citrate may result in hypermagnesemia for a patient with compromised renal function.

21. A patient with severe burns is recovering from his injuries and receiving nutrition through his peripherally inserted central catheter. The nurse should
    a. administer the nutrients over a 5-minute period
    b. monitor the patient for symptoms of hypercalcemia
    c. observe the patient for signs of infection*
    d. assess the patient for symptoms of constipation

    Reference: p. 1305

    Descriptors:

1. 45	2. 07	3. Application
4. IV-3	5. Nursing Process	6. Moderate

    Rationale: The primary responsibility of the nurse is to monitor the patient for any signs of infection, particularly at the site.

22. The nurse is caring for a 70-year-old patient with hyperthyroidism when the patient tells the nurse that he uses a Fleet's enema once or twice per week for constipation. The nurse should assess the patient for symptoms of
    a. hypomagnesemia
    b. hypokalemia
    c. hypernatremia
    d. hyperphosphatemia*

    Reference p. 1300

    Descriptors:

1. 45	2. 07	3. Application
4. IV-3	5. Nursing Process	6. Difficult

    Rationale: Fleet's enemas and other laxatives are high in phosphate and should not be used by a patient with hyperthyroidism.

23. The nurse is caring for an adult patient with pneumonia who has an arterial blood gas that has a pH of 7.30, a $PaCO_2$ of 48 mm Hg, and an HCO_3- of 23 mEq/L. The nurse determines that the patient is experiencing
    a. respiratory acidosis*
    b. respiratory alkalosis
    c. metabolic acidosis
    d. metabolic alkalosis

    Reference: p. 1284

    Descriptors:

1. 45	2. 07	3. Application
4. IV-1	5. Nursing Process	6. Moderate

    Rationale: A patient with pneumonia and blood gases of pH 7.30, $PaCO_2$ of 48 mm Hg, and a normal HCO_3- is experiencing respiratory acidosis.

24. An severely anxious patient visits the emergency room complaining of light-headedness and epigastric pain. The patient's arterial blood gas reveals a pH of 7.49, $PaCO_2$ of 33 mm Hg, and an HCO_3- of 21 mEq/L. The nurse determines that the patient is most likely experiencing
    a. respiratory acidosis
    b. respiratory alkalosis*
    c. metabolic acidosis
    d. metabolic alkalosis

    Reference p. 1284

    Descriptors:

1. 45	2. 07	3. Application
4. IV-1	5. Nursing Process	6. Moderate

    Rationale: Anxiety and the pH of 7.49, $PaCO_2$ of 33 mm Hg, and HCO_3- of 21 mEq/L (low) indicate respiratory alkalosis.

25. The nurse is caring for a postoperative patient who has diabetes mellitus. The nurse observes that the patient appears drowsy and confused with a respiratory rate of 28 breaths per minute. The arterial blood gas reveals a pH of 7.23, a $PaCO_2$ of 33 mm Hg, and an HCO_3- of 20 mEq/L. The nurse notifies the patient's physician of the arterial blood gas results because the patient is most likely experiencing
a. metabolic acidosis*
b. metabolic alkalosis
c. respiratory acidosis
d. respiratory alkalosis

Reference: p. 1284

Descriptors:

1. 45   2. 07   3. Application
4. IV-1   5. Nursing Process   6. Difficult

Rationale: Increased respirations, pH of 7.23, a $PaCO_2$ of 33 mm Hg, and a low HCO_3- indicates metabolic acidosis.

26. The nurse is caring for an adult patient who has gastric suction following surgery. The patient tells the nurse that he has tingling in his fingers and is feeling dizzy. The patient's arterial blood gas reveals a pH of 7.50, a $PaCO_2$ of 48 mm Hg, and an HCO_3- of 27 mEq/L. The nurse notifies the patient's physician because the patient is most likely experiencing
a. metabolic acidosis
b. metabolic alkalosis*
c. respiratory acidosis
d. respiratory alkalosis

Reference p. 1284

Descriptors:

1. 45   2. 07   3. Application
4. IV-1   5. Nursing Process   6. Difficult

Rationale: A blood gas of pH 7.50, a $PaCO_2$ of 48 mm Hg, and an HCO_3- of 27 mEq/L (high) indicates metabolic alkalosis.

27. The nurse is assessing a patient's fluid, electrolyte, and acid–base balance. During the nursing admission interview, an appropriate question for the nurse to ask to gain subjective data from the patient is
a. "Have you had any recent nausea or vomiting?"
b. "Do you take any medications, such as aspirin or vitamins?"
c. "Describe the type of fluid intake and amounts during the last 24 hours."*
d. "Describe how much you perspire on your job."

Reference: p. 1286

Descriptors:

1. 45   2. 08   3. Application
4. IV-1   5. Communication   6. Moderate

Rationale: An appropriate question for the nurse to ask is to have the patient describe the type of fluid intake and amounts in the last 24 hours.

28. During an admission interview with the nurse, the patient tells the nurse that he has experienced a "lot of edema in the past few days." The best response by the nurse is to ask the patient
a. if he adheres to a low-sodium diet
b. if he has had any recent surgery or intravenous solutions
c. when he last had a physical examination
d. what interventions have been attempted with results*

Reference: p. 1286

Descriptors:

1. 45   2. 07   3. Application
4. IV-1   5. Nursing Process   6. Moderate

Rationale: The nurse can obtain significant data if the nurse asks the patient about any interventions that have been attempted and with what results.

29. The nurse is caring for an adult patient with numerous draining wounds from several gunshots. The nurse should assess the patient for
a. third-shift spacing
b. intracellular fluid deficit
c. extracellular fluid deficit*
d. metabolic alkalosis

Reference: p. 1296

Descriptors:

1. 45   2. 08   3. Application
4. IV-3   5. Nursing Process   6. Moderate

Rationale: Extracellular deficit is common with draining wounds.

30. The nurse is caring for an adult patient with hypovolemia and malnutrition. While performing a urine specific gravity on the patient's urine, the nurse anticipates that the specific gravity will be
    a. 1.001 to 1.005
    b. 1.010 to 1.015
    c. 1.016 to 1.020
    d. 1.025 to 1.030*

    Reference: p. 1287

    Descriptors:

1. 45	2. 08	3. Application
4. IV-1	5. Nursing Process	6. Moderate

    Rationale: A patient with hypovolemia will typically have a concentrated urine with a specific gravity of 1.025 to 1.030 or more.

31. A 5-year-old patient is admitted to the hospital with dehydration and hypovolemia. To test the patient's skin turgor, the nurse should pinch the patient's skin over the
    a. sternum
    b. forearm
    c. ankle
    d. abdomen*

    Reference: p. 1288

    Descriptors:

1. 45	2. 08	3. Application
4. IV-1	5. Nursing Process	6. Moderate

    Rationale: For a child, skin turgor is best assessed by pinching the skin over the abdomen.

32. While caring for a 6-year-old child, the nurse observes that the patient has difficulty salivating and complains of a dry mouth. The nurse contacts the child's physician because the nurse determines that the patient is most likely experiencing
    a. metabolic acidosis
    b. fluid volume deficit*
    c. fluid volume excess
    d. sodium excess

    Reference: p. 1288

    Descriptors:

1. 45	2. 08	3. Application
4. IV-3	5. Communication	6. Easy

    Rationale: A child with difficulty salivating and a dry mouth is experiencing fluid volume deficit.

33. The nurse is caring for a patient with congestive heart failure when the patient asks the nurse, "Why are my hands so swollen?" The nurse should explain to the patient that the edema is due to retention of
    a. sodium*
    b. potassium
    c. magnesium
    d. phosphorus

    Reference p. 1282

    Descriptors:

1. 45	2. 07	3. Application
4. IV-1	5. Teach/Learn	6. Moderate

    Rationale: Retention of sodium in congestive heart failure leads to edema.

34. The nurse is preparing to assess the vital signs of a patient with hypovolemia after surgery. The nurse anticipates that the patient's pulse will be
    a. bounding
    b. rapid*
    c. irregular
    d. normal

    Reference: p. 1289

    Descriptors:

1. 45	2. 08	3. Application
4. IV-1	5. Nursing Process	6. Moderate

    Rationale: A patient with hypovolemia will typically have a rapid pulse.

35. The nurse assesses an adult patient who is hospitalized for pneumonia. While assessing the patient's breath sounds, the nurse detects fine, moist crackles. The nurse determines that the patient is experiencing
    a. hyponatremia
    b. hypercalcemia
    c. fluid volume excess*
    d. fluid volume deficit

    Reference: p. 1290

    Descriptors:

1. 45	2. 08	3. Application
4. IV-1	5. Nursing Process	6. Moderate

    Rationale: A patient with moist crackles and pneumonia is experiencing fluid volume excess.

36. While assessing an adult patient's blood pressure, the nurse determines that the blood pressure is 120/82 in the supine position and 100/76 while in the sitting position. The nurse determines that the patient is most likely experiencing
    a. third-shift spacing
    b. increased extracellular fluid
    c. hypomagnesemia
    d. fluid volume deficit*

Reference: p. 1290

Descriptors:

1. 45   2. 08   3. Application
4. IV-1   5. Nursing Process 6. Moderate

Rationale: The drop in the blood pressure is indicative of fluid volume deficit or orthostatic hypotension.

37. The nurse is caring for a patient who tells the nurse that he is a highway engineer and must supervise construction and highway repairs regardless of the weather temperatures. He tells the nurse that he drinks 4 or 5 glasses of water per day. A priority nursing diagnosis for the patient is
    a. Risk for Heat Stroke related to occupation and excessive heat
    b. Risk for Metabolic Acidosis related to occupation
    c. Altered Urinary Elimination related to fluid imbalances
    d. Risk for Fluid Volume Deficit related to insufficient fluid intake*

Reference: p. 1293

Descriptors:

1. 45   2. 07   3. Application
4. IV-1   5. Nursing Process 6. Moderate

Rationale: The average adult should drink 6 to 8 glasses of water per day. The priority diagnosis is Risk for Fluid Volume Deficit related to insufficient fluid intake.

38. The nurse is caring for an 80-year-old patient who is hospitalized with congestive heart failure. A priority nursing diagnosis for the patient is
    a. Risk for Injury related to the patient's age
    b. Impaired Skin Integrity related to edema*
    c. Altered Cardiac Output related to congestive heart failure
    d. Risk for Fluid Volume Deficit related to the patient's age

Reference: p. 1293

Descriptors:

1. 45   2. 07   3. Application
4. IV-1   5. Nursing Process 6. Moderate

Rationale: The priority nursing diagnosis is Impaired Skin Integrity related to edema. The older adult is prone to decubitus ulcers and the edema over the sacrum can make this problem worsen.

39. An adult patient diagnosed with hypovolemia and receiving intravenous therapy needs to have at least 3000 mL of fluid daily. However, her intake has only been 2000 mL during the last 24 hours. An appropriate nursing goal for this patient is: The patient will
    a. increase her fluid intake by selecting juices that she enjoys
    b. have a pitcher of ice water at her bedside at all times
    c. inform the nursing staff when she is thirsty
    d. drink an 8-ounce glass of fluid every hour while awake*

Reference: p. 1295

Descriptors:

1. 45   2. 09   3. Application
4. IV-1   5. Nursing Process 6. Moderate

Rationale: A priority goal is to increase fluid intake. This can best be accomplished by having the patient drink an 8-ounce glass of fluid every hour while awake.

40. The nurse has instructed a caregiver of an 82-year-old patient with fluid volume deficit. Following the instructions, the nurse determines that the caregiver understands the instructions when the caregiver says
    a. "My mother should have at least 3500 mL of fluid daily."
    b. "If I notice that she has edema of her hands, I should increase her potassium intake."
    c. "If my mother has persistent nausea and vomiting, I should call the physician."*
    d. "I should withhold her diuretic medication if she isn't drinking enough fluids."

Reference: p. 1294

Descriptors:

1. 45	2. 09	3. Application
4. IV-3	5. Teach/Learn	6. Moderate

Rationale: The nurse determines that the caregiver understands the instructions when the caregiver says. "If my mother has persistent nausea and vomiting, I should call the physician." The patient can quickly become dehydrated.

41. The nurse is caring for a patient with renal disease who is on restricted fluids. The nurse should plan to
    a. offer small amounts of fluid with meals
    b. use large cups to administer small amounts of fluid
    c. serve the patient ice chips from time to time*
    d. offer the patient soft caramels throughout the day

Reference: p. 1301

Descriptors:

1. 45	2. 09	3. Application
4. IV-3	5. Teach/Learn	6. Moderate

Rationale: The nurse should plan to offer ice chips from time to time during the day.

42. To avoid the potential for a fatality, the nurse should use extreme caution when injecting a patient with
    a. sodium
    b. calcium
    c. magnesium
    d. potassium*

Reference: p. 1302

Descriptors:

1. 45	2. 09	3. Application
4. IV-2	5. Nursing Process	6. Moderate

Rationale: Potassium injections can be lethal and potassium should never be given intravenously.

43. The nurse is caring for a patient who will be receiving intravenous antibiotics through a peripherally inserted central catheter (PICC). Following instructions about the PICC, the nurse determines that the patient needs further instructions when she says
    a. "I can expect to have more pain with this type of catheter."*
    b. "This type of catheter is less costly than multiple intravenous solutions."
    c. "This type of IV access has a decreased risk of pneumothorax."
    d. "The need for multiple venipunctures is unnecessary with this type of catheter."

Reference: p. 1303

Descriptors:

1. 45	2. 09	3. Application
4. IV-2	5. Teach/Learn	6. Moderate

Rationale: Usually the patient can expect to have less pain with this type of catheter because multiple injections are not needed.

44. The nurse is preparing to start an intravenous infusion on an adult patient. The nurse plans to
    a. place the tourniquet 3 inches above the selected site
    b. place an ice pack over the intended vein for greater access
    c. use a circular motion to cleanse from the center of the site outward*
    d. don sterile gloves before inserting the intravenous catheter

Reference: pp. 1307–1308

Descriptors:

1. 45	2. 09	3. Application
4. IV-2	5. Nursing Process	6. Moderate

Rationale: The nurse should place the tourniquet 5 to 6 inches above the site and use a circular motion to cleanse the site from the center outward.

45. The nurse is caring for a patient who is to have an implanted port central venous catheter inserted. The nurse should instruct the patient that the catheter will be placed into which vein?
    a. basalic
    b. antecubital
    c. cephalic
    d. subclavian*

Reference: p. 1310

Descriptors:

1. 45	2. 09	3. Application
4. IV-1	5. Teach/Learn	6. Moderate

Rationale: The vein most likely to be used is the subclavian or jugular.

46. The nurse is caring for a patient who has been receiving intravenous therapy for 48 hours when the nurse observes that the site of the intravenous catheter is cool and swollen. The nurse plans to
   a. tell the patient this is a normal finding
   b. continue to monitor the patient's IV site
   c. flush the tubing with normal saline
   d. discontinue the IV and restart it at another site*

Reference: p. 1313

Descriptors:

1. 45	2. 09	3. Application
4. IV-3	5. Nursing Process	6. Moderate

Rationale: Coolness and swelling are signs of infiltration and requires that the IV line be discontinued and restarted at another site.

47. The nurse is caring for a patient who has been receiving intravenous fluids and intravenous antibiotics for 36 hours. When the nurse observes the patient's blood pressure is elevated and there is neck vein distention, the nurse notifies the physician because the patient is most likely experiencing
   a. an allergic reaction
   b. fluid overload*
   c. speed shock
   d. pulmonary embolism

Reference: p. 1321

Descriptors:

1. 45	2. 09	3. Application
4. IV-2	5. Communication	6. Moderate

Rationale: Elevated blood pressure and neck vein distention is associated with fluid overload.

48. The nurse is caring for a patient who is to have a blood transfusion. The nurse should plan to
   a. use a no. 21 size catheter to start the intravenous therapy
   b. assess the patient's blood pressure every 5 minutes during the first half hour
   c. initiate an intravenous infusion of D_5W solution
   d. ask the patient if he has ever had a reaction to blood in the past*

Reference: p. 1323

Descriptors:

1. 45	2. 10	3. Application
4. IV-3	5. Nursing Process	6. Moderate

Rationale: Before beginning a blood transfusion, the nurse should ask the patient if he has ever had a reaction in the past.

49. A 49-year-old patient is receiving a blood transfusion when the nurse notes that the patient is flushed with a temperature of 100°F. The nurse should
   a. ask another nurse to validate the findings
   b. continue to monitor the patient's blood transfusion
   c. continue to monitor the patient's temperature
   d. discontinue the transfusion and notify the physician*

Reference: p. 1327

Descriptors:

1. 45	2. 10	3. Application
4. IV-3	5. Communication	6. Moderate

Rationale: When the patient develops a febrile reaction to a blood transfusion, the nurse should discontinue the transfusion and notify the physician.

INTRODUCTION

This program includes an expanded list of the clinical skills and steps necessary to appropriately perform this growing number of technologically based procedures required of healthcare providers. Competency with these procedures and equipment is integral to cross training for the continuum of care in all healthcare settings.

The skills and steps associated with each of the procedures represented in this program may be edited and customized to meet the requirements of your institution.

PRODUCT SUPPORT

Lippincott Williams & Wilkins provides technical support for you if you have problems installing and using the Competency Validation Checklist.

Before you call:

- Please call from a phone convenient to your work station

- Write down the sequence of events that leads to the problem

- Write down the exact error message and error number if one is displayed

- If you are having a problem working with another application, be sure you know the version and have the user manual handy.

Hours of Operation are 8:30AM to 6:00PM EST (Monday – Thursday) & 8:30AM to 5:00PM EST (Friday).

(800) 527-5597   US and Canada
(410) 528-4532   outside of the toll-free area
(410) 528-4422   fax

If you need to send information to technical support or wish to submit suggestions for enhancements to the product, please use the following address:
Lippincott Williams & Wilkins
Electronic Media
Technical Support Group
351 W. Camden St.
Baltimore, Maryland 21201-2436
To correspond via E-mail, please use the following address: techsup@LWW.com

ADDING A CHAPTER

You can add a new chapter to your current project by:

- Selecting a chapter from the chapter list by clicking over it to highlight. You should highlight the chapter which is located directly below where you intend to position your new chapter.

THEN

- Clicking the Add Chapter button from the window tool bar.

OR

- Selecting the Add Chapter menu item from the Chapter menu.

The Chapter Maintenance Window will appear to prompt you through your modification.

CHAPTER MAINTENANCE WINDOW

This window appears when a chapter modification command is selected. The window includes the following features to automate and assist you any time you add, edit, or delete a chapter:

- A status bar that prompts you through the steps necessary to carry out the chosen modification.

- A second status bar that displays your current mode of modification (add, edit, or delete).

- When editing or deleting a chapter, the window automatically displays the chapter you have chosen to modify.

- A menu and a button bar that feature edit commands that allow you to cut, copy, and paste text within your entry.

When finished modifying the chapter, you may save your modification and resume CVC by clicking the OK button. To exit the modification process without saving, click the Cancel button.

NOTE: Exiting the window manually by double-clicking the window's control-menu box will not save your modification.

EDITING A CHAPTER

You can edit a previously existing chapter by:

- Selecting the chapter that you intend to edit by clicking over it to highlight.

THEN

- Clicking the Edit Chapter button from the window tool bar.

OR

- Selecting the Edit Chapter menu item from the Chapter menu.

The Chapter Maintenance Window will appear to prompt you through your modification.

DELETING A CHAPTER

You can delete a previously existing chapter by:

- Selecting the chapter you intend to delete by clicking over it to highlight.

THEN

- Clicking the Delete Chapter button from the window tool bar.

OR

- Selecting the Delete Chapter menu item from the Chapter menu.

The Chapter Maintenance Window will appear to prompt you through your modification.

SAVING A CHAPTER

CVC automatically saves any modifications to the checklist as you make them. Simply confirm your modifications in the Chapter Maintenance Window by selecting the OK button upon completion. You will automatically be returned to the checklist with the modifications completed and saved.

VIEWING A CHAPTER

You may view the chapters by clicking over the folder tab labeled Chapter. A list of chapters available will appear.

ADDING A SKILL

You can add a new skill to your current project by:

- Selecting a skill from the list of skills by clicking over it to highlight. You should highlight the skill that is located directly below where you intend to position your new skill.

THEN

- Clicking the Add Skill button from the window tool bar.

OR

- Selecting the Add Skill menu item from the Skill menu.

The Skill Maintenance Window will appear to prompt you through your modification.

SKILL MAINTENANCE WINDOW

This window appears when a skill modification command is selected. The window includes the following features to automate and assist you any time you add, edit, or delete a skill:

- A status bar that offers instructions through your modification and guides you through the functions of the various prompts.

- A second status bar that displays your current mode of modification (add, edit, or delete).

- When editing or deleting a skill, the window automatically displays the skill you have chosen to modify.

- A menu and a button bar that feature edit commands that allow you to cut, copy, and paste highlighted text within your entry.

When you are finished modifying the skill, you may save your modification and resume CVC by clicking the OK button. To exit the modification process without saving, click the Cancel button.

NOTE: Exiting the window manually by double-clicking the window's control-menu box will not save your modification.

EDITING A SKILL

You can edit a previously existing skill by:

- Selecting the skill that you intend to edit by clicking over it to highlight.

THEN

- Clicking the Edit Skill button from the window tool bar.

OR

- Selecting the Edit Skill menu item from the Skill menu.

The Skill Maintenance Window will appear to prompt you through your modification.

DELETING A SKILL

You can delete a previously existing skill by:

- Selecting the skill you intend to delete by clicking over it to highlight.

THEN

- Clicking the Delete Skill button from the window tool bar.

OR

- Selecting the Delete Skill menu item from the Skill menu.

The Skill Maintenance Window will appear to prompt you through your modification.

SAVING A SKILL

CVC automatically saves any modifications to the checklist as you make them. Simply confirm your modifications in the Skill Maintenance Window by selecting the OK button upon completion. You will automatically be returned to the checklist with the modifications completed and saved.

VIEWING A SKILL

You may view the skills for a particular chapter by:

- Selecting a chapter from the list of chapters by clicking over it to highlight.

THEN

- Clicking over the folder tab labeled Skill.

PRINTING A SKILL

You may print a skill by:

- Selecting the skill that you intend to print by clicking over it to highlight.

THEN

- Clicking the Print Skill button from the window toolbar.

OR

- Selecting the Print menu item from the File menu.

The Print Preview Window will appear to prompt you through your print command. After reviewing your document, if satisfied, proceed with the print command by simply clicking the Print button. To continue CVC without printing, click the Close button and you will return to the main screen.

ADDING A STEP

You can add a new step to your current project by:

- Selecting a step from the list of steps by clicking over it to highlight. You should highlight the step located directly below where you intend to position your new step.

THEN

- Clicking the Add Step button from the window tool bar.

OR

- Selecting the Add Step menu item from the Step menu.

The Step Maintenance Window will appear to prompt you through your modification.

STEP MAINTENANCE WINDOW

This window appears when a step modification command is selected. The window includes the following features to automate and assist you anytime you add, edit, or delete a skill:

- A status bar that offers instructions through your modification and guides you through the functions of the various prompts.

- A second status bar that displays your current mode of modification (add, edit, or delete).

- When editing or deleting a step, the window automatically displays the step that you have chosen to modify.

- A menu and a button bar that feature edit commands that allow you to cut, copy, and paste highlighted text within your entry.

When finished modifying the step, you may save your modification and resume CVC by clicking the OK button. To exit the modification process without saving, click the Cancel button.

NOTE: Exiting the window manually by double-clicking the window's control-menu box will not save your modification.

EDITING A STEP

You can edit a previously existing step by:

- Selecting the step that you intend to edit by clicking over it to highlight.

THEN

- Clicking the Edit Step button from the window tool bar.

OR

- Selecting the Edit Step menu item from the Step menu.

The Step Maintenance Window will appear to prompt you through your modification.

DELETING A STEP

You can delete a previously existing step by:

- Selecting the step you intend to delete by clicking over it to highlight.

THEN

- Clicking the Delete Step button from the window tool bar.

OR

- Selecting the Delete Step menu item from the Step menu.

The Step Maintenance Window will appear to prompt you through your modification.

ADDING A SUBSTEP

You can add a new Substep to your current project by:

- Selecting the step you intend to add a substep to by clicking over it to highlight.

THEN

- Clicking the Add Substep button from the window tool bar.

OR

- Selecting the Add Substep menu item from the Step menu.

The Step Maintenance Window will appear to prompt you through your modification.

After adding a substep, you may use the regular step commands to edit and delete.

VIEWING A STEP

In order to view a step you must first be viewing a skill. To view the steps of a particular skill, click over the skill that you would like to see expanded. The steps will appear aligned underneath the selected skill.

SAVING A STEP

CVC automatically saves any modifications to the checklist as you make them. Simply confirm your modifications in the Step Maintenance Window by selecting the OK button upon completion. You will automatically be returned to the checklist with the modifications completed and saved.